CLINICAL ELECTROCARDIOGRAPHY

A Simplified Approach

7 Jan, 1994

To Marla, with
warmest regards and every
best wishes for an outstanding
career.

Ary Goldberger

CLINICAL ELECTROCARDIOGRAPHY

A Simplified Approach

ARY L. GOLDBERGER, M.D.

Associate Professor of Medicine, Harvard Medical School;
Director of Electrocardiography, Beth Israel Hospital
Boston, Massachusetts

EMANUEL GOLDBERGER, M.D., F.A.C.P.

Clinical Associate Professor of Medicine, New York Medical College
Valhalla, New York; Attending Cardiologist
Hospital of the Albert Einstein College of Medicine
Bronx, New York

FOURTH EDITION
With **479** *illustrations*

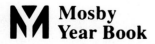
Mosby
Year Book

St. Louis   Baltimore   Boston   Chicago   London   Philadelphia   Sydney   Toronto

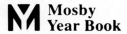
Mosby
Year Book

Dedicated to Publishing Excellence

Acquisition Editor: Stephanie Manning
Assistant Editor: Anne Gunter
Manuscript Editor: George B. Stericker, Jr.
Book and Cover Design: Gail Morey Hudson
Production: Kathleen L. Teal

FOURTH EDITION

Mosby–Year Book, Inc.
11830 Westline Industrial Drive, St. Louis, Missouri 63146

Library of Congress Cataloging-in-Publication Data

Goldberger, Ary Louis, 1949-
    Clinical electrocardiography : a simplified approach / Ary L.
Goldberger, Emanuel Goldberger. — 4th ed.
        p.   cm.
    Includes bibliographical references.
    Includes index.
    ISBN 0-8016-6217-6
    1. Electrocardiography.   I. Goldberger, Emanuel, 1913-
II. Title.
    [DNLM: 1. Electrocardiography.   WG 140 G616c]
    RC683.5.E5G593   1990
    616.1′207547—dc20
    DNLM/DLC
    for Library of Congress   90-5983
                                                                        CIP

CRC/D/D 9 8 7 6 5 4 3 2

For
Ellen, Zach, and Lexy
with love

Preface

This book is an introduction to electrocardiography. It is written particularly for medical students, nurses, and paramedical assistants and assumes no previous instruction in ECG reading. It has been widely used in introductory courses on the subject. Physicians wishing to review basic electrocardiography have also found it useful. The text derives from the cumulative experience of both authors in the field of eletrocardiography, beginning in 1944 with the invention of the aV_R, aV_L, and aV_F leads by one of us (E.G.). It is closely based on a series of lectures given over the past two decades by the other (A.G.) to physician associates, medical students, nurses, house officers, and specialists in emergency medicine.

We have divided the book into three sections. Part I covers the basic principles of electrocardiography, normal ECG patterns, and the major abnormal P-QRS-T patterns. Part II describes the major abnormalities of heart rhythm and conduction. Part III is an extensive collection of practice questions and problems for review. In addition, we have interspersed practice questions throughout the text. In reading ECGs, as in learning a new language, fluency is attained only with repetition and review.

The clinical applications of ECG reading have been stressed throughout the book. Each time an abnormal pattern is mentioned, there is a discussion of the conditions that might have produced it. Although this is not intended as a manual of therapeutics, general principles of treatment and clinical management are briefly discussed. In addition, students are encouraged to approach ECGs in terms of a rational simple differential diagnosis, rather than through the tedium of rote memorization. It is comforting for most students to discover that the number of possible arrhythmias that can produce a heart rate of 170 beats per minute is limited to just a handful of choices. Only three basic ECG patterns are found with cardiac arrest. Similarly, there are only a few causes of low-voltage patterns, of patterns in which the QRS complex is abnormally wide, etc.

In approaching any given ECG, there are always three essential questions. First, what does the ECG show; second, what are the possible causes of this pattern; and, third, what if anything should be done about it? Most conventional ECG books focus on the first question, emphasizing pattern recognition. However, it is only a first step, for example, to diagnose the presence of atrial fibrillation on an ECG. More important questions are . . . what could have caused the arrhythmia and what adverse effects follow it? Treatment, of course, will depend in part on the answers to these questions.

The aim of this book, therefore, is to present the ECG as it is used on the hospital wards, in the outpatient clinics, and in the intensive care units, where recognition of normal and abnormal patterns is only a starting point in patient management.

The fourth edition contains new information on multiple topics, including arrhythmias, conduction disturbances, myocardial ischemia and infarction, and pacemakers. Furthermore, the review questions throughout the text and the self-assessment problems in Part III have been revised and expanded.

We would like to express our special gratitude to Blanche and Ellen Goldberger for their encouragement and support during the preparation of all four editions of this book.

Ary L. Goldberger
Emanuel Goldberger

Contents

CLINICAL ELECTROCARDIOGRAPHY

A Simplified Approach

I

BASIC PRINCIPLES AND PATTERNS

1

Introductory Principles

DEFINITION

An *electrocardiogram* (ECG or EKG) records cardiac electrical currents (voltages, potentials) by means of metal *electrodes* placed on the surface of the body.* As described in Chapter 3, these metal electrodes are placed on the arms, legs, and chest wall (precordium).

BASIC CARDIAC ELECTROPHYSIOLOGY

Before discussing the basic ECG patterns, we will review some elementary aspects of cardiac electrophysiology. Fortunately, only certain simple principles are required for clinical interpretation of ECGs. In addition, it is worth mentioning now that no special knowledge of electronics or electrophysiology is necessary despite the connotations of the term *"electrocardiography."*

In simplest terms the function of the heart is to contract and pump blood to the lungs for oxygenation and then to pump this oxygenated blood into the general (systemic) circulation. The signal for cardiac contraction is the spread of electrical currents through the heart muscle. These currents are produced both by specialized pacemaker cells and conducting tissue within the heart and by the heart muscle itself. The ECG records the currents produced by the heart muscle.

---

*As discussed in Chapter 3, the electrocardiogram actually records the *differences* in potential between these electrodes.

Electrical Stimulation of the Heart

The electrical "wiring" of the heart is outlined in Fig. 1-1. Normally the signal for cardiac electrical stimulation starts in the *sinus node* (also called the sinoatrial or SA node). The sinus node is located in the right atrium near the opening of the superior vena cava. It is a small collection of specialized cells capable of spontaneously generating electrical stimuli (signals). From the sinus node, this electrical stimulus spreads first through the right atrium and then into the left atrium. Thus the sinus node functions as the normal *pacemaker* of the heart.

The first phase of cardiac activation consists of the electrical stimulation of the right and left atria. This stimulation, in turn, signals the atria to contract and to pump blood simultaneously through the tricuspid and mitral valves into the right and left ventricles. The electrical stimulus then spreads to specialized conduction tissues in the *atrioventricular* (AV) *junction* (which includes the *AV node* and *bundle of His*) and then into the *left* and *right bundle branches,* which transmit the stimulus to the ventricular muscle cells.

The AV junction, which acts as a sort of electrical "bridge" connecting the atria and ventricles, is located at the base of the interatrial septum and extends into the ventricular septum (as shown in Fig. 1-1). It has two subdivisions: The upper (proximal) part is the AV node. (In older texts the terms "AV node" and "AV junction" are used synon-

CONDUCTION SYSTEM OF THE HEART

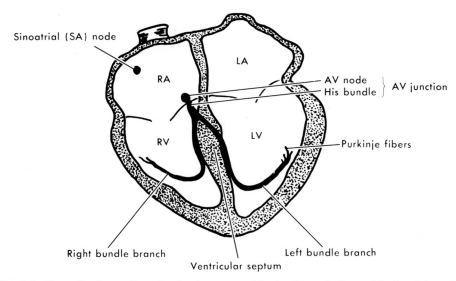

Fig. 1-1. Normally the cardiac stimulus is generated in the *SA node* (located in the right atrium, *RA*). It then spreads through the *RA* and *LA* (right and left atria). Next, it spreads through the *AV node* and *His bundle,* which comprise the *AV junction.* It then passes into the left and right ventricles (*LV* and *RV*) by way of the *left* and *right bundle branches,* which are continuations of the His bundle. Finally, it spreads to the ventricular muscle cells through the *Purkinje fibers.*

ymously.) The lower (distal) segment of the AV junction is called the bundle of His, after the physiologist who described it. The bundle of His then divides into two main branches: the right bundle branch, which brings the electrical stimulus to the right ventricle, and the left bundle branch,* which brings the stimulus to the left ventricle (Fig. 1-1).

The electrical stimulus spreads simultaneously down the left and right bundle branches into the ventricular muscle itself *(ventricular myocardium).* It spreads itself into the ventricular myocardium by way of specialized conducting cells, called *Purkinje fibers,* located in the ventricular muscle.

Under normal circumstances, when the sinus node is pacing the heart (normal sinus rhythm), the AV junction appears to serve primarily as a shuttle, directing the electrical stimulus into the ventricles. However, under some circumstances (described

later) the AV junction can also act as an independent pacemaker of the heart. For example, if the sinus node fails to function properly, the AV junction may act as an *escape* pacemaker. In such cases an AV junctional rhythm (and *not* sinus rhythm) is present. This produces a distinct ECG pattern (described in Chapter 12).

Just as the spread of electrical stimuli through the atria leads to atrial contraction, so the spread of stimuli through the ventricles leads to ventricular contraction with pumping of blood to the lungs and into the general circulation.

In summary: The electrical stimulation of the heart normally follows a repetitive sequence of five steps:

1. Production of a stimulus from pacemaker cells in the sinus node (in the right atrium)
2. Stimulation of the right and left atria
3. Spread of the stimulus to the AV junction (AV node and bundle of His)
4. Spread of the stimulus simultaneously through the left and right bundle branches

---

*The left bundle actually divides into two subbranches called *fascicles* (which are discussed on pp. 85 to 87).

5. Stimulation of the left and right ventricular myocardium

Cardiac Conductivity and Automaticity

The speed with which the electrical impulses are conducted through different parts of the heart varies. For example, conduction speed is *slowest* through the AV node and *fastest* through the Purkinje fibers. The relatively slow conduction speed through the AV node is of functional importance because it allows the ventricles time to fill with blood before the signal for cardiac contraction arrives.

In addition to *conductivity,* the other major electrical feature of the heart is *automaticity.* Automaticity refers to the capacity of certain myocardial cells to function as pacemakers, to spontaneously generate electrical impulses that spread throughout the heart. Normally, as mentioned earlier, the sinus node is the pacemaker of the heart because of its inherent automaticity. Under special conditions, however, other cells outside the sinus node (in the atria, the AV junction, or the ventricles) can also act as independent pacemakers. For example, as mentioned before, if the automaticity of the sinus node is depressed, the AV junction may act as an escape pacemaker.

The term *"sick sinus syndrome"* (Chapter 18) is used clinically to describe patients who have severe depression of sinus node function. Such individuals may experience light-headedness or even syncope due to their excessive bradycardia. The sick sinus syndrome and other causes of bradycardia are discussed in Part II of this book, in the section on cardiac arrhythmias.

In other conditions the automaticity of pacemakers outside the sinus node may be abnormally increased, and these *ectopic* (non-sinus) pacemakers may compete with the sinus node for control of the heartbeat. A rapid run of ectopic beats results in an abnormal *tachycardia.* Ectopy is also discussed in detail in Part II of this book.

If you understand the normal physiologic stimulation of the heart, you have the basis for understanding the abnormalities of heart rhythm and conduction that produce distinctive ECG patterns. For example, as just noted, failure of the sinus node to stimulate the heart properly may result in various rhythm disturbances associated with the sick sinus syndrome. Blockage of the spread of stimulus through the AV junction produces various degrees of AV heart block (Chapter 15). Disease of the bundle branches may produce left or right bundle branch block (Chapter 7). Finally, any disease process that involves the ventricular muscle itself (for example, destruction of the heart muscle by myocardial infarction) also produces marked changes in the normal ECG patterns.

The first part of this book therefore is devoted to explaining the basis of the normal ECG, followed by a detailed look at major conditions causing abnormal P, QRS, and T* patterns. The second part of the book is devoted to describing the various abnormal rhythms (arrhythmias) and AV conduction disturbances that can occur. The third part of the book is a collection of review questions and examples. A short selective bibliography is provided at the end of the text.

---

*P, QRS, and T are defined in Chapter 2.

REVIEW

An *electrocardiogram* (*ECG* or *EKG*) records the electrical voltages (potentials) produced in the heart. It does this by means of metal *electrodes* (connected to an electrocardiograph) placed on the patient's chest wall and extremities. The potentials recorded by the ECG are produced by the atrial and ventricular fibers themselves.

Normally a stimulus starts in the pacemaker cells of the *sinus* (*sinoatrial* or *SA*) *node,* located high in the right atrium near the superior vena cava. From here it spreads downward and to the left, through the right and left atria, and reaches the *atrioventricular (AV) node,* located near the top of the interventricular septum (Fig. 1-1). After a delay, the stimulus spreads through the *AV junction* (*AV node* and *bundle of His*). The bundle of His then subdivides into *right* and *left bundle branches.* The *right* bundle branch runs down the interventricular septum and into the right ventricle. From there, small fibers, the *Purkinje fibers,* bring the stimulus outward into the main muscle mass of the right ventricle. Simultaneously, the *left* main bundle branch carries the stimulus down the interventricular septum to the muscle mass of the left ventricle, also by way of the Purkinje fibers.

This sequence of stimulation of the heart is the normal basic process. Disturbances in it may produce abnormalities of heart rhythm (the cardiac *arrhythmias*) or abnormalities in cardiac conduction (*SA block, AV heart block,* or *bundle branch block).*

Questions

1. Label the major parts of the cardiac conduction system in this diagram and then trace the spread of the normal cardiac stimulus from atria to ventricles.

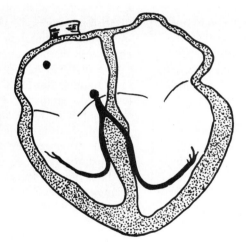

2. What does the electrocardiogram record?

Answers

1. See Fig. 1-1.
2. It records the differences in cardiac electrical potential between electrodes placed on the surface of the body.

2

Basic ECG Waves

DEPOLARIZATION AND REPOLARIZATION

In Chapter 1 we used the general term "electrical stimulation" to refer to the spread of electrical stimuli through the atria and ventricles. The technical term for this cardiac electrical stimulation is *"depolarization."* The return of heart muscle cells to their resting state following stimulation (depolarization) is called *"repolarization."* These terms are derived from the fact that the normal myocardial cells (atrial and ventricular) are *polarized;* that is, they carry electrical charges on their surface. Fig. 2-1, *A,* shows the resting polarized state of a normal heart muscle cell. Notice that the outside of the resting cell is positive and the inside is negative (about −90 mV).

When a heart muscle cell is stimulated, it depolarizes. As a result the outside of the cell, in the area where the stimulation has occurred, becomes negative while the inside of the cell becomes positive. This produces a difference in electrical voltage on the outside surface of the cell between the stimulated depolarized area and the unstimulated polarized area (Fig. 2-1, *B*). As a result a small electrical current is formed. This current spreads along the length of the cell as stimulation and depolarization occur until the entire cell is depolarized (Fig. 2-1, *C*). The path of depolarization can be represented by an arrow, as shown in Fig. 2-1. For individual myocardial cells (fibers) depolarization and repolarization proceed in the same direction. However, for the entire myocardium

depolarization proceeds from innermost layer (endocardium) to outermost layer (epicardium) while repolarization proceeds in the opposite direction. The mechanism of this difference is not well understood.

The depolarizing electrical current is recorded by the ECG as a *P wave* (when the atria are stimulated and depolarize) and as a *QRS complex* (when the ventricles are stimulated and depolarize).

After a time, the fully stimulated and depolarized cell begins to return to the resting state. This is known as repolarization. A small area on the outside of the cell becomes positive again (Fig. 2-1, *D*). The repolarization spreads along the length of the cell until the entire cell is once again fully repolarized. Ventricular repolarization is recorded by the ECG as the *ST segment, T wave,* and *U wave.* (Atrial repolarization is usually obscured by ventricular potentials, as will be discussed later.)

The ECG records the electrical activity of a large mass of atrial and ventricular cells, not that of just a single cell. Since cardiac depolarization and repolarization normally occur in a synchronized fashion, the ECG is able to record these electrical currents as specific waves (P wave, QRS complex, ST segment, T wave, and U wave).

To summarize: Regardless of whether the ECG is normal or abnormal, it merely records two basic events: (1) depolarization, the spread of a stimulus through the heart muscle, and (2) repolarization, the return of the stimulated heart muscle to the resting state.

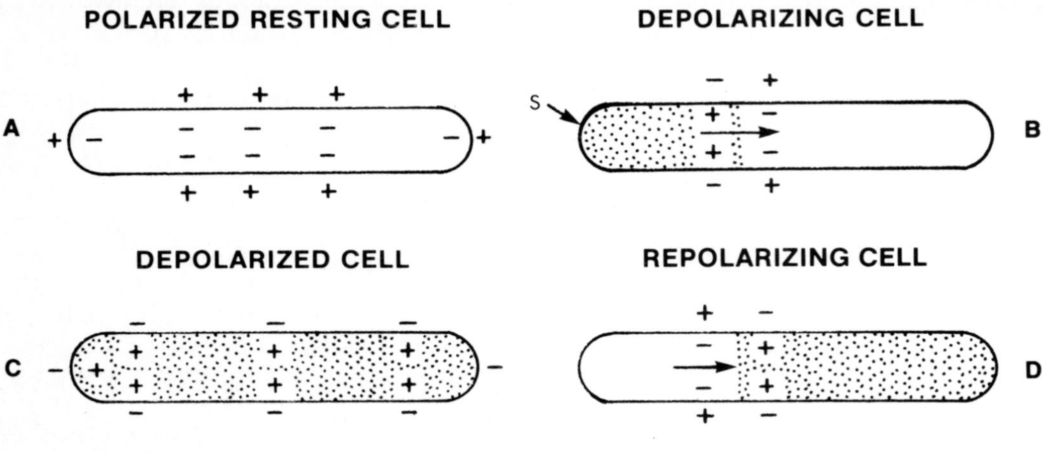

POLARIZED RESTING CELL

A

DEPOLARIZING CELL

B

DEPOLARIZED CELL

C

REPOLARIZING CELL

D

Fig. 2-1. Depolarization and repolarization. The resting heart muscle cell, **A,** is polarized; that is, it carries an electrical charge, with the outside of the cell positively charged and the inside negatively charged. When the cell is stimulated *(S)*, as in **B,** it begins to depolarize *(stippled area)*. The fully depolarized cell, **C,** is positively charged on the inside and negatively charged on the outside. Repolarization, **D,** occurs when the stimulated cell returns to the resting state. The direction of depolarization and repolarization is represented by *arrows*. Depolarization (stimulation) of the atria produces the P wave on the ECG, whereas depolarization of the ventricles produces the QRS complex. Repolarization of the ventricles produces the ST-T complex.

BASIC ECG COMPLEXES

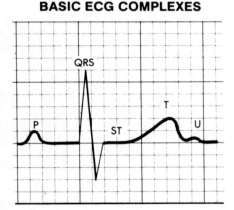

Fig. 2-2. The P wave represents atrial depolarization. The PR interval is the time from initial stimulation of the atria to initial stimulation of the ventricles. The QRS represents ventricular depolarization. The ST segment, T wave, and U wave are produced by ventricular repolarization.

BASIC ECG COMPLEXES: P, QRS, ST, T, AND U WAVES

The spread of stimulus through the atria and ventricles followed by the return of stimulated atrial and ventricular muscle to the resting state produces, as noted previously, the electrical currents recorded on the ECG. Furthermore, each phase of cardiac electrical activity produces a specific wave or complex (shown in Fig. 2-2). These basic ECG waves are labeled alphabetically and begin with the P wave.

P wave:	atrial depolarization (stimulation)
QRS complex:	ventricular depolarization (stimulation)
ST segment ⎫	
T wave ⎬	ventricular repolarization
U wave ⎭	(recovery)

The P wave represents the spread of stimulus through the atria (atrial depolarization). The QRS complex represents the spread of stimulus through the ventricles (ventricular depolarization). The ST segment and T wave represent the return of stimulated ventricular muscle to the resting state (ventricular repolarization). The U wave is a small deflection sometimes seen just after the T wave. It represents the final phase of ventricular repolarization, although its exact significance is not known.

You are probably wondering why there is no wave or complex representing the return of stimulated atria to their resting state. The answer is that the atrial ST segment (STa) and atrial T wave (Ta) are generally not observed on the normal ECG because of their low amplitudes. (An important exception is discussed on p. 135.) Similarly, the routine ECG is not sensitive enough to record any electrical activity during the spread of stimulus through the AV junction (AV node and bundle of His). The spread of electrical stimulus through the AV junction occurs between the beginning of the P wave and the beginning of the QRS complex. This interval, known as the PR interval, is a measure of the time it takes for the stimulus to spread through the atria and pass through the AV junction.

To summarize: The P-QRS-ST-T-U sequence represents the repetitive cycle of the electrical activity in the heart, beginning with the spread of stimulus through the atria (P wave) and ending with the return of stimulated ventricular muscle to its resting state (ST-T-U sequence). As shown in the rhythm strip in Fig. 2-3, this cardiac cycle repeats itself again and again.

ECG PAPER

The P-QRS-T sequence is recorded on special ECG paper (shown in Figs. 2-3 and 2-4). This paper is divided into gridlike boxes. Each of the small boxes is 1 millimeter square (1 mm²). The paper usually moves out of the electrocardiograph at a speed of 25 mm/sec. Therefore, horizontally, each box represents 0.04 second (25 mm/sec × 0.04 sec = 1 mm). Notice also that between every five boxes there are heavier lines, so each of the 5 mm units horizontally corresponds to 0.2 second (5 × 0.04 = 0.2).

The ECG can therefore be regarded as a moving graph that horizontally corresponds to time, with 0.04 and 0.2 second divisions. Vertically the ECG graph measures the voltages, or amplitudes, of the ECG waves or deflections. The exact voltages can be measured because the electrocardiograph is standardized such that a 1 millivolt signal produces a deflection of 10 mm amplitude (1 mV = 10 mm). (In most electrocardiographs the standardization can also be set at one-half or two times normal sensitivity.)

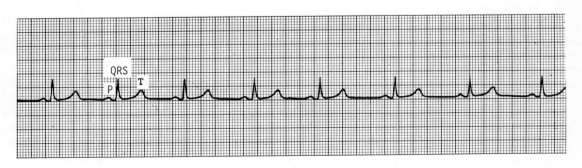

Fig. 2-3. Cardiac cycle. The basic cycle (P-QRS-T) repeats itself again and again.

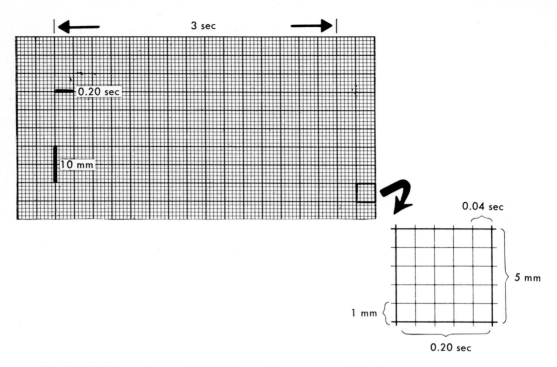

Fig. 2-4. ECG paper is a graph divided into millimeter squares. Time is measured on the horizontal axis. Each small millimeter box equals 0.04 second, and each larger (5 mm) box equals 0.2 second with a paper speed of 25 mm/sec. The amplitude of any wave is measured on the vertical axis in millimeters.

BASIC ECG MEASUREMENTS AND SOME NORMAL VALUES
Standardization Mark

The electrocardiograph must be properly standardized so a 1 mV signal produces a 10 mm deflection. The unit may have a special standardization button that produces a 1 mV wave. As shown in Fig. 2-5, the standardization mark (St) produced when the machine is correctly calibrated is a square wave 10 mm tall. If the machine is not standardized correctly, the 1 mV signal will produce a deflection either more or less than 10 mm and the amplitudes of the P, QRS, and T deflections will be larger or smaller than they should. The standardization deflection is also important because standardization can be varied in most electrocardiographs (Fig. 2-5). When very large deflections are present (as occurs, for example, in some patients who have an electronic pacemaker that produces very large

spikes), it may be advisable to take the ECG at half standardization to avoid damaging the stylus and to get the entire tracing on the paper. If the ECG complexes are very small, it may be advisable to double the standardization (for example, to study a small Q wave more thoroughly). The standardization need be set only once on an ECG—just before the first lead is recorded.*

Because the ECG is calibrated, we can describe any part of the P, QRS, and T deflections in two ways. We can measure the amplitude (voltage) of any of the deflections, and we can also measure the width (duration) of any of the deflections. We can therefore measure the amplitude and width of the P wave, the amplitude and width of the QRS

---

*Some electronic electrocardiographs do not display the calibration pulse. Instead, they print the paper speed and standardization at the bottom of the ECG paper (25 mm/sec, 10 mm/mV).

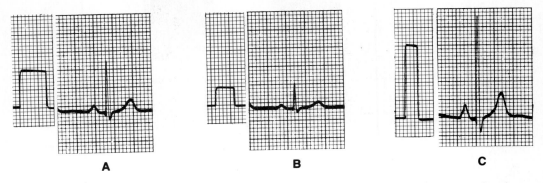

Fig. 2-5. Standardization mark. Before taking an ECG, the operator must check to see that the machine is properly calibrated such that the 1 mV standardization mark is 10 mm tall, **A.** Electrocardiographs can also be set at half standardization, **B,** or 2 × standardization, **C.**

complex, the amplitude of the ST segment deviation (if present), and the amplitude of the T wave. For clinical purposes, if the standardization is set at 1 mV = 10 mm, the height of a wave is usually recorded in millimeters and not in millivolts. For example, in Fig. 2-3, the P wave is 1 mm in amplitude, the QRS complex is 8 mm, and the T wave is about 3.5 mm.

In describing the amplitude of any wave or deflection, it is also necessary to specify if it is positive or negative. By convention, an *upward* deflection or wave is called *positive.* A *downward* deflection or wave is called *negative.* A deflection or wave that rests on the baseline is said to be *isoelectric.* A deflection that is partly positive and partly negative is call *biphasic.* For example, in Fig. 2-6 the P wave is positive, the QRS complex is biphasic (initially positive, then negative), the ST segment is isoelectric (flat on the baseline), and the T wave is negative.

In this chapter we shall look at the P, QRS, ST, T, and U waves in a general way and the measurement of the heart rate, PR interval, QRS width, QT interval, and their normal values in detail.

P Wave

The P wave, which represents atrial depolarization, is a small positive (or negative) deflection before the QRS complex. The normal values for P wave amplitude and width are described in Chapter 6.

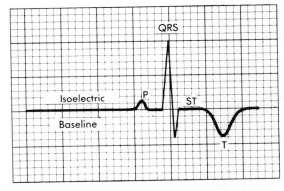

Fig. 2-6. Positive and negative complexes. The P wave here is positive (upward), and the T wave is negative (downward). The QRS complex is biphasic (partly positive, partly negative), and the ST segment isoelectric (neither positive nor negative).

PR Interval

The PR interval is measured from the beginning of the P wave to the beginning of the QRS complex (Fig. 2-7). The PR interval may vary slightly in different leads, and the shortest PR interval should be noted. The PR interval represents the time it takes for the stimulus to spread through the atria and to pass through the AV junction. (This physiologic delay allows the ventricles to fill fully with blood before ventricular depolarization occurs.) *In adults the normal PR interval is between 0.12 and 0.2 second (three to five small boxes).* When con-

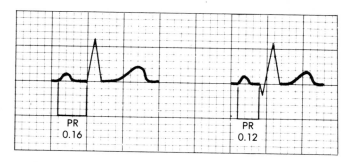

Fig. 2-7. Measurement of the PR interval. See text.

duction through the AV junction is impaired, the PR interval may become prolonged. Prolongation of the PR interval above 0.2 second is called *first-degree heart block* and is discussed in Chapter 15.

QRS Nomenclature

One of the most confusing aspects of electrocardiography for the beginning student is the nomenclature of the QRS complex. The QRS complex, as noted previously, represents the spread of a stimulus through the ventricles. However, not every QRS complex contains a Q wave, an R wave, and an S wave; hence the confusion. This bothersome but unavoidable nomenclature becomes understandable if you remember the following (Fig. 2-8): When the initial deflection of the QRS complex is negative (below the baseline), it is called a Q wave. The first positive deflection in the QRS complex is called an R wave. A negative deflection following the R wave is called an S wave. Thus this QRS complex $\left(\begin{array}{c}R\\ \diagdown\!\!\!\diagup\\ Q\ \ S\end{array}\right)$ contains a Q wave, an R wave, and an S wave. This one $\left(\bigwedge\limits_{}^{R}\right)$ does not. If the entire QRS complex is positive, it is simply called an R wave. However, if the entire complex is negative, it is termed a QS wave (not just a Q wave as you might expect). Occasionally the QRS complex will contain more than two or three deflections, and in such cases the extra waves are called R′ (R prime) waves if they are positive and S′ (S prime) waves if they are negative. Fig.

2-8 shows the various possible QRS complexes and the nomenclature of the respective waves. Notice that capital letters (QRS) are used to designate waves of relatively large amplitude while small letters (qrs) label relatively small waves (Fig. 2-8).

This nomenclature is confusing at first, but it allows you to describe any QRS complex over the phone and to evoke in the mind of the trained listener an exact mental picture of the complex named. For example, in describing an ECG you might say that lead V_1 showed an rS complex $\left(\begin{array}{c}r\\ \diagdown\!\!\!\diagup\\ S\end{array}\right)$ ("small r, capital S") while lead aV_F showed a QS wave $\left(\bigvee\limits_{QS}\right)$.

QRS Width (Interval)

The QRS width (Fig. 2-9) represents the time required for a stimulus to spread through the ventricles (ventricular depolarization) and is normally 0.1 second or less. If the spread of stimulus through the ventricles is slowed, for example, by a block in one of the bundle branches, the QRS width will be prolonged. (The full differential diagnosis of a wide QRS is discussed on p. 143.)

ST Segment

The ST segment is that portion of the ECG cycle from the end of the QRS complex to the beginning of the T wave (Fig 2-10). It represents the beginning of ventricular repolarization. The normal ST segment is usually *isoelectric* (that is, flat on the baseline, neither positive nor negative), but it may

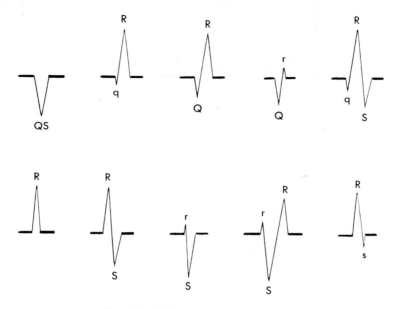

Fig. 2-8. QRS nomenclature. See text.

be slightly elevated or depressed normally (usually by less than 1 mm). Some pathologic conditions, such as myocardial infarction, produce characteristic abnormal deviations of the ST segment. The very beginning of the ST segment (actually the junction between the end of the QRS complex and the beginning of the ST segment) is sometimes called the J point. Fig. 2-10 shows the J point and the normal shape of the ST segment. Fig. 2-11 compares a normal isoelectric ST segment with abnormal ST segment elevation and ST segment depression.

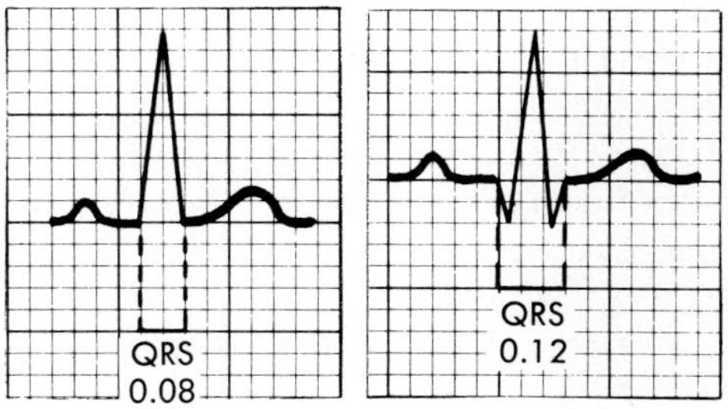

T Wave

The T wave represents part of ventricular repolarization. A normal T wave has an asymmetric shape; that is, its peak is closer to the end of the wave than to the beginning (Fig. 2-10). When the T wave is positive, it normally rises slowly and then abruptly returns to the baseline.* When it is negative, it descends slowly and abruptly rises to the baseline (Fig. 2-10). The *asymmetry* of the

---

*The exact point at which the ST segment ends and the T wave begins is arbitrary and sometimes impossible to define.

Fig. 2-9. Measurement of the QRS width. See text.

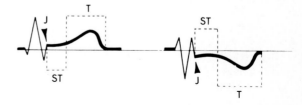

Fig. 2-10 Characteristics of the normal ST segment and T wave. *J,* Junction, marks the beginning of the ST segment.

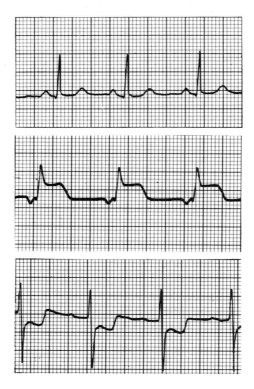

Fig. 2-11. ST segments. *Top,* Normal. *Middle,* Abnormal elevation. *Bottom,* Abnormal depression.

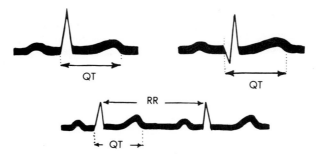

Fig. 2-12. Measurement of the QT interval. *RR* is the interval between two consecutive QRS complexes. See text.

normal T wave contrasts with the symmetry of T waves in certain abnormal conditions, such as myocardial infarction (Chapters 8 and 9) and high serum potassium (Chapter 10).

QT Interval

The QT interval is measured from the beginning of the QRS complex to the end of the T wave (Fig. 2-12). It primarily represents the return of stimulated ventricles to their resting state (ventricular repolarization). The normal values for the QT interval depend on the heart rate. As the heart rate increases (RR interval shortens), the QT normally shortens; as the heart rate decreases (RR interval lengthens), the QT lengthens.

The QT should be measured in ECG leads (Chapter 3) that show the largest-amplitude T waves. You should measure several intervals and use the average value. The QT is often difficult to measure when it is long because the end of the T wave may merge imperceptibly with the U wave. As a result you may be measuring the QU interval rather than the QT.

Table 1 shows the upper normal limits for the QT interval with different heart rates. Unfortunately, there is no simple rule for calculating the normal limits of the QT interval.

Because of this problem, another index of the QT has been devised. It is the *rate-corrected* QT or QT_c. The rate-corrected QT is obtained by dividing the QT that you actually measure by the square root of the RR interval:

$$QT_c = \frac{QT}{\sqrt{RR}}$$

Normally the QT_c is less than or equal to 0.44.

There are a number of factors that can abnormally prolong the QT interval (Fig. 2-13). For example, certain drugs, such as quinidine and procainamide, and electrolyte disturbances, such as a low serum potassium or low serum calcium, can prolong it. Hypothermia also prolongs it, by slowing the repolarization of heart muscle cells. The QT may be prolonged with myocardial ischemia and infarction and with subarachnoid hem-

orrhage. QT prolongation may predispose patients to potentially lethal ventricular arrhythmias (see p. 191).

The QT interval may also be shortened, for example, by digitalis in therapeutic doses or by hypercalcemia (high serum calcium concentration). The lower limits of normal for the QT have not

Table 1. QT Interval: Upper Limits of Normal

Measured RR Interval (sec)	Heart Rate (per min)	QT Interval Upper Normal Limits(sec)
1.50	40	0.50
1.20	50	0.45
1.00	60	0.42
0.86	70	0.40
0.80	75	0.38
0.75	80	0.37
0.67	90	0.35
0.60	100	0.34
0.50	120	0.31
0.40	150	0.25

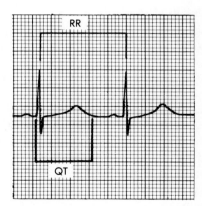

Fig. 2-13. Abnormal QT prolongation in a patient taking quinidine. The QT interval (0.6 sec) is markedly prolonged for the heart rate (65/min). See Table 1. The rate-corrected QT (normally 0.44 or less) is also prolonged (0.63).*

---

*In Fig. 2-13, find the QT_c:

$$\frac{QT}{\sqrt{RR}} = \frac{0.60}{\sqrt{0.92}} = 0.63$$

been well defined, so only the upper limits are given in Table 1.

U Wave

The U wave is a small rounded deflection sometimes seen after the T wave (Fig. 2-2). As noted previously, its exact significance is not known. Functionally U waves represent the last phase of ventricular repolarization. Prominent U waves are characteristic of hypokalemia (low serum potassium, Chapter 10). Very prominent U waves may also be seen in other settings, for example, in patients taking drugs such as quinidine or one of the phenothiazines, or sometimes after cerebrovascular accidents. The appearance of very prominent U waves in such settings, with or without actual QT prolongation, may also predispose patients to ventricular arrhythmias (p. 191).

Normally the direction of the U wave is the same as that of the T wave. Negative U waves sometimes appear with positive T waves. This is abnormal and has been noted in left ventricular hypertrophy and myocardial ischemia.

Calculation of Heart Rate

There are two simple methods for measuring the heart rate (number of heartbeats per minute) from the ECG.

1. The easier way, when the heart rate is regular, is to count the number of large (0.2 sec) boxes between two successive QRS complexes and divide a constant (300) by this. (The number of large time boxes is divided into 300, because 300 × 0.2 = 60 and we are calculating the heart rate in beats per minute or 60 seconds.)

For example, in Fig. 2-14 the heart rate is 100 beats/min, since there are three large time boxes between two successive R waves (300 ÷ 3 = 100). Similarly, if there are two large time boxes between two successive R waves, the heart rate is 150 beats/min. If there are five intervening large time boxes, the heart rate is 60 beats/min.

If it is necessary to measure the heart rate very accurately from the ECG, you can use the following modification of the above rule: Count the number of small

(0.04 sec) boxes between two successive R waves and divide a constant (1500) by this number. For example, in Fig. 2-14 there are 15 small time boxes between two successive QRS complexes. Therefore the heart rate is 1500 ÷ 15 = 100 beats/min. (The constant 1500 is used since 1500 × 0.04 = 60 and the heart rate is calculated in beats per 60 seconds.)

2. If the heart rate is irregular, the first method will not be accurate since the intervals between QRS complexes will vary from beat to beat. In such cases an average rate can be determined simply by counting the number of cardiac *cycles* every 6 seconds and multiplying this number by 10 (Fig. 2-15). (A cardiac cycle is the interval between two successive R waves.) Counting the number of cardiac cycles every 6 seconds can be easily done because the top of the ECG paper, as shown in Fig. 2-14, is generally scored with vertical marks every 3 seconds.

By definition, a heart rate exceeding 100 beats/min is termed "tachycardia" (*tachys,* Greek, swift) while one slower than 60 beats/min is called "bradycardia" (*bradys,* slow). Thus, during exercise you probably develop a sinus tachycardia but during sleep or relaxation your pulse rate may drop into the 50s, or even lower, indicating a sinus bradycardia.

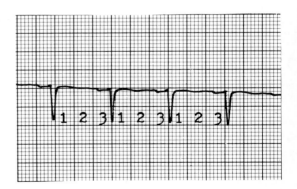

Fig. 2-14. Measurement of heart rate (beats per minute) by counting the number of large (0.2 sec) time boxes between two successive QRS complexes and dividing 300 by this number. In this example the heart rate is 300 ÷ 3 = 100 beats/min.

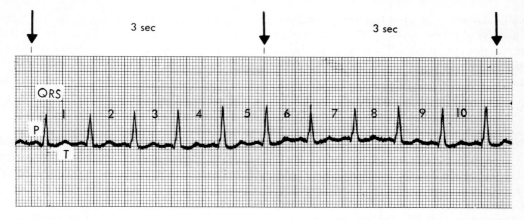

Fig. 2-15. Measurement of heart rate (beats per minute) by counting the number of cardiac cycles in a 6-second interval and multiplying by 10. In this example there are 10 cardiac cycles/6 sec. Therefore the heart rate is 10 × 10 = 100 beats/min.

THE ECG AS A COMBINATION OF ATRIAL AND VENTRICULAR ELECTROCARDIOGRAMS

The ECG we have been discussing really consists of two separate but normally related parts: an atrial ECG, represented by the P wave, and a ventricular ECG, represented by the QRS-T-U sequence. With normal sinus rhythm, when the sinus node is pacing the heart, the P wave (atrial stimulation or depolarization) will always precede the QRS complex (ventricular stimulation or depolarization) because the atria are first to be electrically stimulated. Therefore we normally consider the P-QRS-T cycle as a unit. However, as we shall see later on, in some abnormal conditions the atria and the ventricles can be stimulated by separate pacemakers. For example, suppose that the AV junction is diseased and stimuli cannot pass from the atria to the ventricles. In such cases a new (subsidiary) pacemaker located below the level of the block in the AV junction may take over the task of pacing the ventricles while the sinus node continues to pace the atria. In this case, stimulation of the atria is independent of stimulation of the ventricles, and the P waves and QRS complexes have no relation to each other. This type of arrhythmia is called *complete heart block* and is described in detail in

Chapter 15. Fig. 15-5 shows an example of this abnormal condition, in which the atrial and ventricular ECGs are independent of each other.

THE ECG IN PERSPECTIVE

Up to this point we have considered only the basic components of the ECG. Several general points should be emphasized before we proceed with our discussion of actual ECG patterns:

First, it is always necessary to remember that the ECG is a recording of cardiac *electrical* activity. It does not directly measure the *mechanical* function of the heart, that is, how well the heart is contracting and performing as a pump. Thus a patient with acute pulmonary edema may have a normal ECG. Conversely, a patient with a grossly abnormal ECG may have normal cardiac function.

Furthermore, the ECG does not directly depict abnormalities in cardiac structure, such as ventricular septal defects, or abnormalities of the heart valves. It only records the electrical changes produced by structural defects. However, in some cases it is possible to infer a specific structural diagnosis such as mitral stenosis, pulmonary embolism, or myocardial infarction from the ECG because typical electrical abnormalities may develop in such patients.

Finally, it is necessary to remember that the ECG does not record *all* the heart's electrical activity. The electrodes placed on the surface of the body record only those currents transmitted to the area of electrode placement. Therefore there are actually "silent" electrical areas of the heart. For example, the ECG is not sensitive enough to record depolarization of pacemaker cells *in* the sinus node occurring just before the P wave. Repolarization of the atria, as noted earlier, is generally not recorded by the conventional electrocardiograph. (See p. 135 for an important exception.) Also the spread of stimulus through the AV junction is not detected by the conventional ECG. The electrical activity of the AV junction can be recorded using a special apparatus and a special electrode placed in the heart *(His bundle electrogram)*. In addition, remember that the ECG records the summation of electrical potentials produced by innumerable cardiac muscle cells. Therefore the presence of a normal ECG does not necessarily mean that all these heart muscle cells are being depolarized and repolarized in a normal way.

For these reasons, the ECG must be regarded as any other laboratory test, with proper consideration for both its uses and its limitations (see Chapter 19).

In Chapter 3 we shall look first at the 12 ECG leads and then proceed with a discussion of normal and abnormal ECG patterns.

REVIEW

The ECG, whether normal or abnormal, records the following two basic physiologic processes: (1) *Depolarization* (the spread of stimulus through the heart muscle) produces the P wave from the atria and the QRS complex from the ventricles. (2) *Repolarization* (the return of stimulated muscle to the resting state) produces the atrial ST segment and T wave (which are ordinarily not seen on the ECG) and the ventricular ST segment, T wave, and U wave.

ECGs are recorded on special paper that is divided into gridlike boxes (Fig. 2-4). Each small box is 1 mm². Each millimeter horizontally represents 0.04 second. Each 0.2 second is noted by a heavier vertical line. ECG deflections are usually standardized so a 1 mV signal produces a 10 mm deflection. Therefore, each millimeter vertically represents 0.1 mV. Each 5 mm interval is noted by a heavier horizontal line.

Basic measurements of an ECG should include the following:

1. *Standardization mark.* The ECG needs to be standardized only before the first lead is recorded.
2. *PR interval.* The PR interval is measured from the beginning of the P wave to the beginning of the QRS complex. The normal PR interval varies from 0.12 to 0.2 second.
3. *QRS width.* The normal QRS width is 0.1 second or less. Description of the QRS complex is shown in Fig. 2-8.
4. *QT interval.* The QT interval is measured from the beginning of the QRS complex to the end of the T wave. It varies with the heart rate, becoming shorter as the heart rate increases.
5. *Heart rate.* The heart rate can be calculated in two ways:
   METHOD 1. Count the number of large (0.2 sec) time boxes between two successive R waves and divide the constant 300 by this number (Fig. 2-14). If you want a more accurate measurement of the rate, divide the constant 1500 by the number of small (0.04 sec) time boxes between two successive R waves.

METHOD 2. Count the number of cardiac cycles that occur every 6 seconds and multiply this number by 10 (Fig. 2-15). A vertical mark may be present on the top of the ECG paper every 3 seconds. A cardiac cycle is the interval between two successive R waves.

A heart rate slower than 60 beats/min is called *bradycardia;* a rate faster than 100 beats/min is called *tachycardia.*

Questions

1. Calculate the heart rate in each of the following examples:

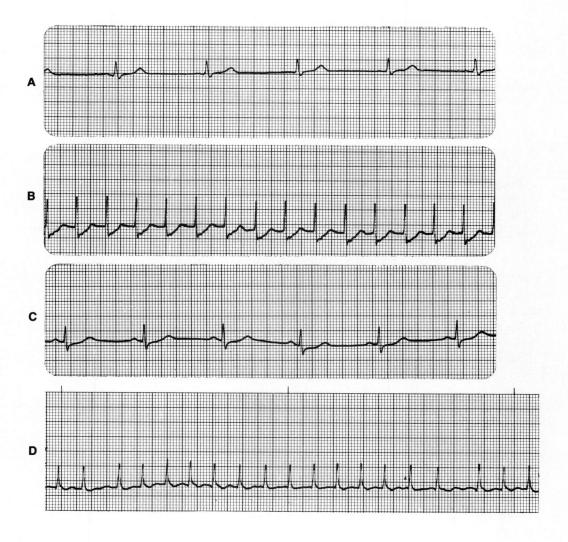

2. Name the major abnormality in each example.

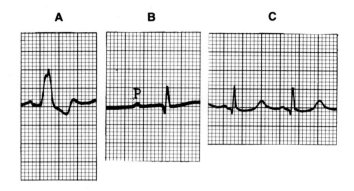

3. A block in the AV node is most likely to do which of the following?
   a. Prolong the PR
   b. Prolong the QRS
   c. Prolong the QT
   d. None of the above

4. A block in the left or right bundle branch is most likely to do which of the following?
   a. Prolong the PR
   b. Prolong the QRS
   c. Shorten the QT
   d. None of the above

5. Name the component waves of the QRS complexes shown below.

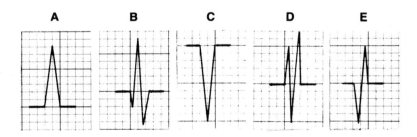

6. Name four factors that may prolong the QT interval.

Answers

1. a. 50 beats/min.
   b. 150 beats/min.
   c. 60 beats/min.
   d. Approximately 160 beats/min. (There are 16 QRS cycles in 6 sec.*)
2. a. Abnormally wide QRS complex (0.14 sec).
   b. Abnormally long PR interval (approximately 0.3 sec).
   c. Abnormally long QT interval (0.4 sec). The RR measures 0.6 second, and the heart rate is 100 beats/min. (See Table 1, p. 15.) The rate-corrected QT ($QT_c = QT/\sqrt{RR}$) is also prolonged, at 0.77 ($0.4/\sqrt{0.6}$). Normal is ≤ 0.44.
3. a.
4. b.
5. a. R wave.
   b. qRS complex.
   c. QS complex.
   d. RSR′ complex.
   e. QR complex.
6. Drugs (quinidine, procainamide, disopyramide), electrolyte abnormalities (hypocalcemia, hypokalemia), hypothermia, myocardial infarction.

---

*Notice the irregularity of the QRS complexes and the absence of P waves. This rhythm is *atrial fibrillation* (Chapter 13).

3

ECG Leads

In Chapter 1 we saw that the heart produces electrical currents similar to the familiar dry cell battery. The strength or voltage of these currents and the way they are distributed throughout the body can be measured by a suitable recording instrument, such as an electrocardiograph.

The body acts as a conductor of electricity. Therefore recording electrodes placed at some distance from the heart, such as on the arms, legs, or chest wall, are able to detect the voltages of the cardiac currents conducted to these locations. The usual way of recording these voltages from the heart is with the 12 standard ECG *leads*. The leads actually show the *differences* in voltage (potential) between electrodes placed on the surface of the body.

Taking an ECG is like drawing a picture or taking a photograph of a person. If we want to know what a person's face really looks like, for example, we have to draw it or take photographs from the front, side, and back. One view is not enough. Similarly, it is necessary to record multiple ECG leads to be able to describe the electrical activity of the heart adequately. Fig. 3-1 shows the various ECG patterns that are obtained when electrodes are placed at varying points on the chest. Notice that each lead presents a different pattern.

Fig. 3-2 is an ECG illustrating the 12 leads. The leads can be subdivided into two groups: the six *extremity* (limb) leads (shown in the top rows) and the six chest (precordial) leads (shown in the bottom rows).

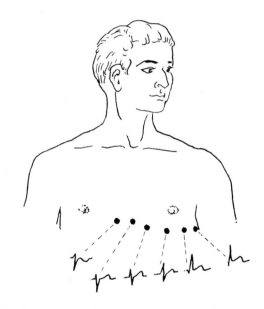

Fig. 3-1. Multiple chest leads give a three-dimensional view of cardiac electrical activity.

The six extremity leads—I, II, III, aV_R, aV_L, and aV_F—record voltage differences by means of electrodes placed on the limbs. They can be further divided into two subgroups: the *bipolar* extremity leads (I, II, and III) and the *unipolar* extremity leads (aV_R, aV_L, and aV_F).

The six chest leads—V_1, V_2, V_3, V_4, V_5, and V_6—record voltage differences by means of electrodes placed at various positions of the chest wall.

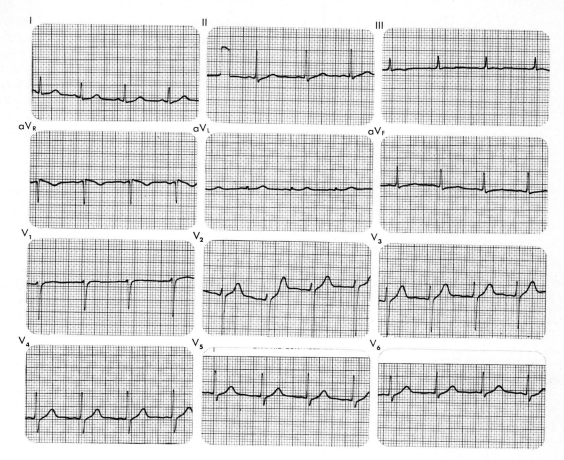

Fig. 3-2. Sample ECG mounted for interpretation showing the 12 standard leads.

The 12 ECG leads can also be viewed as 12 "channels." However, in contrast to television channels (which can be tuned to different events), the 12 ECG channels (leads) are all tuned to the *same* event (the P-QRS-T cycle), with each lead viewing the event from a different angle.

EXTREMITY (LIMB) LEADS
Bipolar Leads (I, II, and III)

We will begin with the extremity leads, since they are recorded first. In connecting a patient to an electrocardiograph, first place metal electrodes on the arms and legs. The right leg electrode functions solely as an electrical ground, so you need concern yourself with it no further. As shown in Fig. 3-3, attach the arm electrodes just above the wrist and the leg electrodes above the ankles.

The electrical voltages of the heart are conducted through the torso to the extremities. Therefore an electrode placed on the right wrist will detect electrical voltages equivalent to those detected below the right shoulder. Similarly, the voltages detected at the left wrist or anywhere else on the left arm will be equivalent to those detected below the left shoulder. Finally, voltages detected by the left leg electrode will be comparable to those at the left thigh or near the groin. In clinical practice the

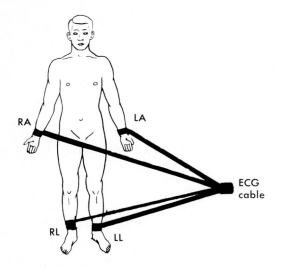

Fig. 3-3. Metal electrodes placed on the patient to take an ECG. The right leg *(RL)* electrode functions solely as ground to prevent alternating current interference.

electrodes are attached to the wrists and ankles simply for convenience.*

As mentioned, the extremity leads consist of two groups: the bipolar (I, II, and III) and the unipolar (aV_R, aV_L, and aV_F) leads. The bipolar leads are so named because the differences in electrical voltage between two extremities are recorded by them.

From lead I, for example, the difference in voltage is recorded between the left arm (LA) and the right arm (RA).

$$Lead\ I = LA - RA$$

From lead II the difference is recorded between the left leg (LL) and the right arm (RA).

$$Lead\ II = LL - RA$$

From lead III the difference is recorded between the left leg (LL) and the left arm (LA).

$$Lead\ III = LL - LA$$

---

*Obviously, if you are taking an ECG on an amputee or someone with a cast, you will have to place the electrodes below or near the shoulders or groin depending on the circumstance.

Consider then what happens when you turn on the electrocardiograph to lead I. The LA electrode detects the electrical voltages of the heart transmitted to the left arm. The RA electrode detects the voltages transmitted to the right arm. Inside the electrocardiograph the RA voltages are subtracted from the LA voltages and the difference appears at lead I. When lead II is recorded, a similar situation occurs between the voltages of LL and RA. When lead III is recorded, the same occurs between the voltages of LL and LA.

Leads I, II, and III can be represented schematically in terms of a triangle, called *Einthoven's triangle* (after the Dutch physician who invented the electrocardiograph). At first the ECG consisted only of recordings from leads I, II, and III. Einthoven's triangle (Fig. 3-4) shows the spatial orientation of the three bipolar extremity leads (I, II, and III). As you can see, lead I points horizontally. Its left pole (LA) is positive and its right pole (RA) is negative. Therefore lead I = LA − RA. Lead II points diagonally downward. Its lower pole (LL) is positive and its upper pole (RA) is negative. Therefore lead II = LL − RA. Lead III also points diagonally downward. Its lower pole (LL) is positive and its upper pole (LA) is negative. Therefore lead III = LL − LA.

EINTHOVEN TRIANGLE

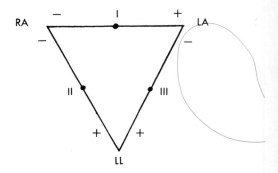

Fig. 3-4. Orientations of leads I, II, and III. Lead I records the difference in electrical potentials between the left arm and the right arm. Lead II records it between the left leg and the right arm. Lead III records it between the left leg and left arm.

Einthoven, of course, could have hooked the leads up differently; but because of the way he arranged them, the bipolar leads are related by the following simple equation:

$$\text{Lead I} + \text{Lead III} = \text{Lead II}$$

In other words, add the voltage in lead I to that in lead III and you get the voltage in lead II.* You can test this equation by looking at Fig. 3-2. Add the voltage of the R wave in lead I (+ 6 mm) to the voltage of the R wave in lead III (+ 5 mm) and you get + 11 mm, the voltage of the R wave in lead II. You can do the same with the voltages of the P waves and T waves.

It is a good custom to scan leads I, II, and III rapidly when you first look at a mounted ECG. If the R wave in lead II does not seem to be the sum of R waves in leads I and III, this may be a clue that the leads have been either recorded incorrectly or mounted improperly.

Einthoven's equation is simply the result of the way the bipolar leads are recorded. (The LA is

---

*This rule is only approximate. It is exact when the three bipolar extremity leads are recorded simultaneously, using a three-channel electrocardiograph, because the peaks of the R waves in the three leads do *not* occur simultaneously. The exact rule is as follows: the voltage at the peak of the R wave (or at any point) in lead II equals the sum of the voltages in leads I and III at points occurring simultaneously.

positive in lead I and negative in lead III and thus cancels out when the two leads are added.)

$$
\begin{array}{l}
\text{I} = \cancel{\text{LA}} - \text{RA} \\
\underline{\text{III} = \text{LL} - \cancel{\text{LA}}} \\
\text{I} + \text{III} = \text{LL} - \text{RA} = \text{II}
\end{array}
$$

In electrocardiography, therefore, one plus three equals two.

To summarize: The first three leads (I, II, and III) are bipolar extremity leads, which historically were the first invented. These leads record the differences in electrical voltage between extremities.

In Fig. 3-5, the Einthoven triangle has been redrawn so leads I, II, and III all intersect at a common central point. This was done simply by sliding lead I downward, lead II rightward, and lead III leftward. The result is the *triaxial* diagram in Fig. 3-5, *B*. This diagram is a useful way of representing the three bipolar leads and will be employed later (in Chapter 5).

Unipolar Extremity Leads (aV_R, aV_L, and aV_F)

Following the invention of the three bipolar extremity leads nine additional leads were added. In the 1930s Dr. Frank N. Wilson and his colleagues at the University of Michigan invented the unipolar limb leads and introduced the six unipolar chest leads, V_1 through V_6. Shortly after this, one of the

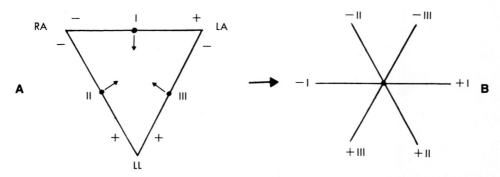

Fig. 3-5. Einthoven's triangle, **A,** has been converted to a triaxial diagram, **B.** This is done simply by shifting leads I, II, and III so they intersect at a common point.

authors of this text (E.G.) invented the three augmented unipolar extremity leads, aV_R, aV_L, and aV_F. The abbreviation *a* refers to *augmented; V, voltage; R, L,* and *F, right arm, left arm,* and *left foot* (leg) respectively. So, today, 12 leads are routinely employed.

A unipolar lead records the electrical voltages at one location relative to zero potential, rather than relative to the voltages at another extremity, as in the case of the bipolar extremity leads. The zero potential is obtained inside the electrocardiograph by joining the three extremity leads to a central terminal. Since the sum of the voltages of RA, LA, and LL equals zero, the central terminal has a zero voltage. The aV_R, aV_L, and aV_F leads are derived in a slightly different way, because the voltages recorded by the electrocardiograph have been augmented 50% over the actual voltages detected at each extremity. This augmentation is also done electronically inside the electrocardiograph.*

Just as we used Einthoven's triangle to represent the spatial orientation of the three bipolar extremity leads, so we can use the diagram in Fig. 3-6 to

---

*Augmentation was developed to make the complexes more readable.

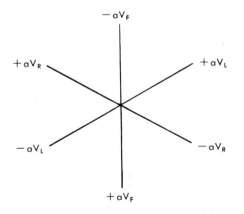

Fig. 3-6. Triaxial lead diagram showing the relationship of the three augmented unipolar leads: aV_R, aV_L, and aV_F. Notice that these leads are represented by axes with positive and negative poles. *Unipolar* means that the leads record the voltage in one location relative to zero potential.

represent the spatial orientation of the three unipolar extremity leads. Notice that each of the unipolar leads can also be represented by a line (axis) with a positive and a negative pole.* Since the diagram has three axes, it is also called a *triaxial diagram.*

The positive pole of lead aV_R, the right arm lead, points upward and to the patient's right arm as you would expect. The positive pole of lead aV_L points upward and to the patient's left arm. The positive pole of lead aV_F points downward toward the patient's left foot.

Furthermore, just as leads I, II, and III are related by Einthoven's equation, so leads aV_R, aV_L, and aV_F likewise are related:

$$aV_R + aV_L + aV_F = 0$$

In other words, when the three unipolar extremity leads are recorded, they should total zero. Thus the sum of the P wave voltages is zero, the sum of the QRS voltages is zero, and the same holds for the T wave voltages. Go back to Fig. 3-2 and test this equation by adding the sum of the QRS voltages in the three unipolar extremtiy leads, aV_R, aV_L, and aV_F.

It is also a good custom to scan leads aV_R, aV_L, and aV_F rapidly when you first look at a mounted ECG. If the sum of the waves in these three leads does not equal zero, this may also be a clue that these leads have either been recorded incorrectly or mounted improperly.

The ECG leads, both bipolar and unipolar, have two major features, which have already been described. They have both a specific *orientation* and a specific *polarity*.

Thus the axis of lead I is oriented horizontally while the axis of lead aV_R points diagonally downward. The orientation of the bipolar leads is shown in Einthoven's triangle (Fig. 3-5) while that of the unipolar extremity leads is diagrammed in Fig. 3-6.

---

*Although unipolar leads (like bipolar leads) are represented by axes with positive and negative poles, the term "unipolar" refers not to these poles but to the fact that unipolar leads record the voltage in *one* location relative to zero potential.

The second major feature of the ECG leads, their polarity, can be represented by a line (axis) with a positive and a negative pole, as shown before. The polarity and spatial orientation of the leads are discussed further in Chapters 4 and 5 (when we consider the normal ECG patterns seen in each of the leads and the concept of electrical axis).

Do not be confused by the difference in meaning between ECG electrodes and ECG leads. An *electrode* is simply the metal plate used to detect the electrical currents of the heart in any location. An ECG *lead,* as we have been discussing, shows the differences in voltage detected by these electrodes. (For example, lead I presents the differences in

voltage detected by the left and right arm electrodes.) Therefore, a lead is a means of recording the differences in cardiac voltages obtained by different electrodes.

Relationship Between Unipolar and Bipolar Extremity Leads

The Einthoven triangle (Fig. 3-4) shows the relationship of the three bipolar extremity leads (I, II, and III). Similarly the triaxial diagram in Fig. 3-7 shows the relationship of the three unipolar extremity leads (aV$_R$, aV$_L$, and aV$_F$). For convenience, we can combine these two diagrams so the axes of all six extremity leads intersect at a common

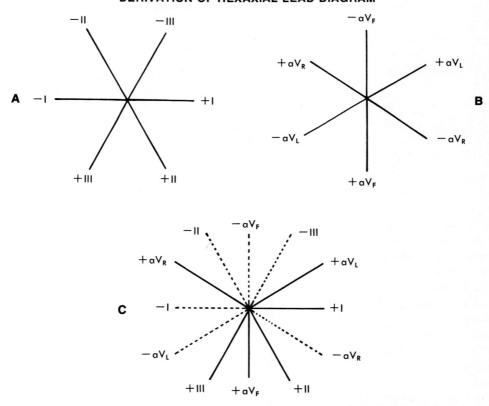

Fig. 3-7. Triaxial diagrams of the bipolar leads (I, II, and III), **A,** and the unipolar leads (aV$_R$, aV$_L$, and aV$_F$), **B,** can be combined into a hexaxial diagram, **C,** showing the relationship of all six extremity leads. The negative pole of each lead is now indicated by a *dashed line.*

point. The result is the *hexaxial* lead diagram shown in Fig. 3-7. The hexaxial diagram shows the spatial orientation of the six extremity leads (I, II, III, aV_R, aV_L, and aV_F).

The exact relationships among the three unipolar extremity leads and the three bipolar extremity leads can also be described mathematically. However, for present purposes, the following simple guidelines allow you to get an overall impression of the similarities between these two sets of leads.

As you might expect by looking at the hexaxial diagram, the pattern in lead aV_L usually resembles that in lead I. The positive poles of lead aV_R and lead II, on the other hand, point in opposite directions. Therefore the P-QRS-T pattern recorded by lead aV_R is generally the reverse of that recorded by lead II. (For example, when lead II shows a

qR $\left(\begin{smallmatrix} R \\ \wedge \\ \neg\!\!\!\wedge\!\!\!\!L \\ q \end{smallmatrix}\right)$ pattern lead aV_R usually shows an

rS $\left(\begin{smallmatrix} r \\ \neg\!\!\!|\!\!\!\Gamma \\ \vee \\ S \end{smallmatrix}\right)$ pattern.) Finally, the pattern shown by

lead aV_F usually but not always resembles that shown by lead III.

CHEST (PRECORDIAL) LEADS

The chest leads (V_1 to V_6) show the electrical currents of the heart detected by electrodes placed at different positions on the chest wall. The chest leads used today are also unipolar leads in that they measure the voltage in any one location relative to zero potential. By convention the six leads are placed as follows*:

Lead V_1 is recorded with the electrode in the fourth intercostal space just to the right of the sternum.

Lead V_2 is recorded with the electrode in the fourth intercostal space just to the left of the sternum.

---

*Sometimes, in special circumstances (such as a patient with suspected congenital heart disease or right ventricular infarction), additional leads are placed on the right side of the chest. For example, lead V_{3R} is equivalent to V_3 but the electrode is placed to the right of the sternum.

Lead V_3 is recorded on a line midway between leads V_2 and V_4.

Lead V_4 is recorded in the midclavicular line in the fifth interspace.

Lead V_5 is recorded in the anterior axillary line at the same level as lead V_4.

Lead V_6 is recorded in the midaxillary line at the same level as lead V_4.

The chest leads are recorded simply by means of electrodes (usually attached to suction cups to hold them in place on the chest) at six designated locations on the chest wall (Fig. 3-8).

Two points are worth mentioning here:

First, how do you locate the fourth intercostal space? Start by placing your finger at the top of the sternum and moving it slowly downward. After moving down about $1\frac{1}{2}$ inches, you will feel a slight horizontal ridge. This is called the *angle of Louis* (Fig. 3-8), where the manubrium joins the body of the sternum. The second intercostal space is just below and lateral to this point. Move down two more spaces and you are in the fourth interspace and ready to place lead V_1.

Second, in females the situation is complicated by breast tissue, which may result in misplacement

CHEST LEAD PLACEMENT

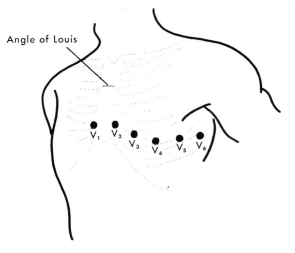

Fig. 3-8. Locations of the electrodes for the chest (precordial) leads.

of the chest leads. In taking ECGs on women you must remember to place the electrode *under* the breast for leads V_3 to V_6. If, as so often happens, the electrode is placed *on* the breast, you will be recording electrical voltages from higher interspaces.

(*Never* use the nipples to locate the position of any of the chest lead electrodes, even in men, because nipple location varies greatly in different persons.)

The chest leads, like the six extremity leads, can be represented diagrammatically as shown in Fig. 3-9. Like the other leads, each of the chest leads has a positive and a negative pole. The positive pole of each chest lead points anteriorly, toward the front of the chest. The negative pole of the chest leads points posteriorly, toward the back (*dashed lines* in Fig. 3-9).

TAKING AN ECG

Now you are ready to take an ECG. The extremity electrodes are attached to the patient. First, the machine is standardized (p. 10). Then the dial on the electrocardiograph is turned to lead I. Several P-QRS-T cycles are run. Next, the dial is advanced to lead II and the ECG records a few more cycles. This is repeated for leads III, aV_R, aV_L, and aV_F. Next the dial is turned to the position for the chest leads. The suction cup is placed in the V_1 position, and so on, until the six V leads have been recorded. The result is a long ECG strip showing the 12 leads recorded sequentially.* The ECGs in this book have been cut and mounted in the usual way for interpretation (Fig. 3-2).

THE 12-LEAD ECG: FRONTAL AND HORIZONTAL PLANE LEADS

You may now be wondering why we use 12 leads in clinical electrocardiography; why not 10 or 22? The reason for exactly 12 leads is partly historical,

---

*Many of the modern electrocardiographs have been designed to record three ECG leads simultaneously; thus four groups of three leads (I, II, III), (aV_R, aV_L, aV_F), (V_1 to V_3), and (V_4 to V_6) can be recorded at the same time. (For example, see Fig. 10-7.)

ORIENTATION OF CHEST LEADS

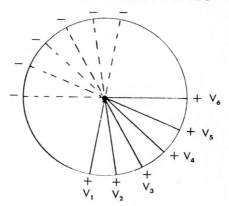

Fig. 3-9. Notice that the positive poles of the chest leads point anteriorly and the negative poles (indicated by *dashed lines*) point posteriorly.

a matter of the way the ECG has evolved over the years since Einthoven's original three bipolar extremity leads. There is nothing sacred about the electrocardiographer's dozen. In some cases, for example, we do record additional leads by placing the chest electrode at different positions on the chest wall. There are good reasons for using multiple leads. The heart, after all, is a three-dimensional structure and its electrical currents spread out in all directions across the body. Recall that the ECG leads were described as being like photographs by which we can see the electrical activity of the heart from different locations. To a certain extent, the more points we record from the more accurate will be our representation of the heart's electrical activity.

The importance of multiple leads is illustrated in the diagnosis of myocardial infarction (MI). An MI typically affects one localized portion of either the anterior or the inferior portion of the left ventricle. The ECG changes produced by an anterior MI are usually best shown by the chest leads, which are close to and face the injured anterior surface of the heart. The changes seen with an inferior MI usually appear only in leads such as II, III, and aV_F, which face the injured inferior surface of the

FRONTAL PLANE LEADS

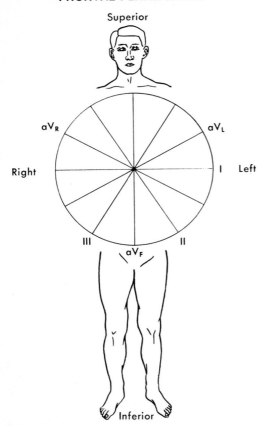

Fig. 3-10. Spatial relationships of the six extremity (frontal plane) leads.

HORIZONTAL PLANE LEADS

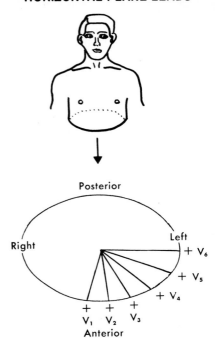

Fig. 3-11. Spatial relationships of the six chest (horizontal plane) leads.

heart. (We discuss this further in Chapters 8 and 9.) The 12 leads therefore provide a three-dimensional view of the electrical activity of the heart.

Specifically, the six extremity leads (I, II, III, aV_R, aV_L, aV_F) will record electrical voltages transmitted onto the *frontal* plane of the body (Fig. 3-10) while the six precordial leads record voltages transmitted onto the *horizontal* plane. For example, if you walk up to and face a large window, the window will be parallel to the frontal plane of your body. Similarly heart voltages directed upward and downward and to the right and left will be recorded by the frontal plane leads. A figure with the frontal

plane leads superimposed would contain the electrocardiographic relationships illustrated in the diagram on the preceding page (see also Fig. 3-10).

The chest leads (V_1 through V_6) record heart voltages from a different viewpoint, on the *horizontal* plane of the body, as shown in Fig. 3-11. The horizontal plane cuts your body into an upper and a lower half. Similarly the chest leads record heart voltages directed anteriorly (front), posteriorly (back), and to the right and left.

We therefore have two sets of ECG leads: the six *extremity* leads (three unipolar and three bipolar), which record voltages on the frontal plane of the body, and the six *chest* (precordial) leads, which record voltages on the horizontal plane. Together these 12 leads provide a three-dimensional picture of atrial and ventricular depolarization and repolarization.

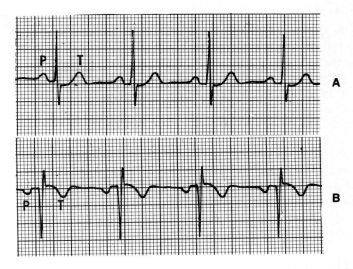

Fig. 3-12. Rhythm strips from a cardiac monitor taken moments apart. Notice that **A** is completely the opposite of **B.** This is because the polarity of the electrodes in **B** was reversed.

CARDIAC MONITORS AND MONITOR LEADS
Bedside Cardiac Monitors

Up to now, we have considered only the standard 12 lead ECG. However, it is not always necessary or feasible to record a full 12-lead ECG. For example, patients in coronary care units require continuous monitoring. In such settings special cardiac monitors are used to give a continuous beat-to-beat record of cardiac activity from one monitor lead.

Fig. 3-12 is a rhythm strip recorded from a monitor lead obtained by means of three disk electrodes on the chest wall. As shown in Fig. 3-13, one of these electrodes (the positive one) is usually pasted in the V_1 position. The other two are placed near the right and left shoulders. One serves as the negative electrode, the other as ground.

When the location of the electrodes on the chest wall is varied, the resultant ECG patterns will also vary. In addition, if the polarity of the electrodes changes (for example, connecting the negative electrode to the V_1 position and the positive electrode to the right shoulder), the ECG will show a completely opposite pattern (Fig. 3-12).

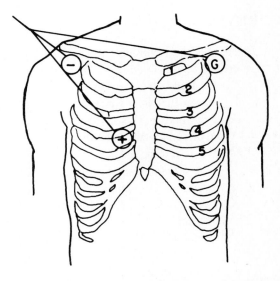

Fig. 3-13. Monitor lead. A chest electrode (+) is placed at the V_1 position. The right shoulder acts as a negative (−) electrode. A ground electrode *(G)* is placed at the left shoulder.

Ambulatory (Holter) Monitors

The cardiac monitors just described are useful in patients confined to bed or chair, but sometimes it is essential to record the heartbeat in ambulatory patients over longer periods. A special portable ECG system, designed in 1961 by N.J. Holter, records the cardiac activity of patients as they go about their daily activities. The Holter monitor currently in use consists of electrodes placed on the chest wall and lower abdomen and a special portable tape recorder to record the ECG. The patient can then be monitored over a long period (for example, 24 hours). Usually two ECG leads are recorded. The tape is played back, and the P-QRS-T complexes are displayed on a special screen. Printouts of any portion of the ECG can be obtained for further study and permanent records.

Holter monitors are invaluable in many settings.

For example, in evaluating patients with unexplained *syncope,* they may reveal serious arrhythmias that are intermittent and may not have been seen on a routine ECG. Holter monitors are also useful for establishing the diagnosis of the *brady-tachy syndrome* (p. 230), in which periods of bradycardia alternate with periods of tachycardia. A Holter monitor may be useful in detecting ST segment shifts associated with *myocardial ischemia* in selected patients (p. 115).

Special ECG Recordings

To help diagnose arrhythmias, special ECG electrodes have been developed for recording inside the esophagus (esophageal leads) or inside the right atrium and right ventricle (intracardiac leads). Discussion of these topics, however, is beyond the scope of this introductory text.

REVIEW

The electrical currents produced during atrial and ventricular depolarization and repolarization are detected by electrodes placed on the extremities and chest wall.

Twelve leads are usually recorded.

1. The six *extremity* (limb) leads record voltages from the heart directed onto the frontal plane of the body. (This divides the body into front and back halves.) These six leads consist of the three bipolar extremity leads (I, II, and III) and three augmented unipolar extremity leads (aV_R, aV_L, and aV_F).

   A *bipolar* lead records the difference between voltages from the heart detected at two extremities. A *unipolar* lead records voltages at one point relative to zero potential. The bipolar extremity leads can be represented by Einthoven's triangle (Fig. 3-4). They are related by the equation II = I + III. The unipolar extremity leads can also be represented by a triaxial diagram (Fig. 3-6). They are related by the equation $aV_R + aV_L + aV_F = 0$.

   The three unipolar extremity leads and the three bipolar extremity leads can be shown on the same diagram, so the axes of all six leads intersect at a common point, producing the *hexaxial lead diagram.*

   As a general rule, the P-QRS-T pattern in lead I resembles that in lead aV_L. Leads aV_R and II usually show reverse patterns. Lead aV_F usually resembles lead III.

2. The six *chest* (precordial) leads (V_1 to V_6) record voltages from the heart directed onto the horizontal plane of the body (dividing the body into an upper and a lower half). They are taken with electrodes in specific anatomic locations (Fig. 3-8).

In addition to the 12 conventional leads, ECGs can be taken in special ways: In cardiac care units (CCUs), monitor leads, in which electrodes are placed on the chest, are generally used. Fig. 3-13 shows the usual location of the chest electrodes for a monitor lead. Continuous ECGs are often recorded with the Holter apparatus for a period of 12 to (preferably) 24 or more hours in ambulatory patients who have transient or unpredictable arrhythmias.

Questions

1. Leads I and II are shown below. Draw the P-QRS-T pattern in lead III.

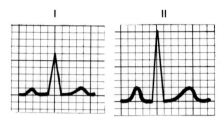

2. Leads I, II, and III are shown below. What is wrong with them?

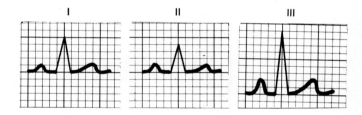

3. Draw the hexaxial lead diagram showing the six frontal plane (extremity) leads.
4. Why does the P-QRS-T pattern in lead aV_R usually show a reverse of the pattern in lead II?

Answers

1. Since lead II = lead I + lead III, then according to Einthoven's equation lead III = lead II − lead I as shown below:

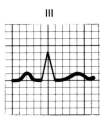

III

Notice that the voltages of the P wave, QRS complex, and T wave in lead II are equal to the sum of the P, QRS, and T voltages in leads I and III

2. The voltages in lead II here do *not* equal those in leads I and III. The reason is that leads II and III were mislabeled. Reverse the labels; now the voltage in II will equal the voltages in I and III.
3. See Fig. 3-7, *C*.
4. The positive poles of lead aV_R and lead II point in opposite directions (Fig. 3-7).

4

The Normal ECG

We have reviewed the cycle of atrial and ventricular depolarization and repolarization detected by the ECG as well as the 12 lead system used to record this electrical activity. This chapter describes the P-QRS-T patterns seen normally in each of the 12 leads. Fortunately, this does not require memorization of 12 or more separate patterns. Rather, knowledge of a few basic ECG principles and understanding of the sequence of atrial and ventricular depolarization will enable us to predict the normal ECG patterns in each lead.

As you can see from the sample ECG in Fig. 3-2, each of the 12 leads appears to be different from the next. In some leads, for example, the P waves are positive (upward); in others they are negative (downward). In some leads the QRS complexes are represented by an rS wave; in other leads they are represented by qR or QS waves. Finally, in some leads the T waves are positive, and in others negative. What determines this variety in the appearance of ECG complexes in the different leads, and how does the repetitive cycle of cardiac electrical activity produce such different patterns in these leads?

THREE BASIC "LAWS" OF ELECTROCARDIOGRAPHY

Answering the preceding questions requires understanding of the following three basic ECG "laws" (Fig. 4-1):

1. A *positive* (upward) *deflection* will appear in any lead if the wave of depolarization spreads toward the positive pole of that lead. Thus, if the path of atrial stimulation is directed downward and to the patient's left, toward the positive pole of lead II, a positive (upward) P wave will be seen in lead II (Figs. 4-2 and 4-3). Similarly, if the ventricular stimulation path is directed to the left, a positive deflection (an R wave) will be seen in lead I (Fig. 4-1, *A*).

2. A *negative* (downward) *deflection* will appear in any lead if the wave of depolarization spreads toward the negative pole of that lead (or away from the positive pole). Thus, if the atrial stimulation path spreads downward and to the left, a negative P wave will be seen in lead aV_R (Figs. 4-2 and 4-3). If the ventricular stimulation path is directed entirely away from the positive pole of any lead, a negative QRS complex (QS deflection) will be seen (Fig. 4-1, *B*).

3. If the mean depolarization path is directed at right angles (perpendicular) to any lead, you will usually see a small *biphasic deflection* (consisting of positive and negative deflections of equal size). If the atrial stimulation path spreads at right angles to any lead, you will see a biphasic P wave in that lead. If the ventricular stimulation path spreads at right angles to any lead, then the QRS complex will be biphasic (Fig. 4-1, *C*). A biphasic QRS complex may consist of either an RS pattern or a QR pattern.

• • •

THREE BASIC LAWS OF ELECTROCARDIOGRAPHY

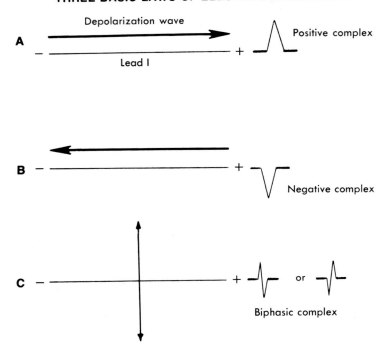

Fig. 4-1. A, A positive complex will be shown in any lead if the wave of depolarization spreads toward the positive pole of that lead. **B,** A negative complex will be shown if the depolarization wave spreads toward the negative pole (away from the positive pole) of the lead. **C,** A biphasic (partly positive, partly negative) complex will be seen if the mean direction of the wave is at right angles (perpendicular) to the lead. These three basic laws apply to both the P wave (atrial depolarization) and the QRS complex (ventricular depolarization).

DIRECTION OF ATRIAL DEPOLARIZATION WITH NORMAL SINUS RHYTHM

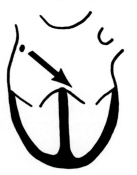

Fig. 4-2. With normal sinus rhythm the atrial depolarization wave will spread from the right atrium downward toward the AV junction and left leg.

To summarize: When depolarization spreads toward the positive pole of any lead it produces a positive (upward) deflection. When it spreads toward the negative pole (away from the positive pole) of any lead, it produces a negative (downward) deflection. When it spreads at right angles to any lead axis, it produces a biphasic deflection.

Mention of repolarization—the return of stimulated muscle to the resting state—has deliberately been omitted. The subject will be touched upon later in this chapter in discussing the normal T wave.

With these three basic ECG laws in mind, all you need to know is the direction in which depolarization spreads through the heart at any time to predict what the P waves and the QRS complexes will look like in any lead.

THE NORMAL P WAVE

Let us begin our description of the normal ECG with the first waveform seen in any cycle, the P wave, which represents atrial depolarization. Atrial depolarization is initiated by the sinus node, in the right atrium (Fig. 1-1). The atrial depolarization path therefore spreads from right to left and downward toward the AV junction. We can represent the spread of atrial depolarization by an arrow* that points downward and to the patient's left (as shown in Fig. 4-2).

Now go back to the diagram we drew in Chapter 3 showing the spatial relationship of the six frontal plane (extremity) leads. This diagram is redrawn in Fig. 4-3. Notice that the positive pole of lead aV_R points upward in the direction of the right shoulder. The normal path of atrial depolarization, as described, spreads downward toward the left leg (away from the positive pole of aV_R). *Therefore, with normal sinus rhythm, lead aV_R will always show a negative P wave.* Conversely, lead II is oriented with its positive pole pointing downward in the direction of the left leg (Fig. 4-3). Therefore the normal atrial depolarization path will be directed toward the positive pole of that lead. *When normal sinus rhythm is present, lead II will always record a positive (upward) P wave.*

To summarize: When normal sinus rhythm is

---

*The arrows used to represent cardiac electrical potentials have both specific direction and specific magnitude and are, therefore, ''vectors.'' The details of *vectorcardiography* lie outside the scope of this book, although vectorial principles are used throughout the discussions.

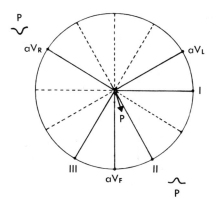

Fig. 4-3. With sinus rhythm the normal P wave will be negative (downward) in lead aV_R and positive (upward) in lead II. Recall that with normal atrial depolarization the arrow points down toward the patient's left (Fig. 4-2), away from the positive pole of lead aV_R and toward the positive pole of lead II.

DIRECTION OF ATRIAL DEPOLARIZATION WITH AV JUNCTIONAL RHYTHM

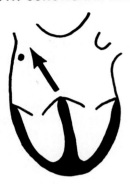

Fig. 4-4. When the AV junction acts as the cardiac pacemaker (junctional rhythm), the atria will be depolarized in a retrograde (backward) fashion. An *arrow* representing atrial depolarization in such cases will point upward toward the right atrium, just opposite the pattern seen with sinus rhythm.

present, the P wave will always be negative in lead aV_R and positive in lead II.

Using the same principles of analysis, can you predict what the P wave will look like in leads II and aV_R if the heart is being paced not by the sinus node but by the AV junction (AV junctional rhythm)? When the AV junction is pacing the heart, atrial depolarization will have to spread up the atria in a *retrograde* direction, just the opposite of what happens with normal sinus rhythm. Therefore an arrow representing the spread of atrial depolarization with AV junctional rhythm will point upward and to the right (Fig. 4-4), just the opposite of what occurs with normal sinus rhythm. Spread of atrial depolarization upward and to the right will result in a positive P wave in lead aV_R, since the stimulus is spreading toward the positive pole of that lead (Fig. 4-5). Conversely, lead II will show a negative P wave. We will discuss AV junctional rhythms in detail in Part II. The topic was introduced here simply to show how the polarity of the P wave in lead aV_R and lead II depends on the direction of atrial depolarization and how the pat-

terns can be predicted using simple basic principles.

You need not be concerned with the polarity of the P waves in the other 10 leads. You can get all the clinical information you need to determine whether or not the sinus node is pacing the atria by simply looking at the P wave in leads II and aV_R. The size and shape of the P waves in other leads may be of importance in determining whether left or right atrial enlargement is present (which will be discussed in Chapter 6).

THE NORMAL QRS COMPLEX

The same principles as those used above can be applied in deducing the shape of the QRS waveform in the various leads. The QRS, which represents ventricular depolarization, is somewhat more complex than the P wave, but the same basic ECG rules apply to both.

To predict what the QRS will look like in the different leads, you must first know the direction of ventricular depolarization. Although the spread of atrial depolarization can be represented by a single arrow, the spread of ventricular depolarization consists of two major sequential phases:

The *first* phase is of relatively brief duration

ORIENTATION OF P WAVES WITH AV JUNCTIONAL RHYTHM

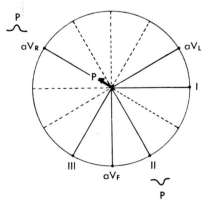

Fig. 4-5. With AV junctional rhythm the P waves will be upward (positive) in lead aV_R and downward (negative) in lead II.

NORMAL VENTRICULAR DEPOLARIZATION

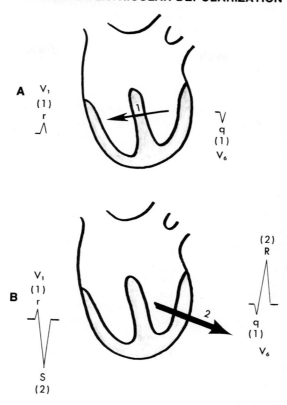

Fig. 4-6. Ventricular depolarization consists of two sequential phases. Phase one, **A,** proceeds from the left wall of the septum to the right. An *arrow* representing this phase points through the septum from the left to the right side. Phase two, **B,** is depolarization of the main bulk of the ventricles. The *arrow* points through the left ventricle, because this is normally electrically predominant. The two phases will produce an rS complex in the right chest lead (V_1) and a qR complex in the left chest lead (V_6).

(shorter than 0.04 sec) and small amplitude. It results from the spread of stimulus through the ventricular septum. The ventricular septum is the first part of the ventricles to be stimulated. Furthermore, the left side of the septum is stimulated first (by a branch of the left bundle of His); thus depolarization spreads from the left ventricle to the right across the septum. Phase one of ventricular depolarization, septal stimulation, can therefore be represented by a small arrow pointing from the left septal wall to the right (Fig. 4-6, *A*).

The *second* phase of ventricular depolarization involves simultaneous stimulation of the main mass of both the left and the right ventricles from the inside (endocardium) to the outside (epicardium) of the heart muscle. In the normal heart the left ventricle is electrically predominant. In other words, it electrically overbalances the right ventricle. Therefore an arrow representing phase two of ventricular stimulation will point toward the left ventricle (Fig. 4-6, *B*).

To summarize: The ventricular depolarization

process can be divided into two main phases. The first phase, stimulation of the ventricular septum, is represented by a short arrow pointing through the septum into the right ventricle. The second phase, simultaneous left and right ventricular stimulation, is represented by a larger arrow pointing through the left ventricle and toward the left chest.

Now that the ventricular stimulation sequence has been outlined, we can begin to predict what types of QRS patterns this sequence will produce in the different leads. For the moment, we will discuss only the QRS patterns normally seen in the chest leads (the horizontal plane leads).

Chest Leads

We will talk first about leads V_1 and V_6. As discussed in Chapter 3, lead V_1 shows voltages detected by an electrode placed on the right side of the sternum (fourth intercostal space). Lead V_6, a left chest lead, shows voltages detected in the left midaxillary line (as shown in Fig. 3-8). What will the QRS complex look like in these leads (Fig. 4-6)?

The first phase of ventricular stimulation, septal stimulation, is represented by an arrow pointing to the right, reflecting the left-to-right spread of depolarization stimulus through the septum (Fig. 4-6, A). This small arrow will point toward the positive pole of lead V_1. Therefore the spread of stimulation to the right during the first phase produces a small positive deflection (r wave) in lead V_1. What will lead V_6 show? The left-to-right spread of septal stimulation will produce a small negative deflection (q wave) in lead V_6. Thus the same electrical event, septal stimulation, produces a small positive deflection (or r wave) in lead V_1 and a small negative deflection (q wave) in a left precordial lead like V_6. (This situation is analogous to the one described for the P wave, which is normally positive in lead II but always negative in lead aV_R.)

The second phase of ventricular stimulation is represented by an arrow pointing in the direction of the left ventricle (Fig. 4-6, B). This arrow will point away from the positive pole of lead V_1 and toward the negative pole of V_6. Therefore the spread of stimulation to the left during the second phase results in a negative deflection in the right precor-

dial leads and a positive deflection in the left precordial leads. Lead V_1 will show a deep negative (S) wave, lead V_6 a tall positive (R) wave.

To summarize what we have learned about the normal QRS pattern in leads V_1 and V_6: Normally lead V_1 will show an rS type of complex. The small initial r wave represents the left-to-right spread of septal stimulation. This wave is sometimes referred to as the *septal r wave* because it reflects septal stimulation. The negative (S) wave reflects the spread of ventricular stimulation forces during phase two, away from the right and toward the dominant left ventricle. Conversely, the same electrical events, septal and ventricular stimulation, viewed from an electrode in the V_6 position will produce a qR pattern. The q wave is a *septal q wave,* reflecting the left-to-right spread of the stimulus through the septum away from lead V_6. The positive (R) wave reflects the leftward spread of ventricular stimulation voltages through the left ventricle.

Once again, to reemphasize, the same electrical event, whether depolarization of the atria or depolarization of the ventricles, will produce very different-looking waveforms in different leads because the spatial orientation of the leads is different.

We have discussed the patterns normally seen in leads V_1 and V_6. What happens *between* these leads? The answer is that as you move across the chest (in the direction of the electrically predominant left ventricle) the R wave tends to become relatively larger and the S wave becomes relatively smaller. This increase in height of the R wave, which usually reaches a maximum around lead V_4 or V_5, is called *normal R wave progression.* Fig. 4-7 shows examples of normal R wave progression.

At some point, generally around the V_3 or V_4 position, the R/S ratio becomes 1. This point, where the amplitude of the R wave equals that of the S wave, is called the *transition zone* (Fig. 4-7). In some normal people the transition may be seen as early as lead V_2. This is called *early transition.* In other cases the transition zone may be delayed to leads V_5 and V_6, and is called a *delayed transition.*

Examine the set of normal chest leads in Fig. 4-8. Notice the rS complex in lead V_1 and the qR

NORMAL R WAVE PROGRESSION

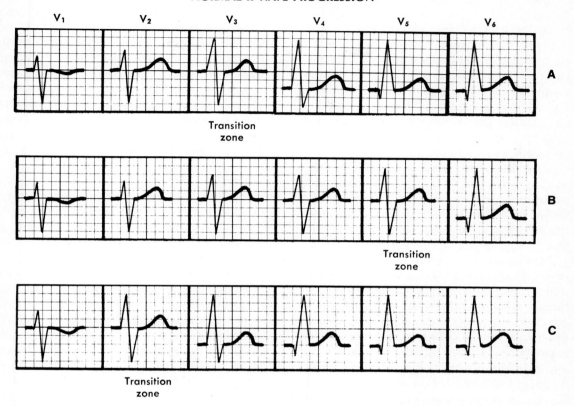

Transition zone

Transition zone

Transition zone

Fig. 4-7. Normally R waves in the chest leads become relatively taller from lead V_1 to the left chest leads. **A,** Notice the transition in lead V_3. **B,** Somewhat delayed R wave progression, with the transition in lead V_5. **C,** Early transition in lead V_2.

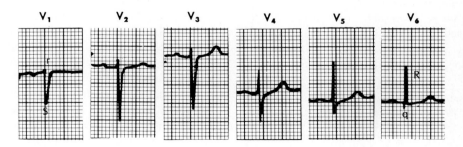

Fig. 4-8. Normal chest leads. The transition is in lead V_4. Notice the normal septal r wave in lead V_1 (as part of an rS complex) and the normal septal q in lead V_6 (part of a qR complex).

complex in lead V_6. The R wave tends to get gradually larger here as you move toward the left chest leads. The transition zone, where the R wave and S wave are about equal, is in lead V_4. In normal chest leads the R wave voltage need not get literally larger as you go from leads V_1 and V_6. However, the overall trend should show a relative increase. For example, notice that in this example there is not much difference between the complexes in leads V_2 and V_3, and that the R wave in lead V_5 is taller than the R wave in lead V_6.

In summary: The normal chest lead ECG shows an rS-type complex in lead V_1 with a steady increase in the relative size of the R wave toward the left chest and a decrease in S wave amplitude. Leads V_5 and V_6 generally show a qR-type complex.*

The concept of *normal R wave progression* is key in distinguishing normal and abnormal ECG patterns. For example, imagine the effect that an anterior wall myocardial infarction would have on normal R wave progression. Anterior wall infarction results in the death of myocardial cells and the loss of normal positive (R wave) voltages. Therefore one of the major ECG signs of an anterior wall infarction will be the loss of normal R wave progression in the chest leads. (The topic of myocardial infarction is discussed in detail in Chapters 8 and 9.)

Understanding normal R wave progression in the chest leads also sets the basis for recognizing other basic ECG abnormalities. For example, consider the effect of left or right ventricular hypertrophy (enlarged muscle mass) on the chest lead patterns. As mentioned before, the left ventricle is normally electrically predominant; and left ventricular depolarization produces deep (negative) S waves in

the right chest leads with tall (positive) R waves in the left chest leads. With left ventricular hypertrophy, these left ventricular voltages will be further increased, resulting in very tall R waves in the left chest leads and very deep S waves in the right chest leads. On the other hand, right ventricular hypertrophy would be expected to shift the balance of electrical forces to the right, producing tall positive (R) waves in the right chest leads. (These patterns of left and right ventricular hypertrophy are described in detail in Chapter 6.)

Extremity Leads

We have discussed the normal QRS patterns in the chest leads. All that remains is to describe the normal QRS patterns in the extremity leads: I, II, III, aV_R, aV_L, and aV_F.

We will begin with lead aV_R, which is the easiest to visualize. The positive pole of lead aV_R is oriented upward and toward the right shoulder. The ventricular stimulation forces are oriented primarily toward the left ventricle. Therefore lead aV_R normally shows a predominantly negative QRS complex. You may see any of the QRS-T complexes shown in Fig. 4-9 in lead aV_R. In all cases, the QRS is predominantly negative. The T wave in lead aV_R is also normally negative. The QRS patterns in the other five extremity leads are somewhat more complicated. The reason is that there is considerable normal variation in the QRS patterns seen in the extremity leads. For example, some normal people will have an ECG that shows one pattern (Fig. 4-10) in the extremity leads (qR-type complexes in leads I and aV_L, rS-type complexes in leads III and aV_F) while other people will have just the opposite picture (Fig. 4-11) (qR complexes in leads II, III, and aV_F, RS complexes in lead aV_L and sometimes lead I).

How can we account for this marked normal variability in the QRS patterns shown in the extremity leads? The patterns seen depend on the *electrical position* of the heart. The term "electrical position" is virtually synonymous with "*mean QRS axis*," which is described in greater detail in Chapter 5.

---

*Normal chest lead patterns may show slight variation from the patterns we have been discussing. For example, some people will have a QS and not an rS pattern in lead V_1. In other cases the septal q wave in the left chest leads may not be seen and thus leads V_5 and V_6 will show an R wave and not a qR complex. On other normal ECGs, leads V_5 and V_6 may show a narrow qRs complex as a normal variant and lead V_1 may show a narrow rSr'.

LEAD aV$_R$: NORMAL PATTERNS

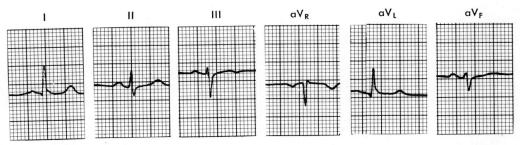

Fig. 4-9. Normally lead aV$_R$ shows one of three basic negative patterns: an rS complex, a QS complex, or a Qr complex. The T wave also is normally negative.

NORMAL HORIZONTAL QRS AXIS

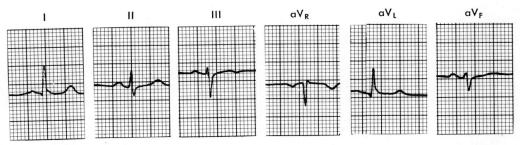

Fig. 4-10. With a horizontal QRS position (axis) leads I and aV$_L$ show qR complexes while lead II shows RS and leads III and aV$_F$ show rS complexes.

NORMAL VERTICAL QRS AXIS

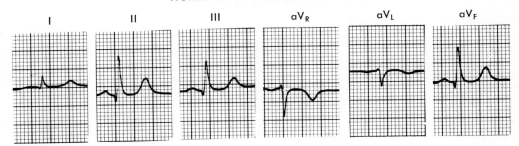

Fig. 4-11. With a vertical QRS position (axis) leads II, III, and aV$_F$ show qR complexes while lead aV$_L$ (and sometimes lead I) shows an RS complex. This is just the reverse of the pattern with a normal horizontal axis.

In simplest terms the electrical position of the heart may be described as either *horizontal* or *vertical.*

1. When the heart is electrically horizontal *(horizontal QRS axis)*, ventricular depolarization is directed mainly horizontally and to the left in the frontal plane. Looking at the frontal plane diagram (Fig. 3-10), you can see that the positive poles of leads I and aV_L are oriented horizontally and to the left. Therefore, when the heart is electrically horizontal, the QRS voltages will be directed toward leads I and aV_L, producing a tall R wave (usually as part of a qR complex) in these leads.

2. When the heart is electrically vertical *(vertical QRS axis)*, ventricular depolarization is directed mainly downward. Looking at the frontal plane diagram (Fig. 3-10), you can see that the positive poles of leads II, III, and aV_F are oriented downward. Therefore, when the heart is electrically vertical, the QRS voltages will be directed toward leads II, III, and aV_F, producing a tall R wave (usually as part of a qR complex) in these leads.

The concepts of electrically horizontal and electrically vertical heart positions can be expressed in another way. When the heart is electrically horizontal, leads I and aV_L will show qR complexes similar to the qR complexes seen normally in the left chest leads (V_5 and V_6). Leads II, III, and aV_F will show rS complexes similar to those seen in the right chest leads normally. Therefore, when the heart is electrically horizontal, the patterns in leads I and aV_L will resemble those in leads V_5 and V_6 while the patterns in leads II, III, and aV_F resemble those in the right chest leads. Conversely, when the heart is electrically vertical, just the opposite patterns will be seen in the extremity leads. With a vertical heart leads II, III, and aV_F will show qR complexes, similar to those seen in the left chest leads, while leads I and aV_L show rS-type complexes, resembling those in the right chest leads.

Dividing the electrical position of the heart into vertical and horizontal variants is obviously an oversimplification. For example, look at Fig. 4-12. Here leads I, II, aV_L, and aV_F all show positive QRS complexes. Therefore, this tracing has features of *both* the vertical and the horizontal variants. (Sometimes this pattern is referred to as an ''intermediate'' heart position.)

For present purposes, however, you can regard the QRS patterns in the extremity leads to be basically variants of either the horizontal or the vertical QRS patterns described.

To summarize: The extremity leads in normal people can show a variable QRS pattern. Lead aV_R normally always records a predominantly negative QRS complex (Qr, QS, or rS). The QRS patterns in the other extremity leads will vary depending on the ''electrical position'' (QRS axis) of the heart.

NORMAL INTERMEDIATE QRS AXIS

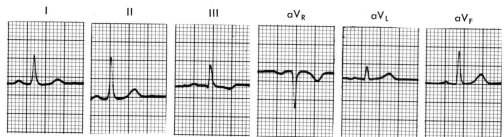

Fig. 4-12. Sometimes extremity leads show patterns that are hybrids of vertical and horizontal variants, with R waves in leads I, II, III, aV_L, and aV_F. This represents an intermediate QRS axis and is also a normal variant.

With an electrically vertical axis, leads II, III, and aV_F will show qR type complexes. With an electrically horizontal axis, leads I and aV_L will show qR complexes. Therefore it is not possible to define a single normal ECG pattern; rather, there is a normal variability. Students and clinicians must familiarize themselves with the normal variants in both the chest leads and the extremity leads.

THE NORMAL ST SEGMENT

As noted in Chapter 2, the normal ST segment, representing the early phase of ventricular repolarization, is usually isoelectric (flat on the baseline). Slight deviations (generally of less than 1 mm) may be seen normally. As described in Chapter 10, certain normal people will have more marked ST segment elevations as a normal variant (early repolarization pattern). Finally, examine the ST segments in the right chest leads (V_1 to V_3) of Figs. 3-2 and 6-10. Notice that they are short and the T waves appear to take off almost from the J point (junction of the QRS complex and the ST segment). This pattern of an early takeoff of the T wave in the right chest leads is not an uncommon finding in normal persons.

THE NORMAL T WAVE

Up to this point, we have deferred discussion of ventricular repolarization—the return of stimulated muscle to the resting state, which produces the ST segment, T wave, and U wave. Deciding whether the T wave in any lead is normal or not is generally straightforward. As a rule, the T wave follows the direction of the main QRS deflection. Thus, when the main QRS deflection is positive (upright), the T wave is normally positive. We can also make some more specific rules about the direction of the normal T wave.

The normal T wave in lead aV_R is always negative, while in lead II it is always positive. Left-sided chest leads, such as V_4 to V_6, normally always show a positive T wave.

The T wave in the other leads may be variable. In the right chest leads (V_1 and V_2) it may be normally negative, isoelectric, or positive but it is almost always positive by lead V_3.* Furthermore, if the T wave is positive in any chest lead, it must remain positive in all chest leads to the left of that lead. Otherwise, it is abnormal. For example, if the T wave is negative in leads V_1 and V_2 and becomes positive in V_3, it should normally remain positive in V_4 to V_6.

The polarity of the T wave in the extremity leads depends on the electrical position of the heart. With a horizontal heart the main QRS deflection is positive in I and aV_L and the T wave is also positive in these leads. With an electrically vertical heart the QRS is positive in II, III, and aV_F and the T wave is also positive in these leads. However, on some normal ECGs with a vertical axis the T wave may be negative in lead III.

---

*In children and in some normal adults, a downward T wave may extend as far left as V_3 or V_4. This is known as the *juvenile T wave pattern.*

REVIEW

The three basic ''laws'' of electrocardiography are as follows:

1. A positive *(upward)* deflection will be seen in any lead if depolarization spreads toward the positive pole of that lead.
2. A negative *(downward)* deflection will be seen if depolarization spreads toward the negative pole (or away from the positive pole) of any lead.
3. If the mean depolarization path is directed at right angles *(perpendicular)* to any lead, a small biphasic (RS or QR) deflection will be seen.

Atrial depolarization starts in the sinus node and spreads downward and to the patient's left, toward the positive pole of lead II and away from the positive pole of lead aV_R. Therefore, with normal sinus rhythm, the P wave will always be positive in lead II and negative in lead aV_R.

Ventricular depolarization consists of two sequential phases:

1. The first phase is stimulation of the ventricular septum from left to right. This produces a small (septal) r wave in the right chest leads and a small (septal) q wave in the left chest leads.

2. During the second major phase of ventricular depolarization, the stimulus spreads simultaneously outward through the right and left ventricles. Since the mass of the normal left ventricle overbalances the mass of the right ventricle, the spread of depolarization through the left ventricle predominates on the normal ECG. This spread of stimulus through the left ventricle produces a tall R wave in the left chest leads (such as V_5 and V_6) (in association with a small initial q wave) and a deep S wave in the right chest leads (V_1 and V_2) (associated with a small initial r wave).

Chest leads between these extreme positions show a transitional pattern with tall R waves and deep S waves.

In the extremity leads the shape of the QRS complex varies with the electrical position (axis) of the heart:

1. When the heart is electrically horizontal, leads I and aV_L show a qR pattern.

2. When the heart is electrically vertical, leads II, III, and aV_F show a qR pattern.

The normal T wave generally follows the direction of the main deflection of the QRS complex in any lead. In the chest leads the T may normally be negative in leads V_1 and V_2. In most adults it becomes positive by lead V_2 and remains positive in the left chest leads. In the extremity leads the T wave is always positive in lead II and negative in lead aV_R. When the heart is electrically horizontal, the QRS and the T are positive in leads I and aV_L. When the heart is electrically vertical, the QRS and T are positive in leads II, III, and aV_F.

Questions

1. Examine the following 12-lead ECG and lead II rhythm strip. Then answer these questions:
   a. Is normal sinus rhythm present?
   b. In the extremity leads, is the QRS axis electrically vertical or electrically horizontal?
   c. In the chest leads, where is the transition zone?
   d. Is the PR interval normal?
   e. Is the QRS interval normal?
   f. Are the T waves in the chest leads normal?

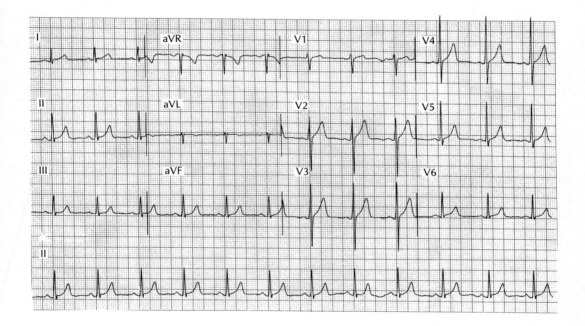

2. Answer these questions about the following ECG:
   a. Is the heart electrically vertical or horizontal?
   b. What is the approximate heart rate?
   c. What is the major abnormality of the QRS complexes in the chest leads?
   d. Are the T waves in leads I and aV_L normal?

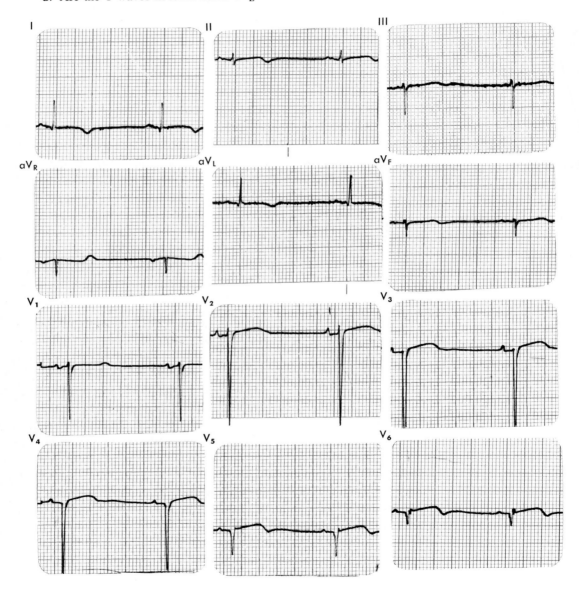

3. On the following ECG, is sinus rhythm present?

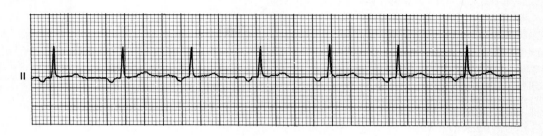

Answers

1. a. Yes. The P waves are positive (upright) in lead II and negative in aV_R, with a rate of about 75/min.
   b. Electrically vertical. The R waves are most prominent in leads II, III, and aV_F.
   c. The transition zone is in lead V_3. Notice that the RS complexes have the R wave approximately equal to the S wave.
   d. The PR interval is about 0.16 second. This is within normal range (0.12 to 0.2 sec).
   e. The QRS width is 0.08 second. This is normal (less than or equal to 0.1 sec).
   f. Yes.
2. a. Electrically horizontal. The R waves are most prominent in leads I and aV_L. (Contrast this with 1a above.)
   b. 50 beats/min.
   c. Loss of R wave progression. Normally there is a steady increase in R wave amplitude as you move from lead V_1 to the left. On this ECG there are small r waves in leads V_1 and V_2 with complete loss of R waves in leads V_3 to V_6. Loss of R wave progression in this case was caused by an extensive anterior wall infarction (Chapter 8).
   d. No. The T waves are abnormally inverted (negative) in leads I and aV_L. Recall that with an electrically horizontal heart the T waves are normally upright in leads I and aV_L.
3. No. Although there is a P wave before each QRS complex, notice that it is negative in lead II. With sinus rhythm the P should be positive (upright) in lead II. Thus in this patient the pacemaker must be outside the sinus node (ectopic), either in the AV junction or low in one of the atria. Inverted P waves such as these are called *retrograde* because the atria are depolarized in the opposite direction from normal, that is, from the bottom to the top rather than from the top (sinus node) to the bottom (AV junction). See also Chapters 11 and 12.

5

Electrical Axis and Axis Deviation

In the previous chapter we discussed normal ECG patterns in the chest and extremity leads. The general terms *"horizontal heart"* (or horizontal QRS axis) and *"vertical heart"* (or vertical QRS axis) were used to describe the normal variations in QRS patterns seen in the extremity leads. In this chapter we will refine this concept of electrical axis and see how the electrical axis of the QRS pattern can be determined in a simple way.

MEAN QRS AXIS: DEFINITION

The depolarization stimulus spreads through the ventricles in different directions from instant to instant. For example, it may be directed toward lead I at one moment and toward lead III the next. We can also talk about the mean direction of the QRS complex, or *mean QRS electrical axis*. If you could draw an arrow to represent the general, or mean, direction in which the QRS complex is pointed *in the frontal plane* of the body, you would be drawing the electrical axis of the QRS complex.

The term *"mean QRS axis"* therefore describes the general direction in the frontal plane toward which the QRS complex is predominantly pointed.

Since we are defining the QRS axis in the frontal plane, we are describing the QRS only in reference to the six extremity leads (the six frontal plane leads). (See Fig. 5-1.) Therefore the scale of reference used to measure the mean QRS axis is the diagram of the frontal plane leads (described in Chapter 3). We also discussed the Einthoven triangle in Chapter 3 and saw how the triangle can

easily be converted into a triaxial lead diagram by simply having the three axes (leads I, II, and III) intersect at a central point (Fig. 5-1, *A*). Similarly we saw how the axes of the three unipolar extremity leads (aV_R, aV_L, and aV_F) also form a triaxial lead diagram (Fig. 5-1, *B*). These two triaxial lead diagrams were combined to produce a hexaxial lead diagram (Fig. 5-1, *C*). This is the lead diagram we will use in determining the mean QRS axis and in describing axis deviation.

As noted in Chapter 3, each of the leads has a positive and a negative pole (Fig. 5-1, *C*). As a wave of depolarization spreads toward the positive pole, an upward (positive) deflection occurs. As a wave spreads toward the negative pole, a downward (negative) deflection is inscribed.

Finally, to determine or calculate the mean QRS axis, we need a scale. By convention, the positive pole of lead I is said to be at $0°$; all points below the lead I axis are positive; all points above that axis are negative (Fig. 5-2). Thus, as we move toward the positive pole of lead aV_L ($-30°$), the scale becomes negative; and as we move downward toward the positive poles of leads II, III, and aV_F, the scale becomes more positive—lead II at $+60°$, lead aV_F at $+90°$, lead III at $+120°$.

Fig. 5-2 is the completed hexaxial diagram used to measure the QRS axis. By convention again, we can say that an electrical axis that points toward lead aV_L is *leftward* or *horizontal*. An axis that points toward leads II, III, and aV_F is *rightward* or *vertical*.

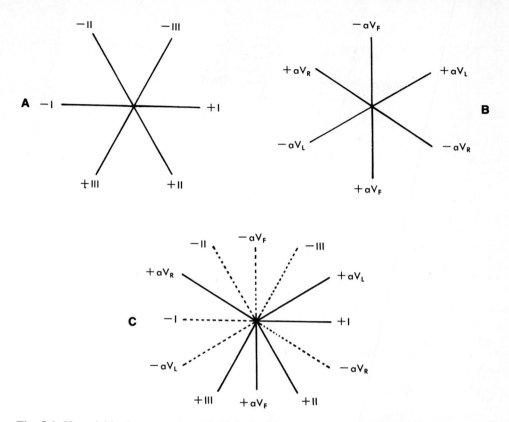

Fig. 5-1. Hexaxial lead system. **A** and **B,** Relationship of leads I, II, and III and of aV_R, aV_L, and aV_F. **C,** These diagrams have been combined to form a hexaxial lead diagram. Notice that each lead has both a positive and a negative pole (the latter designated by *dashed lines*).

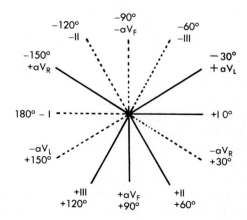

Fig. 5-2. Hexaxial lead diagram. Notice that each lead has an angular designation—with the positive pole of lead I at 0° and all leads above it having negative angular values while those below it have positive values.

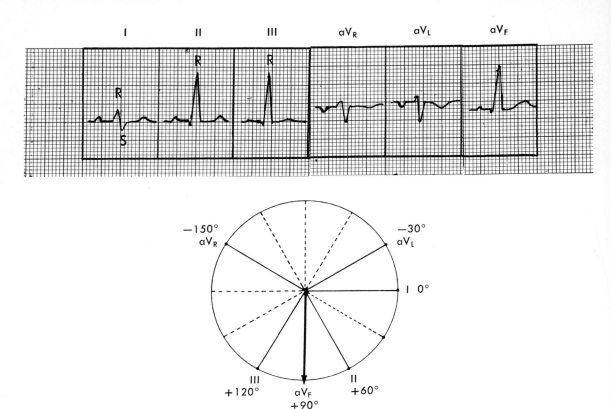

Fig. 5-3. Mean QRS axis of +90°. See text.

MEAN QRS AXIS: CALCULATION

In calculating the mean QRS axis you are answering the question: in what general direction or toward which lead axis is the QRS complex predominantly oriented? For example, consider Fig. 5-3. Notice that there are tall R waves in leads II, III, and aV_F, indicating that the heart is electrically vertical (vertical electrical axis). Furthermore, the R wave is equally tall in leads II and III.* Therefore, by simple inspection, the mean electrical QRS axis can be seen to be directed between leads II and III and toward aV_F. Lead aV_F on the hexaxial diagram is at +90°.

---

*In this case there are actually three leads (II, III, and aV_F) with R waves of equal height. In such cases the electrical axis will point toward the middle lead, that is, toward aV_F or at +90°.

As a general rule: *The mean QRS axis will point midway between any two leads that show tall R waves of equal height.*

In the preceding example the mean electrical axis could have been calculated a second way. Recall from Chapter 3 that if a wave of depolarization is oriented at right angles to any lead axis a biphasic complex (RS or QR) will be recorded in that lead. Reasoning in a reverse manner, if you find a biphasic complex in any of the extremity leads, then the mean QRS axis must be directed at 90° to that lead. Now look at Fig. 5-3 again. Are there any biphasic QRS complexes? Obviously lead I is biphasic and shows an RS pattern. Therefore, the mean electrical axis must be directed at right angles to lead I. Since lead I on the hexaxial lead scale is at 0°, the mean electrical axis must be at right

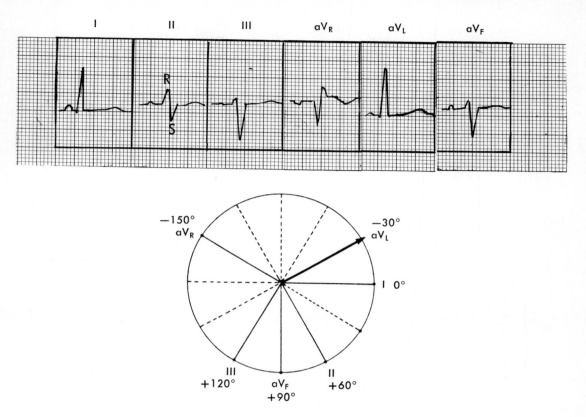

Fig. 5-4. Mean QRS of −30°. See text.

angles to 0° or at either −90° or +90°. If the axis were −90°, then the depolarization forces would be oriented away from the positive pole of lead aV_F and that lead would show a negative complex. In this case lead aV_F shows a positive complex (tall R wave), so the axis must be +90°.

Fig. 5-4 presents another example. In this case, by inspection, the mean QRS axis is obviously horizontal since leads I and aV_L are positive and leads II, III, and aV_F are predominantly negative. The precise electrical axis can be calculated by looking at lead II, which shows a biphasic RS complex. Therefore, using the same logic as before, we can say that the axis must be at right angles to lead II. Since lead II is at +60° on the hexaxial scale (Fig. 5-2), the axis must be either −30° or +150°. If it were +150°, then leads II, III, and

aV_F would be positive. Clearly in this case the axis is −30°.

Another example is given in Fig. 5-5. The QRS complex is positive in leads II, III, and aV_F. Therefore we can say that the axis is relatively vertical. Since the R waves are of equal magnitude in leads I and III, the mean QRS axis must be oriented between these two leads, or at +60°.

Alternatively, we could have calculated the axis by looking at lead aV_L (in Fig. 5-5), which shows a biphasic RS-type complex. The axis must be at right angles to lead aV_L (−30°), that is, either −120° or +60°. Obviously, in this case the answer is +60°. The electrical axis must be oriented toward lead II, which shows a tall R wave.

We can now describe a second general rule: *The mean QRS axis will be oriented at right angles to*

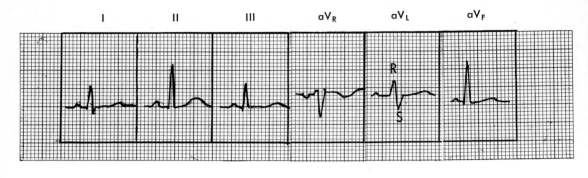

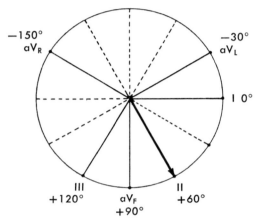

Fig. 5-5. Mean QRS axis of $+60°$. See text.

any lead showing a biphasic complex. In such cases the mean QRS axis will point in the direction of leads showing tall R waves.

Still another example is given in Fig. 5-6. By inspection, the electrical axis can be seen to be oriented away from leads II, III, and aV_F and toward leads aV_R and aV_L, which show positive complexes. Since the R waves are of equal magnitude in leads aV_R and aV_L, the axis must be oriented precisely between these leads, or at $-90°$. Alternatively, look at lead I, which shows a biphasic RS complex. In this case the axis must be directed at right angles to lead I ($0°$); that is, it must be either $-90°$ or $+90°$. Since the axis is oriented away from the positive pole of lead aV_F and toward the negative pole of that lead, it must be $-90°$.

Again, look at Fig. 5-7. There are two ways of approaching the calculation of the mean QRS in this case. Since lead aV_R shows a biphasic RS-type complex, the electrical axis must be at right angles to the axis of that lead; and since the axis of aV_R is at $-150°$, the electrical axis in this case must be either $-60°$ or $+120°$. Clearly it is $-60°$ since aV_L is positive and III shows a negative complex.*

These basic examples should establish the ground rules for calculating the mean QRS axis. It is worth emphasizing that such calculations are generally only an estimate or a near approximation. An error

---

*The QRS axis can also be calculated by looking at lead I, in Fig. 5-7. It shows an R wave of equal amplitude with the S wave in lead II. The mean QRS axis must be oriented between the axis of lead I ($0°$) and the negative axis of lead II ($-120°$). Therefore it must be $-60°$.

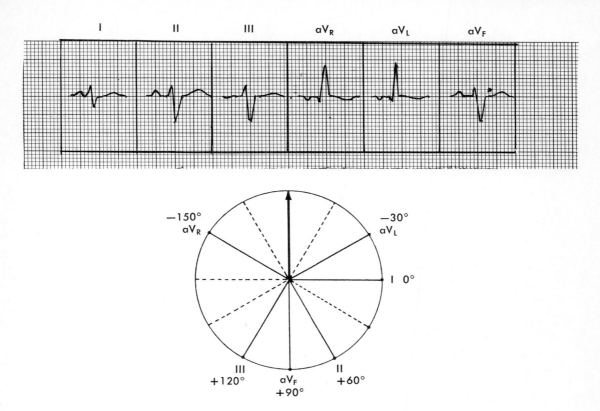

Fig. 5-6. Mean QRS axis of $-90°$. See text.

of 10° or 15° is not clinically significant. Thus it is perfectly acceptable to calculate the axis from leads in which the QRS is nearly biphasic or from two leads where the R (or S) waves are of approximately equal amplitude.*

---

*For example, when the R (or S) waves in two leads have similar but not identical voltages, the mean QRS axis will not lie exactly between these two leads. Instead, it will point more toward the lead with the larger amplitude.

Similarly, if a lead shows a biphasic (RS or QR) deflection where the R and S (or Q and R) waves are *not* of identical amplitude, then the mean QRS axis will *not* be pointed exactly perpendicular to that lead. If the R wave is larger than the S (or Q) wave, the axis will point slightly less than 90° away from the lead. If the R wave is smaller than the S (or Q) wave, the axis will point slightly more than 90° away from that lead.

To summarize: The mean QRS axis can be determined on the basis of one or both of the following rules:

1. It will point midway between the axes of two extremity leads that show tall R waves of equal amplitude.
2. It will point at 90° (right angles) to any extremity lead that shows a biphasic (QR or RS) type complex and in the direction of leads showing relatively tall R waves.

AXIS DEVIATION

The mean QRS axis is a basic measurement that should be made on every ECG. In most normal people it will lie between $-30°$ and $+100°$. An axis of $-30°$ or more negative is described as *left axis deviation (LAD),* and one that is $+100°$ or

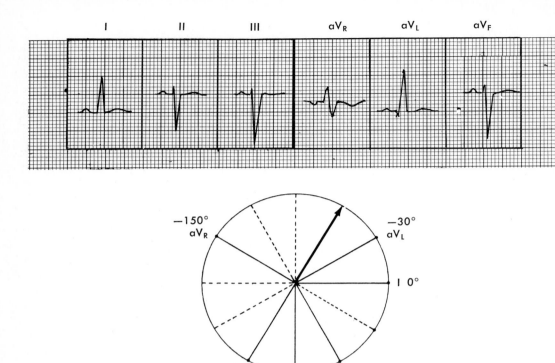

Fig. 5-7. Mean QRS axis of $-60°$. See text.

more positive *right axis deviation (RAD)*. In other words, LAD is abnormal extension of the mean QRS axis found in persons with an electrically horizontal heart while RAD is abnormal extension of the mean QRS axis in persons with an electrically vertical heart.

The mean QRS axis is determined by two major factors: (1) the anatomic position of the heart and (2) the direction in which the stimulus spreads through the ventricles (that is, the direction of ventricular depolarization).

The influence of *cardiac anatomic position* on the electrical axis can be illustrated by the effects of respiration. When a person breathes in, the diaphragm descends and the heart becomes more vertical in the chest cavity. This change generally shifts the QRS electrical axis vertically (to the right). (Patients with emphysema and chronically hyperinflated lungs will usually have anatomically vertical hearts and electrically vertical QRS axes.) Conversely, when the person breathes out, the diaphragm ascends and the heart assumes a more horizontal position in the chest. This generally shifts the QRS electrical axis horizontally (to the left).

The influence of the *direction of ventricular depolarization* can be illustrated by left anterior hemiblock (Chapter 7), in which the spread of stimuli through the more superior and leftward portions of the left ventricle is delayed and the mean QRS axis shifts to the left. By contrast, with right ventricular hypertrophy the QRS axis shifts to the right.

Recognition of right and left axis deviation is quite simple.

RAD exists if the QRS axis is found to be $+100°$ or more positive.

Recall that if leads II and III show tall R waves of equal height then the axis must be $+90°$. As an approximate rule: *If leads II and III show tall R waves and the R wave in lead III exceeds that in lead II then right axis deviation is present.* In addition, lead I will show an RS pattern with the S wave deeper than the R wave is tall (Figs. 5-8 and 5-10).

LAD exists if the QRS axis is found to be $-30°$ or more negative.

Fig. 5-4 presents an ECG in which the QRS axis is exactly $-30°$. Notice that lead II shows a biphasic (RS) complex. Remember that the location of lead II is at $+60°$ (Fig. 5-2) and a biphasic complex indicates that the electrical axis must be at right angles to that lead (at either $-30°$ or $+150°$). Thus, with an axis of $-30°$, lead II will show an RS complex with the R and S of equal amplitude. *If the electrical axis is more negative than $-30°$ (LAD) then lead II will show an RS complex with the S wave deeper than the R wave is tall* (Figs. 5-9 and 5-11).

The rules for recognition of axis deviation can be summarized as follows:
1. *Right axis deviation* is present if the R wave in lead III is taller than the R wave in lead II. Notice that with right axis deviation lead I shows an RS-type complex with the S wave deeper than the R wave is tall (Figs. 5-8 and 5-10).
2. *Left axis deviation* is present if lead I shows a tall R wave, lead III shows a deep S wave, and lead II shows a biphasic rS complex (with the amplitude of the S wave exceeding the height of the r wave) (Figs. 5-9 and 5-11) or a QS complex. Leads I and aV_L will both show tall R waves.

In Chapter 3 the terms *"electrically vertical"* and *"electrically horizontal"* heart positions (mean QRS axis) were introduced. Now in this chapter *"left axis deviation"* and *"right axis deviation,"* have been added. What is the difference between these terms? As mentioned, "electrically vertical" and "electrically horizontal" heart positions are qualitative. With an electrically vertical mean QRS axis, leads II, III, and aV_F will show tall R waves. With an electrically horizontal mean QRS axis, leads I and aV_L will show tall R waves. With an electrically vertical heart, the actual mean QRS axis may be normal (for example, $+80°$) or ab-

RIGHT AXIS DEVIATION

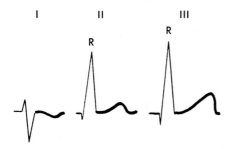

Fig. 5-8. Right axis deviation (RAD)—mean QRS axis more positive than $+100°$—can be determined by simple inspection of leads I, II, and III. Notice that lead III shows an R wave taller than the R wave in lead II.

LEFT AXIS DEVIATION

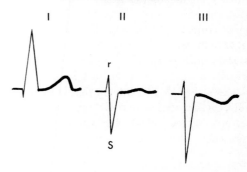

Fig. 5-9. Left axis deviation (LAD)—mean QRS axis more negative than $-30°$—can also be determined by simple inspection of leads I, II, and III. Notice that lead II shows an rS complex (with the S wave of greater amplitude than the r wave).

RIGHT AXIS DEVIATION

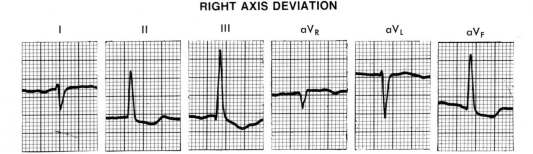

Fig. 5-10. Notice the R waves in leads II and III, with the one in lead III greater than the one in lead II, from a patient with RAD.

LEFT AXIS DEVIATION

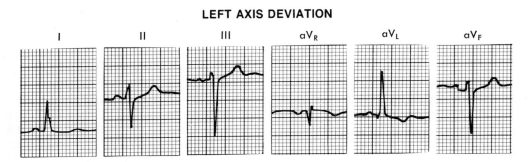

Fig. 5-11. Notice the rS complex in lead II from a patient with LAD.

normally rightward (such as +120°). Similarly, with an electrically horizontal heart, the actual axis may be normal (0°) or abnormally leftward (−50°).

RAD, therefore, is simply an extreme form of a vertical mean QRS axis (Fig. 5-12). LAD, similarly, is an extreme form of a horizontal mean QRS axis (Fig. 5-13). Saying that the patient has an electrically vertical or horizontal mean QRS axis does not, in fact, tell whether actual axis deviation is present.

Clinical Significance

Right and left axis deviations may be encountered in a variety of settings:

RAD, with the mean QRS axis +100° or more, is sometimes seen in normal people. Right ventricular hypertrophy (Chapter 6) is an important

cause of RAD. Another cause is myocardial infarction of the lateral wall of the left ventricle. Loss of the normal leftward depolarization forces in this setting may lead "by default" to a rightward axis (Fig. 8-11). Left posterior hemiblock (Chapter 7) is a much rarer cause of RAD. Patients with chronic lung disease (emphysema or chronic bronchitis) often have electrocardiograms showing RAD. Finally, a sudden shift in the mean QRS axis to the right (not necessarily causing actual RAD) may occur with acute pulmonary embolism (Chapter 10).

LAD, with the mean QRS axis −30° or more, may also be seen in several settings. Patients with left ventricular hypertrophy (Chapter 6) sometimes, but not always, have it. Left anterior hemiblock (Chapter 7) is a fairly common cause of marked deviation (more negative than −45°). LAD

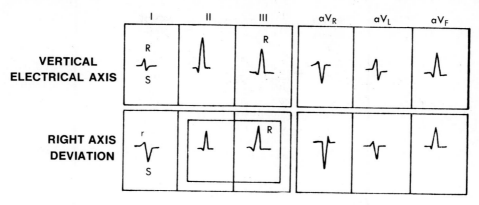

Fig. 5-12. Comparison of a normal vertical axis with actual RAD. See text.

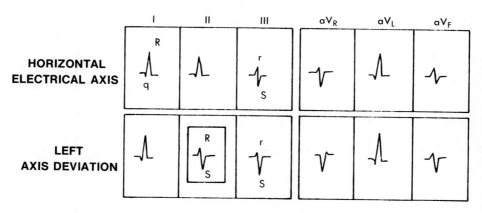

Fig. 5-13. Comparison of a normal horizontal axis with actual LAD. See text.

may be seen in association with left bundle branch block (Chapter 7). It may even occur in the absence of apparent cardiac disease.

However, axis deviation, right or left, does not necessarily imply significant underlying heart disease. Nevertheless, its recognition (Fig. 5-14) often provides supportive evidence for left or right ventricular hypertrophy, ventricular conduction disturbance (left anterior or posterior hemiblock), or one of the other disorders just listed.

Finally, it should be realized that the limits for left and right axis deviation (−30° to +100°) used in this book are necessarily arbitrary. Some authors

use different criteria (for example, 0° to +90°). These apparent discrepancies reflect the important fact that there are no absolute parameters in clinical electrocardiography. The best we can do is apply general criteria. The same problems will be found in the next chapter, on left and right ventricular hypertrophy, in which different voltage criteria have been described by different authors.

On rare occasion, all six extremity leads will show biphasic (QR or RS) complexes, making it impossible to calculate the mean frontal plane QRS axis. In such cases the term *"indeterminate axis"* is used (Fig. 5-15). An indeterminate QRS axis

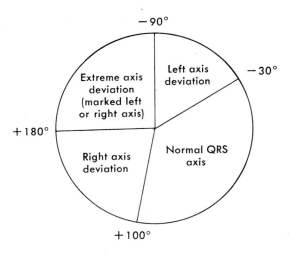

Fig. 5-14. Normal QRS axis and axis deviation. Most electrocardiograms will show either a normal axis or a left or right axis deviation. (Occasionally the QRS axis will be between −90° and 180°. Such an extreme shift may be caused by marked left or marked right axis deviation.)

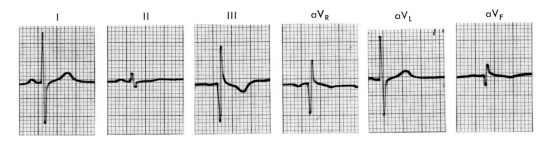

Fig. 5-15. Indeterminate axis. Notice the biphasic complexes (RS or QR) in all six frontal plane leads.

may occur as a normal variant or be seen in a variety of pathologic settings.

MEAN ELECTRICAL AXIS OF THE P WAVE AND T WAVE

Up to now, only the mean electrical axis of the QRS complex in the frontal plane has been considered. Using the same principles, we can also discuss the mean electrical axes of the P wave and T wave in the frontal plane.

For example, when sinus rhythm is present, the normal P wave is always negative in lead aV_R and positive in lead II. Therefore, normally, the P wave is generally directed toward lead II (Fig. 4-3), making the normal mean P wave axis about +60°. On the other hand, if the AV junction (and not the sinus node) is pacing the heart, then the atria will be stimulated in a retrograde way. When AV junctional rhythm is present, atrial depolarization spreads upward, toward lead aV_R and away from lead II (Fig. 4-5). In such patients lead aV_R may show a positive P wave and lead II a negative P wave, and the mean P wave axis may be about −150°.

Using the same principles, we can also calculate the mean electrical axis of the T wave in the frontal plane. As a rule the mean T wave axis and the mean QRS axis normally point in the same general (but not identical) direction. In other words, when the electrical position of the heart is horizontal, the T waves will normally be positive in leads I and aV_L, in association with tall R waves in these leads; and when the electrical position is vertical, the T waves will normally be positive in leads II, III, and aV_F, in association with tall R waves in these leads. (However, the T wave is often negative in lead III normally, regardless of the electrical position of the heart.)

To summarize: The concept of mean electrical axis can be applied to the QRS complex, P wave, or T wave. In each case the mean electrical axis describes the general or overall direction in which depolarization or repolarization is directed in the frontal plane.

REVIEW

The term *"mean QRS axis"* describes the general direction toward which the QRS axis is directed in the frontal plane of the body. Therefore the mean QRS axis is measured in reference to the six extremity (frontal plane) leads. These leads can be arranged in the form of a hexaxial (six axes) diagram (Fig. 5-1, *C*).

The approximate mean QRS axis can be determined by using one of the following rules:

1. The mean QRS axis will be pointed midway between any two leads that show tall R waves of equal height.
2. The mean QRS axis will be pointed at right angles (perpendicular) to any lead showing a biphasic complex and toward other leads showing tall R waves.

The normal mean QRS axis lies between $-30°$ and $+100°$. An axis more negative than $-30°$ is defined as *left axis deviation* (LAD). An axis more positive than $+100°$ is defined as *right axis deviation* (RAD). LAD is an extreme form of a "horizontal" electrical axis. RAD is an extreme form of a "vertical" electrical axis.

LAD can be readily recognized if *lead II* shows an RS complex in which the S wave is deeper than the R wave is tall. In addition, *lead I* will show a tall R wave and *lead III* a deep S wave. LAD can be seen in cases of left ventricular hypertrophy, left anterior hemiblock, and other pathologic conditions and is sometimes seen in normal people.

RAD is present if the R wave in *lead III* is taller than the R wave in *lead II*. In addition, *lead I* will show an rS complex. RAD can be seen in several conditions, including right ventricular hypertrophy, lateral wall myocardial infarction, chronic lung disease, and left posterior hemiblock, and sometimes in normal people.

In rarer cases the QRS will be biphasic in all six extremity leads, making the mean electrical axis *indeterminate*.

The mean electrical axis of the P wave and T wave can also be estimated in the same manner as the mean QRS axis. With normal sinus rhythm the normal P wave will be about $+60°$ (positive P wave in lead II). Normally the T wave axis in the frontal plane will be similar to the QRS axis, so the T waves will normally be positive in leads with a predominantly positive QRS complex.

Questions

1. The six extremity leads (I, II, III, aV_R, aV_L, and aV_F) from a patient are shown. The standardization mark *(St)* in lead I is 10 mm, indicating proper standardization. What is the approximate mean QRS axis?

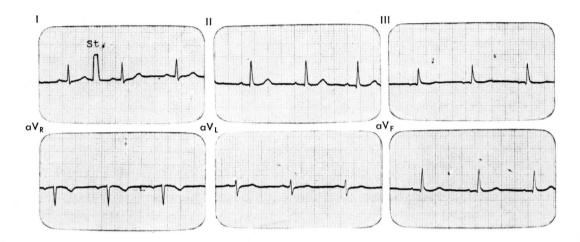

2. *A, B,* and *C* are, in mixed order, leads I, II, and III from a patient with a mean QRS axis of $-30°$. This information should allow you to sort out which lead is which.

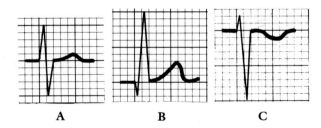

3. Examine Fig. 6-5, p. 67. What is the approximate mean QRS axis on that ECG?

4. Examine the following ECG:
   a. Is sinus rhythm present?
   b. What is the mean QRS axis?

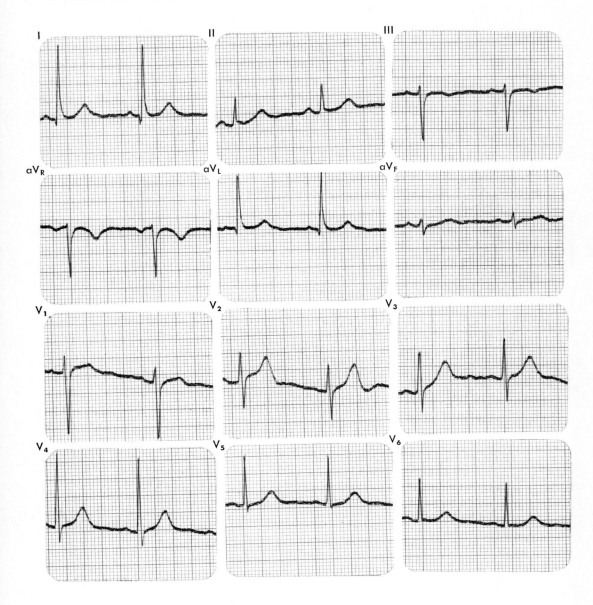

Answers

1. The QRS axis is about $+60°$. Notice that the QRS complex in lead aV_L is biphasic. Therefore the mean QRS axis must point at right angles to $-30°$. In this case, the axis is obviously $+60°$ since leads II, III, and aV_F are positive. You could also calculate the axis here by noting that leads I and III show R waves of approximately equal amplitude. Therefore the axis must be directed between lead I ($0°$) and lead III ($+120°$), or at $+60°$. (You may have tried to calculate the axis by noting that the R waves in leads II and aV_F were about equal, which would make the axis $+75°$. However, recall that leads aV_R, aV_L, and aV_F are *augmented* leads and are not on the same scale as leads I, II, and III. Therefore, in calculating the electrical axis, it is more accurate to compare QRS voltages in leads aV_R, aV_L, and aV_F *or* in leads I, II, and III.)

2. *A,* lead II; *B,* lead I; *C,* lead III. Explanation: You are told that the mean QRS axis is $-30°$. Therefore, you know that the QRS axis is pointed toward lead I (which is at $0°$) and away from lead III (which is at $+120°$). Obviously lead I must be *B* and lead III must be *C*. Lead II is *A*, which is biphasic. Lead II is at $+60°$ on the hexaxial diagram; and if the mean QRS axis is $-30°$, then lead II will have to show a biphasic complex since the mean QRS axis is at right angles to that lead.

3. $+90°$. There are R waves of approximately equal magnitude in leads II and III, and lead I shows a biphasic RS complex.

4. a. Yes, sinus rhythm is present. Notice that the P waves are negative in lead aV_R and positive in lead II.

   b. The mean QRS axis is about $0°$. Notice that the QRS complex is biphasic in lead aV_F. In this case, since the QRS axis in lead I is positive, the QRS axis is oriented at right angles to lead aV_F, toward lead I or at $0°$.

6

Atrial and Ventricular Enlargement

The basics of the normal ECG have been described in the first five chapters. From this point on, we will be concerned primarily with abnormal ECG patterns, beginning in this chapter with a consideration of the effects on the ECG of enlargement of the four cardiac chambers.

Several basic terms must first be defined. "Cardiac enlargement" refers to either *dilation* of a heart chamber or *hypertrophy* of the heart muscle.

In dilation of a chamber the heart muscle is *stretched* and the chamber becomes enlarged. For example, with acute congestive heart failure, dilation of the cardiac chambers occurs and is shown by an increase in the size of the cardiac x-ray silhouette.

In cardiac hypertrophy the heart muscle fibers actually *increase in size,* with resulting enlargement of the chamber. For example, aortic stenosis, which obstructs the outflow of blood from the left ventricle, leads to hypertrophy of the left ventricular muscle. The atria and the right ventricle can also become hypertrophied in other situations (described later in this chapter). When cardiac hypertrophy occurs, the total number of heart muscle fibers does not increase; rather, each individual fiber becomes larger. One obvious ECG effect of cardiac hypertrophy will be an increase in voltage of the P wave or QRS complex. Not uncommonly hypertrophy and dilation occur together.

Both dilation and hypertrophy usually result from some type of chronic pressure or volume load on the heart muscle. We will proceed with a discussion of the ECG patterns seen with enlargement of each of the four cardiac chambers, beginning with the right atrium.

RIGHT ATRIAL ENLARGEMENT (RAE)

Enlargement of the right atrium (either dilation or actual hypertrophy) may increase the voltage of the P wave. To recognize a large P wave, you must know the dimensions of the normal P wave.

When the P wave is positive, its amplitude is measured in millimeters from the upper level of the baseline, where the P wave begins, to the peak of the P wave. A negative P wave is measured from the lower level of the baseline to the lowest point of the P wave (Fig. 6-1). Measurement of the width of the P wave is also shown in Fig. 6-1.

Normally the P wave in every lead is less than or equal to 2.5 mm (0.25 mV) in amplitude and less than 0.12 second (three small boxes) in width. A P wave exceeding either of these dimensions in any lead is abnormal.

Enlargement of the right atrium may produce an abnormally tall P wave (greater than 2.5 mm). However, because pure RAE does not generally increase the total duration of atrial depolarization, the width of the P wave will be normal (less than 0.12 sec) (Fig. 6-2). The abnormal P wave in RAE

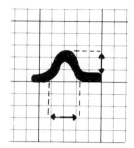

Fig. 6-1. The normal P wave does not exceed 2.5 mm in height and is less than 0.12 second in width.

P pulmonale

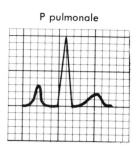

Fig. 6-2. Tall narrow P waves indicate right atrial enlargement (P pulmonale pattern).

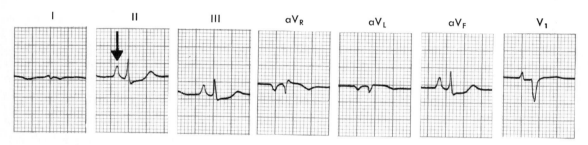

I   II   III   aV$_R$ aV$_L$ aV$_F$ V$_1$

Fig. 6-3. Notice the tall P waves, best seen in leads II, III, aV$_F$, and V$_1$, from a patient with chronic lung disease. This is the *P pulmonale pattern.*

is sometimes referred to as *P pulmonale* because the atrial enlargment that it signifies is often seen with severe pulmonary disease. Fig. 6-3 shows an actual example of RAE with a P pulmonale pattern.

The tall narrow P waves characteristic of RAE can usually be seen best in leads II, III, aV$_F$, and sometimes V$_1$. The ECG diagnosis of P pulmonale can be made by finding a P wave exceeding 2.5 mm in any of these leads. *Echocardiographic* evidence, however, suggests that the finding of a tall peaked P wave does not always correlate with RAE. On the other hand, patients may have RAE and not tall P waves.

RAE can be seen in a variety of clinical settings. Usually it is associated with right ventricular enlargement. Two of the most common clinical causes of RAE are pulmonary disease and congenital heart disease. The pulmonary disease may be either acute

(bronchial asthma, pulmonary embolism) or chronic (emphysema, bronchitis). Congenital heart lesions producing RAE include pulmonic valve stenosis, atrial septal defects, and tetralogy of Fallot.

LEFT ATRIAL ENLARGEMENT (LAE); LEFT ATRIAL ABNORMALITY (LAA)

Enlargement of the left atrium (either by dilation or by actual hypertrophy) also produces distinctive changes in the P wave. Normally the left atrium depolarizes after the right atrium. Thus left atrial enlargement should prolong the total duration of atrial depolarization, indicated by an abnormally wide P wave. LAE characteristically produces a wide P wave of 0.12 second (three small boxes) or more duration. The amplitude (height) of the P wave with LAE may be either normal or increased.

Fig. 6-4 illustrates the characteristic P wave changes seen in LAE. Sometimes, as shown, the

LEFT ATRIAL ENLARGEMENT (ABNORMALITY)

P mitrale   **Biphasic P wave in lead V₁**

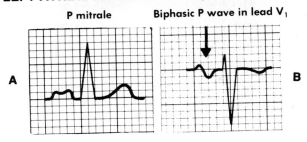

A   **B**

Fig. 6-4. Left atrial enlargement may produce, **A,** wide humped P waves in one or more extremity leads (*P mitrale* pattern) and/or, **B,** wide biphasic P waves in lead V₁.

I   II   III   aV_R   aV_L   aV_F   V₁

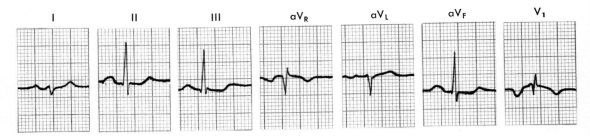

Fig. 6-5. Broad humped P waves from a patient with left atrial enlargement (P mitrale pattern).

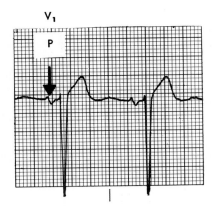

Fig. 6-6. Wide biphasic (initially positive, then negative) P waves from a patient with left atrial enlargement.

P wave will have a distinctive "humped" or "notched" appearance (Fig. 6-4, *A*). The second hump corresponds to the delayed depolarization of the left atrium. These humped P waves are usually best seen in one or more of the extremity leads (Fig. 6-5). The term *"P mitrale"* is sometimes used to describe wide P waves seen with LAE because they were first described in patients with rheumatic mitral valve disease.

In cases of LAE, lead V₁ sometimes shows a distinctive biphasic P wave (Figs. 6-4, *B,* and 6-6). This wave has a small initial positive deflection and a prominent wide negative deflection. The negative component will be of >0.04 second duration or ≥1 mm depth. The prominent negative deflection corresponds to the delayed stimulation of the enlarged left atrium. Remember that, anatomically, the left atrium is situated posteriorly, up against the esophagus, while the right atrium lies anteriorly, against the sternum. The initial positive deflection of the P wave in lead V_1 therefore indicates right atrial depolarization while the deep negative deflection is a result of left atrial depolarization voltages directed posteriorly (away from the positive pole of lead V_1).

In some cases of LAE you will see both the broad often humped P waves in leads I and II and the biphasic P wave in lead V_1. In other cases only the broad bumped P waves will be seen. Sometimes a biphasic P wave in lead V_1 will be the only ECG evidence of left atrial enlargement.

Clinically LAE may occur in a variety of settings:

1. Dilation of the left ventricle and left atrium associated with congestive heart failure of multiple causes (ischemic heart disease, cardiomyopathy)
2. Valvular heart disease, particularly aortic stenosis, aortic regurgitation, mitral regurgitation, and mitral stenosis (With mitral stenosis there is valvular obstruction to the emptying of the left atrium into the left ventricle. This will eventually result in a backup of pressure through the pulmonary vessels to the right ventricle. Therefore with advanced mitral stenosis the ECG may show a combination of LAE with signs of right ventricular hypertrophy, as shown in Fig. 19-1.)

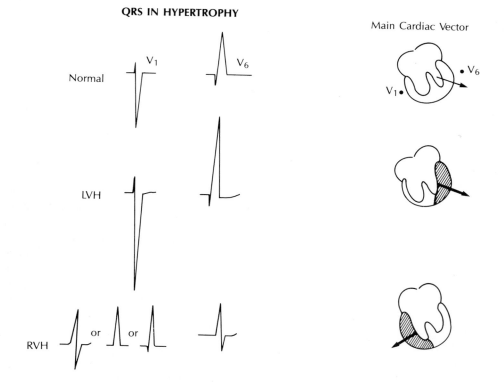

Fig. 6-7. The QRS patterns with left and right ventricular hypertrophy (*LVH* and *RVH*) can be anticipated based on the abnormal physiology. Notice that LVH exaggerates the normal pattern, causing deeper right precordial S waves and taller left precordial R waves. By contrast, RVH shifts the QRS vector to the right, causing increased right precordial R waves.

3. Hypertensive heart disease, which causes left ventricular enlargement and eventually LAE

Some patients, particularly those with coronary artery disease, may have broad P waves without actual LAE. The abnormal P waves in these cases probably represent an atrial conduction delay. Therefore, the more general term *"left atrial abnormality"* is used by some authors in preference to left atrial "enlargement" to describe abnormally broad P waves.

RIGHT VENTRICULAR HYPERTROPHY (RVH)

Although atrial enlargement (dilation or hypertrophy) produces characteristic changes in the P wave, the QRS complex will be modified primarily by ventricular *hypertrophy*. The effects to be described indicate actual hypertrophy of the ventricular muscle and not simply ventricular dilation.

The ECG changes produced by both right and left ventricular hypertrophy can be predicted on the basis of what you already know about the normal QRS patterns. Normally (as described in Chapter 4) the left and right ventricles depolarize simultaneously and the left ventricle is electrically predominant because it has greater mass. As a result, leads placed over the right side of the chest (such as V_1) will record rS-type complexes $\left(\overset{r}{\underset{S}{\wedge}} \right)$, in which the deep negative S wave indicates the spread of depolarization voltages away from the right and toward the left side. Conversely, leads placed over the left chest (such as V_5 or V_6) will record a qR-type complex $\left(\overset{R}{\underset{q}{\wedge}} \right)$, in which the tall positive R wave indicates the predominant depolarization voltages that point to the left generated by the left ventricle.

Now, if the right ventricle becomes sufficiently hypertrophied, this normal electrical predominance of the left ventricle can be overcome. In such cases,

what type of QRS complex might you expect to see in the right chest leads? With RVH, the right chest leads will show tall R waves, indicating the spread of positive voltages from the hypertrophied right ventricle toward the right (Fig. 6-7). Figs. 6-8 and 6-9 show actual examples of RVH. Instead of the rS complex normally seen in lead V_1, we now see a tall positive (R) wave, indicating marked hypertrophy of the right ventricle.

How tall an R wave in lead V_1 do you have to see to make a diagnosis of RVH? As a general rule the normal R wave in lead V_1 in adults will be smaller than the S wave in that lead. An R wave exceeding the S wave in lead V_1 is suggestive, but not diagnostic, of RVH. Sometimes, as shown in Fig. 6-8, a small q wave will precede the tall R wave in lead V_1 in cases of RVH.

Along with tall right chest R waves, RVH often produces two additional ECG signs: right axis deviation and right ventricular "strain" T wave inversions.

As noted in Chapter 5, the normal mean QRS axis in adults lies approximately between $-30°$ and $+100°$. A mean QRS axis of $+100°$ or more is called *right axis deviation*. One of the most common causes of right axis deviation is RVH. Therefore, whenever you see an ECG with right axis deviation, you should search carefully for other confirmatory evidence of RVH (Figs. 6-8 and 6-9). (Remember the simple rule of thumb: *Right axis deviation is present if the R wave in lead III is taller than the R wave in lead II.*)

RVH, however, not only produces depolarization (QRS) changes, it also affects repolarization (the ST-T complex). For reasons not fully understood, hypertrophy of the heart muscle alters the normal sequence of repolarization. With RVH the characteristic repolarization change is the appearance of inverted T waves in the right and middle chest leads, as shown in Figs. 6-8 and 6-9. These right chest T wave inversions are referred to as a right ventricular *strain* pattern. (Strain is a descriptive term. The exact mechanism for the strain pattern is not understood.)

To summarize: With RVH, the ECG may show tall R waves in the right chest leads, with the R

RIGHT VENTRICULAR HYPERTROPHY

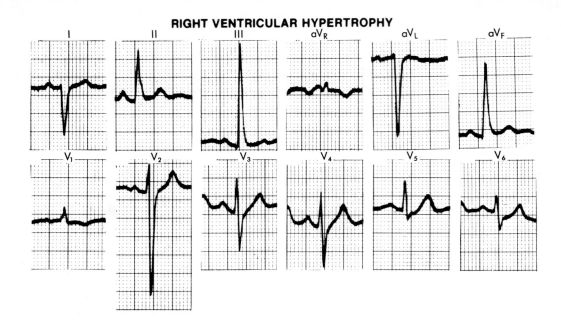

Fig. 6-8. Notice the tall R wave in lead V_1 (with an inverted T wave caused by right ventricular strain). There is also right axis deviation (R wave in lead III taller than that in lead II). This patient had tetralogy of Fallot.

wave greater than the S wave in lead V_1.* Right axis deviation and right ventricular strain T wave inversions are also often present. Some cases of RVH are more subtle, and the ECG may show only one of these patterns. The appearance of all three patterns (tall right precordial R waves, right axis deviation, and right ventricular strain), however, firmly establishes the diagnosis of RVH, although the absence of these patterns does not necessarily exclude RVH.

RVH may occur in a variety of clinical settings. An important cause is congenital heart disease (for example, pulmonic stenosis, atrial septal defect,†

*With RVH the chest leads to the left of leads showing tall R waves may show a variable pattern. Sometimes the middle and left chest leads show poor R wave progression, with rS or RS complexes all the way to lead V_6 (Fig. 6-9). In other cases normal R wave progression is preserved and the left chest leads also show R waves (Fig. 6-8).

†Patients with right ventricular enlargement from the atrial septal defect often exhibit a right bundle branch block pattern (RSR′) in lead V_1 with a vertical or rightward QRS axis.

tetralogy of Fallot, or the Eisenmenger syndrome). Patients with long-standing severe pulmonary disease may have pulmonary artery hypertension and RVH. Mitral stenosis, as mentioned previously, can produce a combination of LAE and RVH. Right ventricular strain T wave inversions (in V_1 to V_3) may also occur without other ECG signs of RVH, as in acute pulmonary embolism (p. 139).

In patients with RVH associated with emphysema the ECG may not show any of the patterns just described. Instead of tall R waves in the right precordial leads, there will be poor R wave progression. Right axis deviation is also commonly present (p. 57). (See Fig. 10-17.)

LEFT VENTRICULAR HYPERTROPHY (LVH)

The ECG changes produced by LVH, like those from RVH, are predictable (Fig. 6-7). Normally the left ventricle is electrically predominant over the right ventricle, producing prominent S waves in the right chest leads and tall R waves in the left

RIGHT VENTRICULAR HYPERTROPHY

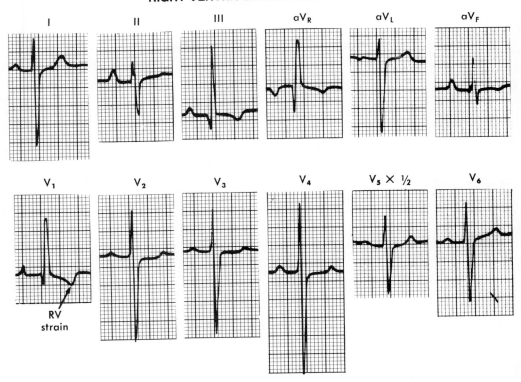

Fig. 6-9. Sometimes lead V_1 will show a tall R wave as part of the qR complex. Notice the peaked P waves (leads II, III, and V_1) because of right atrial enlargement. T wave inversion in V_1 and ST depressions in V_2 and V_3 are due to right ventricular strain. There is also a prolonged PR interval (0.24 sec), indicating first-degree AV block.

chest leads. When LVH is present, the balance of electrical forces is tipped even further to the left. Thus, when LVH is present, abnormally tall R waves will be seen in the left chest leads and abnormally deep S waves in the right chest leads.

The following criteria and guidelines have been established to help in the ECG diagnosis of LVH:

1. If the depth of the S wave in lead V_1 (S_{V_1}) added to the height of the R wave in either lead V_5 or V_6 (R_{V_5} or R_{V_6}) exceeds 35 mm (3.5 mV), then consider LVH (Fig. 6-10).

2. You should also realize that high voltage in the chest leads is commonly seen as a normal finding, particularly in young adults with thin chest walls. Consequently, high voltage in the chest leads (S_{V_1} + R_{V_5} or R_{V_6} > 35 mm) is not a *specific* indicator of LVH (Fig. 6-11).

3. In some cases LVH will produce tall R waves in lead aV_L. An R wave of 13 mm or more in lead aV_L (Fig 6-9) is another sign of LVH.* Occasionally a tall R wave in lead aV_L will be the only ECG sign of LVH and the voltage in chest leads may be normal. In other cases

*Occasionally LVH will develop with an electrically vertical axis. In such cases a qR pattern with a tall R wave (exceeding 20 mm) may appear in lead aV_F.

LEFT VENTRICULAR HYPERTROPHY

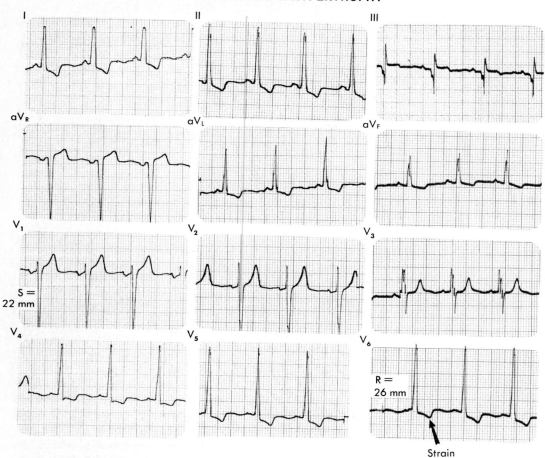

Fig. 6-10. This patient had severe hypertension. Notice the pattern of left ventricular hypertrophy: tall voltage in the chest leads and aV$_L$ (R = 16 mm) with strain pattern in these leads. In addition, there is the pattern of left atrial enlargement, including a biphasic P wave in lead V$_1$ and a broad notched P wave in lead II.

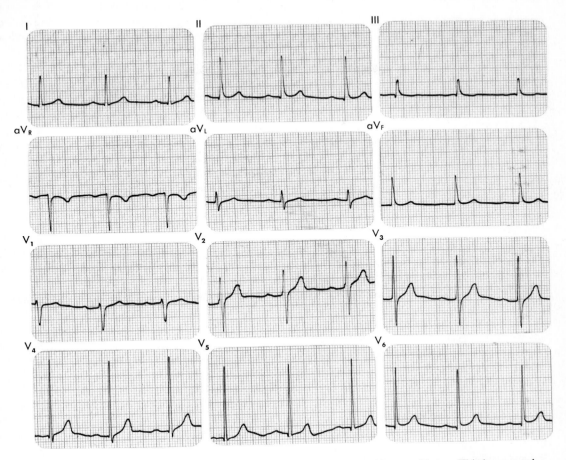

Fig. 6-11. Tall voltage in chest leads ($R_{v_1} + S_{v_5} = 36$ mm) in a 20-year-old man. This is a normal variant caused by the patient's thin chest wall. The ST-T complexes are normal, without evidence of left ventricular strain.

LEFT VENTRICULAR "STRAIN" PATTERN

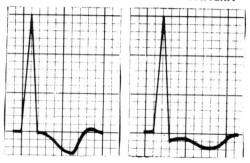

Fig. 6-12. Notice the characteristic wavy ST-T pattern with T wave inversion in leads showing tall R waves.

the chest voltages may be abnormally high, with a normal R wave in lead aV_L.

4. Furthermore, just as RVH is associated with a right ventricular strain pattern, so left ventricular strain ST-T changes are often seen in LVH. Fig. 6-12 illustrates the characteristic shape of the ST-T complex with left ventricular strain. Notice that it has a distinctively asymmetric appearance, with slight ST segment depression followed by a broadly inverted T wave. In some cases these T wave inversions will be very deep. The left ventricular strain pattern is seen in leads with tall R waves (Fig. 6-10).

5. With LVH the electrical axis is usually horizontal. Actual left axis deviation (axis $-30°$ or more negative) may also be seen. In addition, the QRS complex may become wider. Not uncommonly LVH will eventually develop in patients with complete left bundle branch block. (See Chapter 7.)

6. Finally, the signs of LAE (broad notched P waves in the extremity leads or wide biphasic P waves in lead V_1) are often seen in patients with ECG evidence of LVH. Most conditions that lead to LVH ultimately produce LAE as well.

A variety of clinical conditions may be associated with LVH. In adults three of the most common

are (1) valvular heart disease (such as aortic stenosis, aortic regurgitation, or mitral regurgitation), (2) systemic hypertension, and (3) cardiomyopathies (p. 140).

To summarize: The diagnosis of LVH can be made with reasonable certainty from the ECG if you find high QRS voltages with characteristic ST-T changes ("strain" pattern). High voltage in the chest or extremity leads can sometimes be seen in normal subjects, so the diagnosis of LVH should not be made on this finding alone.* T wave inversion resulting from left ventricular overload can also occur without other evidence of LVH.

• • •

We have discussed the patterns of RVH with right ventricular strain and LVH with left ventricular strain. However, the subject is somewhat more complicated than this, because the ST-T changes of ventricular "strain" can also occur in the absence of actual ventricular hypertrophy.

For example, you can see right ventricular strain (T wave inversions in the right to middle chest leads) without actual RVH. Acute right ventricular strain, for example, is sometimes seen with massive pulmonary embolism (Fig. 10-16), in which there is a sudden severe stress on the right side of the heart.

Left ventricular strain can also occur without actual LVH. In such cases the ECG will show the characteristic ST-T changes of Fig. 6-12 *without* high QRS voltages. Acute left ventricular strain may occur, for example, with sudden increases in systemic blood pressure.

ECG IN CARDIAC ENLARGEMENT: A PERSPECTIVE

The ECG findings associated with enlargement of each of the four cardiac chambers have been presented. In some cases combined patterns will be seen on the same tracing (for example, LAE and RVH in cases of mitral stenosis or LAE and

---

*The voltage criteria used here for diagnosing LVH in the chest and extremity leads are by no means absolute numbers. Some authors use somewhat different voltage criteria.

LVH with hypertension). You may be wondering what the ECG shows if both left and right ventricles become hypertrophied (biventricular hypertrophy). In such cases it usually shows mainly evidence of LVH.

Finally, always remember that in the assessment of cardiac size the ECG is only an indirect laboratory test and not an absolute measurement. A person may have underlying cardiac enlargement that does not show up on the ECG. Conversely, hight voltage may be present in normal persons without cardiac enlargement. When the degree of cardiac chamber enlargement must be determined with more precision, an *echocardiogram* should be obtained. (For further discussion of the diagnostic limitations of the ECG, see Chapter 19.)

REVIEW

Cardiac *dilation* refers to stretching of muscle fibers, with enlargement of one or more of the cardiac chambers. Cardiac *hypertrophy* refers to an abnormal increase in the actual size of the heart muscle fibers. The ECG can indicate either right or left atrial dilation or hypertrophy but generally only right or left ventricular hypertrophy.

Right atrial enlargement is manifested by tall peaked P waves *(P pulmonale pattern)* greater than 2.5 mm in height, usually best seen in leads II, III, aV_F, and sometimes V_1.

Left atrial enlargement (abnormality) is manifested by wide, sometimes humped, P waves *(P mitrale pattern)* of 0.12 second or more duration in one or more of the extremity leads. A biphasic P wave with a prominent wide negtive deflection may be seen in lead V_1.

Right ventricular hypertrophy shows any or all of the following:

1. Tall R wave in lead V_1, equal to or larger than the S wave in that lead
2. RAD often present
3. Right ventricular ''strain'' pattern (T wave inversions in the right to middle chest leads)

Left ventricular hypertrophy may show any or all of the following:

1. The voltage of the S wave in lead V_1 plus the voltage of the R wave in lead V_5 or V_6 exceeding 35 mm ($S_{V_1} + R_{V_5}$ or $R_{V_6} > 35$ mm)
2. A high-voltage R wave in lead aV_L (13 mm or more) when the heart is electrically horizontal (When the axis is vertical, lead aV_F may show a tall R wave [>20 mm] as part of a qR complex.)
3. A left ventricular strain pattern (inverted T waves in leads with a qR pattern)

The diagnosis of LVH should *not* be made solely on the basis of high voltage in the chest leads, since this may occur normally, particularly in young adults and thin-chested people.

T wave inversions in both left ventricular and right ventricular ''strain'' may also occur without LVH or RVH. Furthermore, enlargement of any of the four cardiac chambers can be present without diagnostic ECG changes. (See Chapter 19 for additional discussion of the diagnostic limitations of the ECG.)

Questions

1. Answer these questions about the following ECG:
   a. What is the approximate heart rate?
   b. Is sinus rhythm present?
   c. Where is the transition zone in the chest leads?
   d. Mention three signs of LVH.

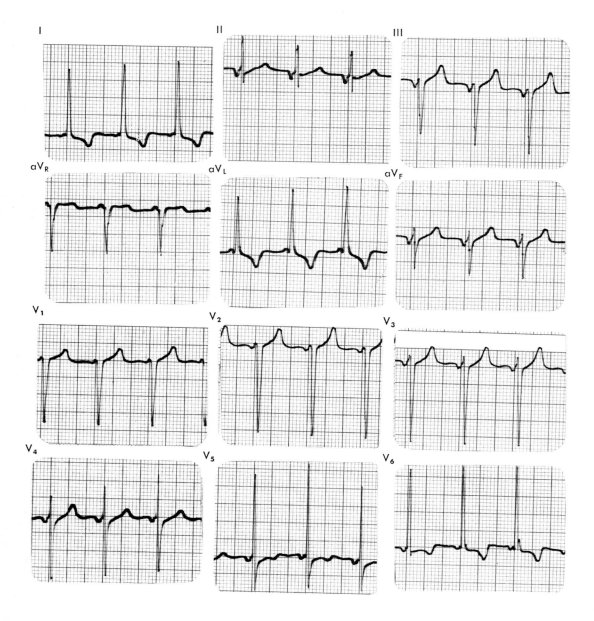

2. On the following ECG
   a. What is the heart rate?
   b. Name two abnormal findings.

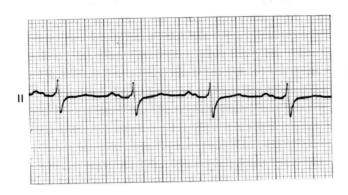

Answers

1. a. About 100 beats/min.
   b. No. Notice the retrograde P waves, positive in lead aV_R and negative in lead II, owing to an AV junctional (or ectopic atrial) rhythm.
   c. Around lead V_4.
   d. Tall voltage in chest leads ($S_{V_1} + R_{V_6} > 35$ mm); tall voltage in lead aV_L (R wave > 13 mm); left ventricular strain pattern in leads I, aV_L, and V_5 and V_6.

2. a. About 75 beats/min.
   b. The PR interval is prolonged (about 0.22 sec) because of first-degree AV block (Chapter 15). Also, the P wave in lead II is abnormally wide and notched (notice the two humps) as a result of left atrial enlargement (abnormality).

7

Ventricular Conduction Disturbances

BUNDLE BRANCH BLOCKS

Recall that in the normal process of ventricular activation (Chapter 4) the electrical stimulus reaches the ventricles from the atria by way of the AV junction. The first part of the ventricles stimulated (depolarized) is the left side of the ventricular septum. Soon after, the depolarization spreads to the main mass of the left and right ventricles by way of the left and right bundle branches. Normally the entire process of ventricular depolarization is completed within 0.1 second. Therefore the normal width of the QRS complex is less than or equal to 0.1 second (two and a half small boxes on the ECG graph paper). Any process that interferes with the normal stimulation of the ventricles may prolong the QRS width. In this chapter we will be concerned primarily with the effects of blocks within the bundle branch system on the QRS complex.

RIGHT BUNDLE BRANCH BLOCK (RBBB)

Consider, first, the effect of cutting the right bundle branch. Obviously this will delay right ventricular stimulation and widen the QRS complex. Furthermore, the shape of the QRS with a right bundle branch block (RBBB) can be predicted on the basis of some familiar principles.

Normally the *first* part of the ventricles to be depolarized is the interventricular septum (Fig. 4-6, *A*). The left side of the interventricular septum is stimulated first (by a branch of the left bundle).

This septal depolarization produces the small septal r wave in lead V_1 and the small septal q wave in lead V_6 seen on the normal ECG (Fig. 7-1, *A*). Clearly, RBBB should not affect this first septal phase of ventricular stimulation, since the septum is stimulated by a part of the left bundle.

The *second* phase of ventricular stimulation is the simultaneous depolarization of the left and right ventricles (Fig. 4-6, *B*). RBBB should not affect this phase either, since the left ventricle is normally electrically predominant, producing deep S waves in the right chest leads and tall R waves in the left chest leads (Fig. 7-1, *B*). The change in the QRS complex produced by RBBB is a result of the delay in the total time needed for stimulation of the right ventricle. This means that following the completion of left ventricular depolarization, the right ventricle continues to depolarize.

This delayed right ventricular depolarization produces a *third* phase of ventricular stimulation. The electrical voltages in the third phase are directed to the right, reflecting the delayed depolarization and slow spread of the depolarization wave outward through the right ventricle. Therefore a lead placed over the right side of the chest (for example, lead V_1) will record this third phase of ventricular stimulation as a positive wide deflection (R' wave). The same delayed and slow right ventricular depolarization voltages spreading to the right will produce a wide negative (S wave) deflection

RIGHT BUNDLE BRANCH BLOCK

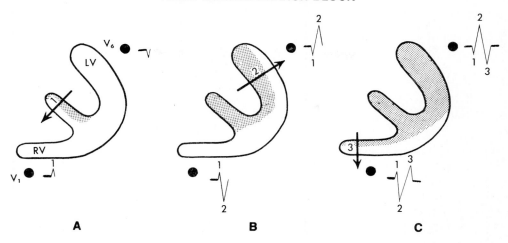

Fig. 7-1. Step-by-step sequence of ventricular depolarization in RBBB. See text.

in the left chest leads (for example, lead V_6) (Fig. 7-1, *C*).

Putting together in step-by-step fashion what has been explained, we can now derive the pattern seen in the chest leads with RBBB. Lead V_1 will show an rSR' complex with a broad R' wave. Lead V_6 will show a qRS-type complex with a broad S wave. The tall wide R wave in the right chest leads and the deep terminal S wave in the left chest leads represent the same event viewed from opposite sides of the chest—the slow spread of delayed depolarization voltages through the right ventricle.

To make the initial diagnosis of RBBB, look at leads V_1 and V_6 in particular. The characteristic appearance of QRS complex in these leads makes the diagnosis simple.

Fig. 7-1 shows how the delay in ventricular depolarization with RBBB produces the characteristic ECG patterns we have been discussing.

To summarize: In RBBB the ventricular stimulation process can be divided into three phases. The first two consist of normal septal and ventricular depolarization. The third phase is delayed stimulation of the right ventricle. These three phases of ventricular stimulation with RBBB are represented on the ECG by the triphasic complexes seen

in the chest leads—V_1 showing an rSR' complex with a wide R' wave, V_6 showing a qRS pattern with a wide S wave.

We have seen that with an RBBB the QRS complex in lead V_1 generally shows an rSR' pattern. Occasionally, however (Fig. 7-3), the S wave never quite makes its way below the baseline, giving the complex in lead V_1 the appearance of a large notched R wave.

Figs. 7-2 and 7-3 show some typical examples of RBBB. Do you notice anything abnormal about the ST-T complexes in these tracings? If you look carefully, you will see that the T waves in the right leads are inverted. Right chest lead T wave inversions are a characteristic finding with RBBB. They are referred to as *secondary changes* because they reflect just the delay in ventricular stimulation. By contrast, *primary T wave abnormalities* reflect an actual change in repolarization, independent of any QRS change. For example, T wave inversions resulting from ischemia (Chapters 8 and 9), hypokalemia (Chapter 10), or drugs such as digitalis (Chapter 10) are all examples of primary T wave abnormalities.

Some ECGs will show both primary and secondary ST-T changes. In Fig. 7-3 the T wave in-

RIGHT BUNDLE BRANCH BLOCK

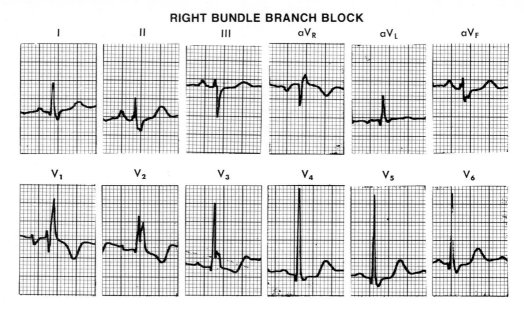

Fig. 7-2. Notice the wide rSR′ complex in lead V_1 and the qRS complex in lead V_6. Inverted T waves in the right precordial leads (V_1 to V_3 in this case) are common with RBBB and are called *secondary* T wave inversions.

RIGHT BUNDLE BRANCH BLOCK

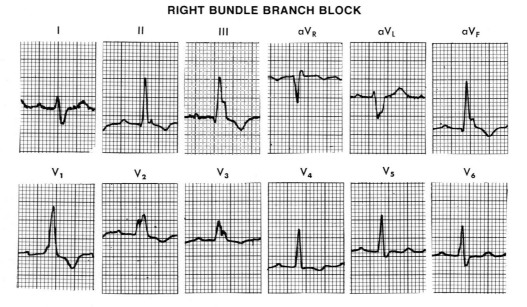

Fig. 7-3. Sometimes, with RBBB, instead of the classic rSR′ pattern, the right precordial leads will show a wide notched R wave (seen here in leads V_1 to V_3). Notice the *secondary* T wave inversions in leads V_1 to V_3, II, III, and aV_F, all of which show rSR′-type complexes. However, the abnormal ST-T changes in V_4 and V_5 are *primary* since they are present in leads without an R′ wave.

versions in leads V_1 to V_3 and in II, III, and aV_F can be explained solely on the basis of the RBBB since they occur in leads with an rSR'-type complex. However, the T wave inversions or ST depressions in other leads (V_4 and V_5) represent a primary change, perhaps resulting from ischemia or a drug effect.

Complete vs Incomplete RBBB

RBBB can be subdivided into complete and incomplete forms depending on the width of the QRS complex. Complete RBBB is defined by a QRS that is 0.12 second or more in duration with an rSR' in lead V_1 and a qRS in V_6. Incomplete RBBB shows the same QRS patterns but its duration is between 0.1 and 0.12 second.

Clinical Significance

RBBB may be caused by a number of factors. First, some normal people will have it without any underlying heart disorder. Therefore RBBB per say is not necessarily abnormal. In many people, however, it is associated with organic heart disease. It may be caused by a condition that affects the right side of the heart (atrial septal defect with left-to-right shunting of blood, chronic pulmonary disease with pulmonary artery hypertension, or a valvular lesion such as pulmonic stenosis). In some individuals (particularly older people) it follows chronic degenerative changes in the conduction system. It may also occur with myocardial ischemia or infarction.

Pulmonary embolism, which produces acute right-sided heart strain, may cause right ventricular conduction delay. When RBBB occurs following coronary artery bypass graft surgery, it does not seem to have any special clinical implications.

RBBB may be permanent or transient, appearing only when the heart rate exceeds a certain critical value (*tachycardia-dependent* RBBB).

Blockage of the right bundle branch does not, in itself, require any specific treatment.

LEFT BUNDLE BRANCH BLOCK (LBBB)

Left bundle branch block (LBBB) also produces a pattern with a widened QRS complex. However, the complex with LBBB is very different from that with RBBB. The reason for this difference is that RBBB affects mainly the terminal phase of ventricular activation while LBBB affects the early phase as well.

Recall that the first phase of ventricular stimulation—depolarization of the left side of the septum—is started by a branch of the left bundle. LBBB therefore will block this normal pattern. When LBBB is present, the septum depolarizes from *right* to *left* and not from left to right. Thus the first major change on the ECG produced by LBBB will be a loss of the normal septal r wave in lead V_1 and the normal septal q wave in lead V_6 (Fig. 7-4, *A*). Furthermore, the total time for left ventricular depolarization will be prolonged with LBBB, resulting in an abnormally wide QRS complex. Lead V_6 will show a wide entirely positive (R) wave (Fig. 7-4, *B*). The right chest leads (such as V_1) record a negative QRS (QS) complex because the left ventricle is still electrically predominant with LBBB and produces greater voltages than the right ventricle. The major change is that the total time for completion of left ventricular depolarization is delayed. Therefore, with LBBB the entire process of ventricular stimulation is oriented toward the left chest leads—the septum depolarizing from right to left, with stimulation of the electrically predominant left ventricle prolonged. Fig. 7-4 illustrates the sequence of ventricular activation in LBBB.*

Sometimes the QS wave in lead V_1 with LBBB will show a small notching at its point, giving it a characteristic **W** shape. Similarly the R wave in lead V_6 may show a notching at its peak, giving it a distinctive **M** shape. An actual example of an LBBB pattern is shown in Fig. 7-5.

Just as there are *secondary* T wave inversions with RBBB, so there are also secondary T wave inversions with LBBB. As you can see from Fig. 7-5, the T waves in the leads with tall R waves are inverted (for example, the left precordial leads),

---

*A variation of this pattern that sometimes occurs is for lead V_1 to show an rS complex with a very small r wave and a wide S wave. This superficially suggests that the septum is being stimulated normally from left to right. However, lead V_6 in such cases will show an abnormally wide and notched R wave *without* an initial q wave.

LEFT BUNDLE BRANCH BLOCK

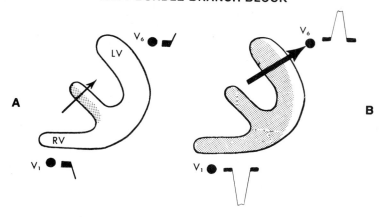

Fig. 7-4. The sequence of ventricular depolarization in LBBB produces a wide QS complex in lead V_1 and a wide R wave in lead V_6.

LEFT BUNDLE BRANCH BLOCK

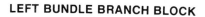

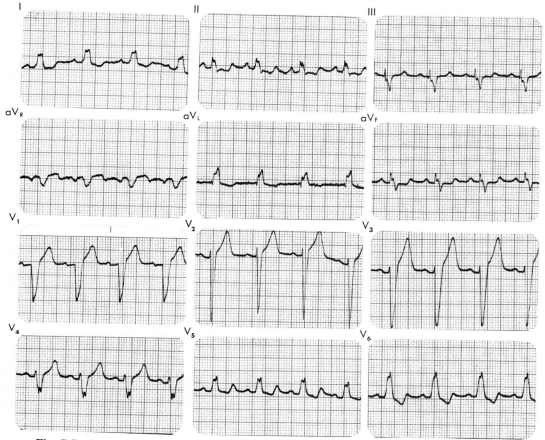

Fig. 7-5. Notice the characteristic wide QS complex in lead V_1 and the wide R wave in lead V_6 with slight notching at the peak. The inverted T waves in leads V_5 and V_6 are also characteristic of LBBB (secondary T wave inversions).

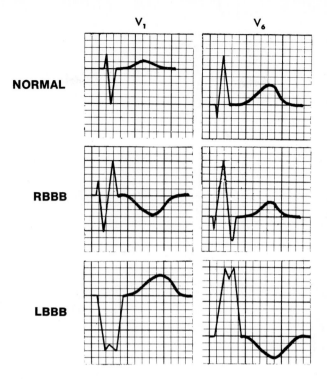

Fig. 7-6. Comparison of leads V_1 and V_6, with normal conduction, right bundle branch block, and left bundle branch block. Normally lead V_1 shows an rS complex and lead V_6 a qR complex. With RBBB, lead V_1 shows a wide rSR′ complex and lead V_6 a qRS complex. With LBBB, lead V_1 shows a wide QS complex and lead V_6 a wide R wave.

characteristic of LBBB. However, T wave inversions in the right precordial leads cannot be explained solely on the basis of LBBB and, if present, reflect some *primary* abnormality, such as ischemia (Fig. 8-21).

To summarize: The diagnosis of LBBB can be made simply by inspection of leads V_1 and V_6. Lead V_1 usually shows a wide, entirely negative, QS complex (rarely a wide rS complex) while V_6 shows a wide tall R wave without a q wave. You should have no problem differentiating left and right bundle branch block patterns. Fig. 7-6 compares the complexes seen. Occasionally an ECG will show wide QRS complexes that are not typical of an RBBB or LBBB pattern. In such cases, the general term *"intraventricular delay"* is used (Fig. 7-7).

Complete vs Incomplete LBBB

As with RBBB, there are complete and incomplete forms of LBBB. With complete LBBB the QRS complex has the characteristic appearance described previously and is 0.12 second or wider. With incomplete LBBB the QRS is between 0.1 and 0.12 second wide.

Clinical Significance

Unlike RBBB, which is occasionally seen in normal people, LBBB is usually a sign of organic heart disease. It often occurs in elderly patients with chronic degenerative changes in their myocardial conduction system. It may develop in patients with long-standing hypertensive heart disease, a valvular lesion (such as aortic stenosis or aortic re-

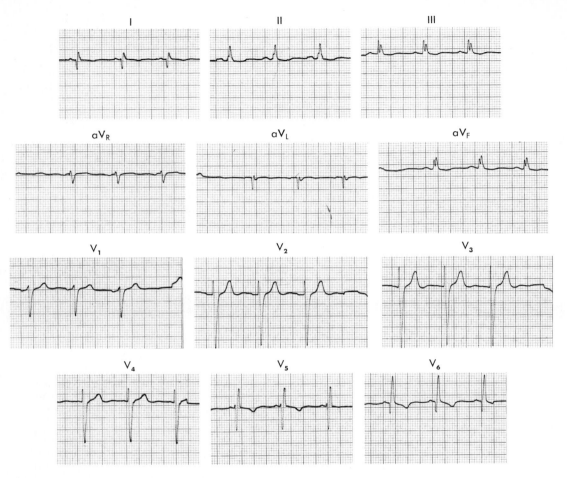

Fig. 7-7. Nonspecific intraventricular conduction delay. The QRS here is abnormally wide (0.11 sec). However, such a pattern is not typical of LBBB or RBBB. In this case it was caused by a lateral infarction. (See Chapter 8.)

gurgitation), or different types of cardiomyopathy (p. 140). It is also seen in patients with coronary artery disease. Most patients with LBBB have underlying left ventricular hypertrophy (Chapter 6). When LBBB occurs with an acute myocardial infarction, it is often a forerunner of complete heart block. In rare instances some otherwise normal individuals will have an LBBB pattern.

If you find LBBB in a patient, it usually does not require any specific treatment. The major exception is patients with acute myocardial infarction

in whom a *new* LBBB pattern develops (p. 110). In the patient who has LBBB *without* acute infarction, the risk of complete heart block is very small. However, if a patient with LBBB complains of dizziness or fainting, a clinical evaluation (usually including a Holter monitor study) should be performed to exclude intermittent AV block.

Like RBBB, LBBB may be a permanent condition or transient. It may appear only when the heart rate exceeds a certain critical value (*tachycardia-dependent* LBBB). In some cases its presence may be a valuable clue to previously undiagnosed but clinically important abnormalities—for example, coronary artery disease, hypertensive heart disease, or cardiomyopathy.

PACEMAKER PATTERNS

Pacemakers are battery-operated devices that are capable of electrically stimulating the heart. They are used primarily when the patient's own heart rate is not adequate (for example, in complete heart block). In most cases the pacemaker electrode is inserted into the right ventricle. Therefore the ECG will show an LBBB pattern, reflecting delayed activation of the left ventricle. Fig. 7-8 is an example of a pacemaker tracing. The vertical spike preceding each QRS complex is the pacemaker spike, followed by a wide QRS with an LBBB morphology (QS in lead V_1 with a wide R wave in lead V_6). Pacemakers are discussed in greater detail in Chapter 20.

Up to this point, we have considered major causes of a wide QRS complex: RBBB, LBBB, and pacemaker patterns. Later (p. 143) the list will be expanded to include hyperkalemia, the Wolff-Parkinson-White preexcitation syndrome, and toxicity due to certain drugs (for example, quinidine or procainamide).

HEMIBLOCKS

A slightly more complex but important topic is the hemiblocks. Up to now we have discussed the left bundle branch system as if it were a single pathway. Actually it has been known for many years to be subdivided into two major branches, or *fascicles* (*fasciculus*, Latin, small bundle). It consists of an anterior fascicle and a posterior fascicle. The right bundle branch, by contrast, is a single pathway and consists of just one main fascicle or bundle.

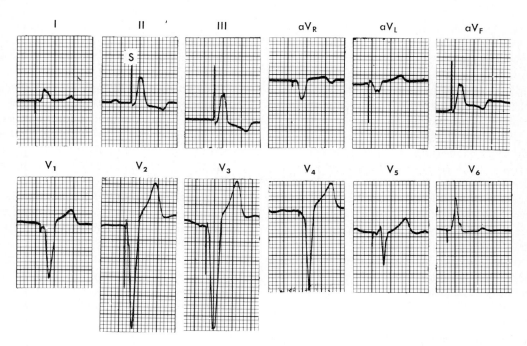

Fig. 7-8. A pacemaker inserted into the right ventricle generally produces a pattern resembling that produced by LBBB, with a wide QS in lead V_1 and a wide R wave in V_6, caused by delayed depolarization of the left ventricle. Notice the pacemaker spike in each lead preceding the QRS complex. In some leads (such as lead II) the spike *(S)* is positive; in others (V_1 to V_6) it is negative.

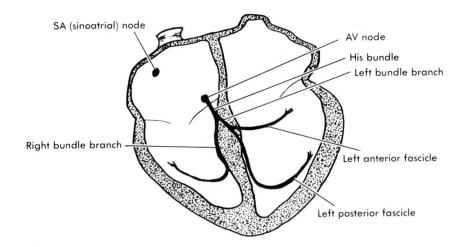

SA (sinoatrial) node

AV node

His bundle

Left bundle branch

Right bundle branch

Left anterior fascicle

Left posterior fascicle

Fig. 7-9. Trifascicular conduction system. Notice that the left bundle branch subdivides into a left anterior fascicle and a left posterior fascicle. This diagram is a revision of the original drawing of the conduction system in Fig. 1-1.

This revised concept of the bundle branch system as a trifascicular highway (one right, two left) is illustrated in Fig. 7-9.

To summarize: The bundle of His divides into a right bundle branch and a left main bundle branch. The left main bundle branch then subdivides into an anterior and a posterior fascicle.

It makes sense to suppose that a block can occur at any single point (or at multiple points) in this trifascicular system. We have already seen the ECG pattern with a block in the right bundle branch. The pattern of LBBB can obviously occur in one of two ways: by a block in the left main bundle before it divides or by blocks in both subdivisions (anterior and posterior fascicles).

The next question is, what happens if a block occurs in just the anterior or just the posterior fascicle of the left bundle? A block in either fascicle of the left bundle branch system is called a *hemiblock*. Recognition of hemiblocks on the ECG is intimately related to the subject of axis deviation, presented in Chapter 5. Somewhat surprisingly, a hemiblock (unlike a full left or right bundle branch block) does not widen the QRS complex markedly. It has been found experimentally that the main effect of cutting these fascicles is to change the QRS

axis. Specifically, *left anterior* hemiblock results in marked left axis deviation ($-45°$ or more); *left posterior* hemiblock produces right axis deviation ($+120°$ or more).*

To summarize: Hemiblocks are partial blocks in the left bundle branch system and involve either the anterior or the posterior fascicle. The diagnosis of a hemiblock is made from the mean QRS axis in the extremity (frontal plane) leads. This is in contrast to the diagnosis of complete (or incomplete) right or left bundle branch block, which is made primarily from the QRS patterns in the chest (horizontal plane) leads. Complete bundle branch blocks, unlike hemiblocks, do not cause a characteristic shift in the mean QRS axis.

Left anterior hemiblock. Isolated left anterior hemiblock is diagnosed by finding a mean QRS axis of $-45°$ or more and a QRS width of less than 0.12 second. A mean QRS axis of $-45°$ or more can be easily recognized because left axis

---

*Left anterior hemiblock shifts the QRS axis to the left by delaying activation of the more superior and leftward portions of the left ventricle. Left posterior hemiblock shifts it to the right by delaying activation of the more inferior and rightward portions of the left ventricle. In both cases therefore the QRS axis is shifted *toward* the direction of delayed activation.

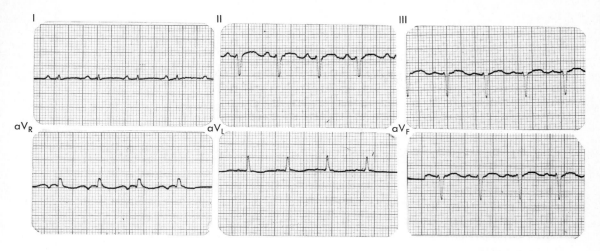

Fig. 7-10. Left anterior hemiblock. Notice the marked left axis deviation, without significant widening of the QRS duration. Compare with Fig. 9-8, *B,* showing left posterior hemiblock.

deviation is present and the S wave in lead aV_F equals or exceeds the R wave in lead I (Fig 7-10).

Left posterior hemiblock. Isolated left posterior hemiblock (Fig. 9-8, *B*) is diagnosed by finding a mean QRS axis of $+ 120°$ or more, with a QRS width of less than 0.12 second. *However, the diagnosis of left posterior hemiblock can be considered only if other, more common, causes of right axis deviation* (such as right ventricular hypertrophy, normal variant, emphysema, lateral wall infarction [Fig. 8-11], and pulmonary embolism) *are first excluded.*

Although left anterior hemiblock is relatively common, isolated left posterior hemiblock is rare. In general, the finding of *isolated* left anterior or left posterior hemiblock is not of much clinical significance.

We will consider the hemiblocks and *bifascicular* and *trifascicular* blocks further in the section on complete heart block (Chapter 15).

DIAGNOSIS OF HYPERTROPHY IN THE PRESENCE OF BUNDLE BRANCH BLOCKS

The ECG diagnosis of hypertrophy (Chapter 6) in the presence of bundle branch blocks may pose special problems. Therefore a few general guidelines will be discussed.

When right ventricular hypertrophy (RVH) occurs with RBBB, right axis deviation is often present. A tall peaked P wave (P pulmonale, p. 65) with RBBB should also suggest underlying RVH.

The usual voltage criteria for left ventricular hypertrophy (LVH) can be used in the presence of RBBB. Unfortunately, RBBB often masks these typical voltage increases.

The finding of LBBB, regardless of the QRS voltage, is highly suggestive of underlying LVH. Finding LBBB with prominent QRS voltages (p. 71) and evidence of left atrial abnormality (p. 66) virtually assures the diagnosis of LVH.

Finally, it should be emphasized that the *echocardiogram* is more accurate than the ECG in the diagnosis of cardiac enlargement (see p. 75).

DIAGNOSIS OF MYOCARDIAL INFARCTION IN THE PRESENCE OF BUNDLE BRANCH BLOCKS

The ECG diagnosis of myocardial infarction in the presence of bundle branch blocks is discussed in Chapter 8.

REVIEW

RBBB shows the following characteristic patterns: an rSR' with a prominent wide final R' wave in V_1, a qRS with a wide final S wave in V_6, and a QRS width of 0.12 second (three small time boxes) or more. *Incomplete RBBB* shows the same chest lead patterns, but the QRS width is between 0.1 and 0.12 second.

LBBB shows the following characteristic patterns: a deep wide QS (occasionally an rS with a wide S wave) in V_1, a prominent (often notched) R wave *without* a preceding q wave in V_6, and a QRS width of 0.12 second or more. *Incomplete LBBB* shows the same chest lead patterns as LBBB, but the QRS width is between 0.1 and 0.12 second.

Pacemaker patterns produced by an electrode in the right ventricle generally resemble LBBB but have a pacemaker spike before each QRS complex.

Hemiblocks can occur because the left bundle divides into two smaller fascicles (bundles): the left anterior fascicle and the left posterior fascicle. Conduction through either or both of these fascicles can be blocked.

Left anterior hemiblock is characterized by a mean QRS axis of $-45°$ or more. (When the mean QRS axis is $-45°$, left axis deviation is present and the height of the R wave in lead I [R_I] is equal to the depth of the S wave in lead aV_F [S_{aV_F}]. When the mean QRS axis is more negative than $-45°$, S_{aV_F} becomes larger than R_I.)

Left posterior hemiblock is characterized by right axis deviation. However, in making the diagnosis of left posterior hemiblock the other more common causes of right axis deviation (such as right ventricular hypertrophy, lateral wall infarction, chronic lung disease, or normal variants) must first be excluded.

Questions

1. Draw the shape of the QRS complexes in leads V_1 and V_6 that would be expected with RBBB and LBBB.
2. Examine the following set of chest leads:
   a. What is the approximate QRS width?
   b. What conduction disturbance is present?
   c. Why are the T waves in leads V_1 to V_3 inverted?

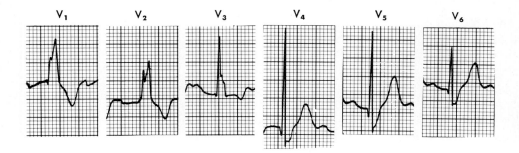

3. Answer these questions about the following ECG:
   a. What is the QRS width?
   b. What type of axis deviation is present?
   c. What ventricular conduction disturbance is present?
   d. What evidence is there of left ventricular hypertrophy?

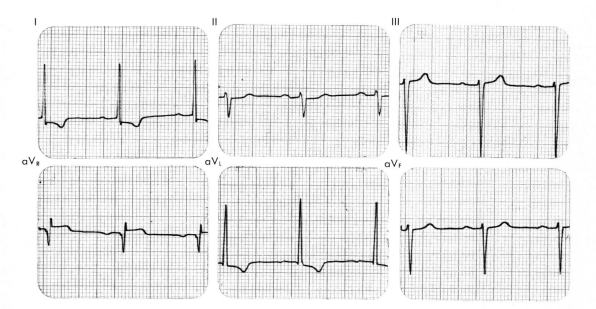

4. Examine the following 12-lead ECG and lead II rhythm strip carefully. Can you identify two conduction abnormalities?

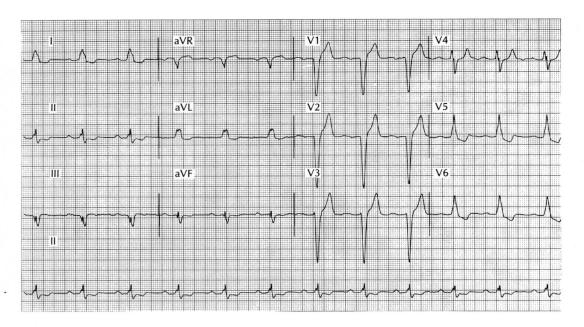

5. Define the terms *"primary"* and *"secondary"* T wave abnormality.

True or false (6 to 8):

6. Left anterior hemiblock does not markedly widen the QRS complex.
7. LBBB is generally seen in patients with organic heart disease.
8. Bundle branch blocks may occur transiently.

Answers

1. See p. 83.
2. a. 0.12 second
   b. RBBB.
   c. Secondary T wave inversions may be seen in the right chest leads with RBBB. (See p. 79 and question 5 below.)
3. a. 0.08 second (normal).
   b. Left axis deviation.
   c. Left anterior hemiblock.
   d. Tall R wave in lead aV_L (18 mm) with "strain" pattern in that lead. (See p. 74.)
4. First-degree AV block (PR interval 0.24 sec) and LBBB.
5. *Primary* T wave abnormalities are due to actual changes in ventricular repolarization caused, for example, by drugs, ischemia, or electrolyte abnormalities. These abnormalities are independent of changes in the QRS complex. *Secondary* T wave changes, by contrast, are related entirely to alterations in the timing of ventricular depolarization and are seen in conditions in which the QRS is wide. For example, with bundle branch block a change in the sequence of depolarization also alters the sequence of repolarization, causing the T wave to point in a direction opposite the last deflection of the QRS complex. Thus, with RBBB the T waves will be secondarily inverted in leads with an rSR' configuration (such as V_1, V_2, and sometimes V_3). With LBBB the secondary T wave inversions will be seen in leads with tall wide R waves (V_5 and V_6). Secondary T wave inversions are also seen with ventricular paced beats (Fig. 7-8) and the Wolff-Parkinson-White preexcitation pattern (Fig. 10-20). Sometimes primary and secondary T wave changes are seen on the same ECG, as when ischemia develops in a patient with a bundle branch block (Fig. 8-21).
6. True.
7. True.
8. True.

Myocardial Ischemia and Infarction—I

TRANSMURAL ISCHEMIA AND INFARCT PATTERNS

In this chapter and the next we will be looking at one of the most important topics of clinical electrocardiography—the diagnosis of myocardial ischemia and infarction (ischemic heart disease). We begin with a discussion of basic terms.

MYOCARDIAL ISCHEMIA

Myocardial cells require oxygen and other nutrients to function. Oxygenated blood is supplied by the coronary arteries. If severe narrowing or complete blockage of a coronary artery causes the flow to become inadequate, ischemia of the heart muscle will develop. The term *"ischemia"* means literally "to hold back blood." Myocardial ischemia may occur transiently. For example, patients who experience angina pectoris with exercise are having transient myocardial ischemia. If the ischemia is more severe, actual necrosis of a portion of heart muscle may occur. The term *"myocardial infarction"* (MI) refers to myocardial necrosis usually caused by severe ischemia.

In this discussion we will be considering primarily ischemia and infarction of the left ventricle, the predominant chamber of the heart. Right ventricular infarction will be discussed briefly.

TRANSMURAL AND SUBENDOCARDIAL ISCHEMIA

Fig. 8-1 diagrams a cross section of the left ventricle. Notice that it consists of an outer layer, the

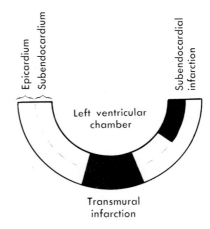

Fig. 8-1. Cross section of the left ventricle showing the difference between a *subendocardial* infarct, which involves the inner half of the ventricular wall, and a *transmural* infarct, which involves the full thickness of the wall.

epicardium, and an inner layer, the *subendocardium.* This distinction is important because myocardial ischemia or infarction may be limited to just the inner layer or may affect the entire thickness of the ventricular wall (transmural ischemia or infarction).

MYOCARDIAL BLOOD SUPPLY

It is also important to understand certain basic facts about the blood supply to the left ventricle.

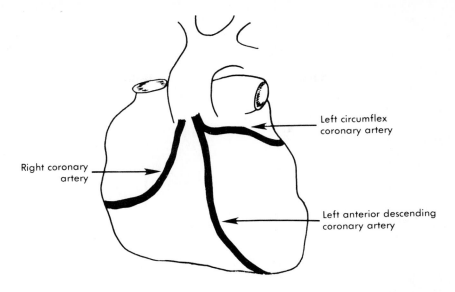

Fig. 8-2. Three major coronary arteries that supply blood to the heart.

The cardiac blood supply is delivered by the three main coronary arteries (Fig. 8-2). The right coronary artery supplies the inferior (diaphragmatic) portion of the heart. The left anterior descending coronary artery generally supplies the ventricular septum and part of the left ventricular wall. The left circumflex coronary artery supplies the lateral wall of the left ventricle. This circulation pattern may be variable. For example, in some cases the circumflex artery also supplies the inferior portion of the left ventricle. MIs tend to be *localized* to the portion (anterior or inferior) of the left ventricle supplied by one of these arteries.

TRANSMURAL MI

We will begin by considering the effect of a transmural MI on the ECG. In the next chapter we will consider the ECG patterns of subendocardial ischemia and infarction.

Transmural infarction is characterized by ischemia and, ultimately, by necrosis of a portion of the entire thickness of the left ventricular wall. Not surprisingly, it produces changes in both myocardial depolarization (QRS complex) and myocardial repolarization (ST-T complex).

The earliest changes seen with an acute transmural infarction occur in the ST-T complex. There are two sequential phases to these ST-T changes: the *acute* and the *evolving*. The acute phase is marked by the appearance of ST segment elevations and sometimes tall positive (hyperacute) T waves in certain leads. The evolving phase (occurring after hours or days) is characterized by deep T wave inversions in those leads that previously showed ST elevations.

Transmural MI can also be described in terms of the location of the infarct: *anterior* means involving the anterior and/or lateral wall of the left ventricle; *inferior* means involving the inferior (diaphragmatic) wall of the left ventricle (Fig. 8-3). The anatomic location of the infarct determines the leads in which the typical ECG patterns appear. For example, with an acute anterior wall MI the ST segment elevations and tall hyperacute T waves appear in one or more of the anterior leads (chest leads V_1 to V_6, limb leads I and aV_L) (Fig. 8-4). With an inferior wall MI the ST segment elevations and tall hyperacute T waves are seen in inferior leads II, III, and aV_F (Fig. 8-5).

One of the most important characteristics of the

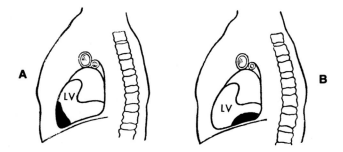

Fig. 8-3. Myocardial infarcts are generally localized to either the anterior, **A,** or the inferior (diaphragmatic), **B,** portions of the left ventricle.

ECG SEQUENCE WITH ANTERIOR WALL INFARCTION

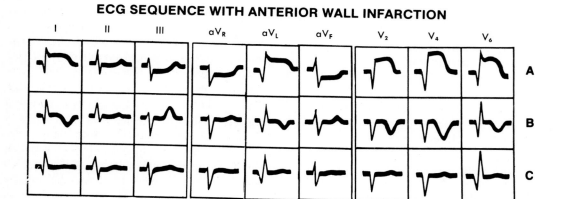

Fig. 8-4. Notice the reciprocal ST-T changes in the inferior leads (II, III, and aV_F). **A,** Acute phase: ST elevations and new Q waves. **B,** Evolving phase: deep T wave inversions. **C,** Resolving phase: partial or complete regression of ST-T changes (and sometimes of Q waves).

ECG SEQUENCE WITH INFERIOR WALL INFARCTION

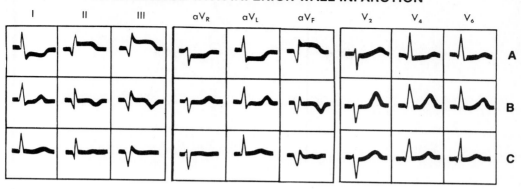

Fig. 8-5. Notice the reciprocal ST-T changes in the anterior leads (I, aV_L, V_2, V_4). **A,** Acute phase: ST elevations and new Q waves. **B,** Evolving phase: deep T wave inversions. **C,** Resolving phase: partial or complete regression of ST-T changes (and sometimes of Q waves).

ST-T changes seen with MI is their *reciprocity.* The anterior and inferior leads tend to show inverse patterns. Thus, with an anterior infarction with ST segment elevations in leads V_1 to V_6, I, and aV_L, leads II, III, and aV_F will often show ST segment depression. Conversely, with an acute inferior wall infarction, leads II, III, and aV_F will show ST segment elevation, with reciprocal ST depressions often seen in one or more of leads V_1 to V_3, I, and aV_L. (These reciprocal changes are illustrated in Figs. 8-4 and 8-5.)

The ST segment elevation seen with acute MI is called a "current of injury" and indicates that damage has occurred to the epicardial layer of the heart with a transmural infarction. The exact reasons why acute MI produces ST segment elevation are complex and not fully understood. Normally the ST segment is isoelectric (neither positive nor negative) because there is no net current flow at this time. Myocardial infarction alters the electrical charge on the myocardial cell membranes. As a result there is an abnormal current flow (current of injury) that produces the ST segment deviations.

The ST segment elevation seen with acute MI may have a variable appearance. The different shapes and appearances are shown in Fig. 8-6. In some cases, notice that the ST segment is plateau shaped and in others dome shaped; sometimes it is obliquely elevated.

The ST segment elevations (and reciprocal ST depressions) are the *earliest* ECG signs of infarction and are generally seen within minutes of the infarct. Tall positive (hyperacute) T waves may also be seen at this time (Figs. 8-7 and 8-8) and have the same significance as the ST elevations. In some cases hyperacute T waves actually precede the ST elevations.

After a variable time lag (hours to days) the elevated ST segments start to return to the baseline. At the same time the T waves become inverted in leads that previously showed ST segment elevations. This phase of T wave inversions is called the evolving phase of the infarct. Thus, with an anterior wall infarction the T waves become inverted in one or more of the anterior leads (V_1 to V_6, I, aV_L). With an inferior wall infarction the T waves become inverted in one or more of the inferior leads (II, III, aV_F). These T wave inversions are illustrated in Figs. 8-4 and 8-5.

QRS Changes: Q Waves of Transmural Infarction

Transmural infarctions also produce distinctive changes in the QRS (depolarization) complex. The

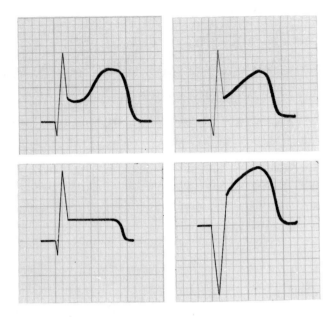

Fig. 8-6. ST segment elevations seen with acute infarction may have variable shapes.

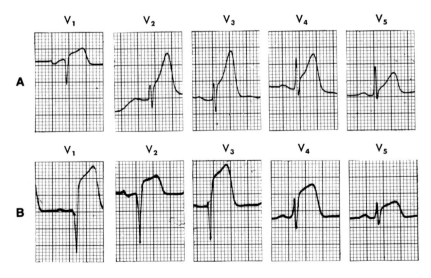

Fig. 8-7. Chest leads from a patient with acute anterior wall infarction. **A,** Notice the tall positive (hyperacute) T waves in leads V_2 to V_5 in the earliest phase of the infarction. **B,** Recorded several hours later. There is marked ST segment elevation in the same leads (current of injury pattern) with abnormal Q waves in leads V_1 and V_2.

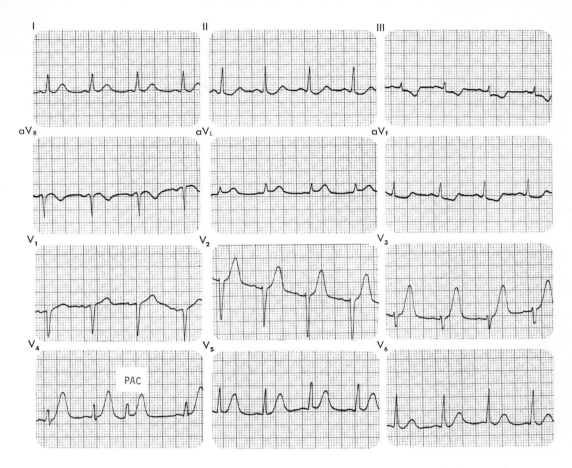

Fig. 8-8. Hyperacute T waves with anterior wall infarction. This patient was complaining of severe chest pain. Notice the very tall (hyperacute) T waves in the chest leads. There are also slight ST segment elevations in lead aV$_L$ with reciprocal ST depressions in leads II, III, and aV$_F$. In lead V$_4$, note the premature atrial contraction *(PAC)*.

characteristic sign of a transmural infarct is the appearance of new Q waves.

Why do transmural MIs lead to Q waves? Recall that a Q wave is simply an initial negative deflection of the QRS complex. If the entire QRS complex is negative $\left(\bigvee\right)$, we call it a *QS complex*.

A Q wave (negative deflection) in any lead indicates that the electrical voltages are directed away from that particular lead. When transmural infarction occurs, there is necrosis of heart muscle in a localized area of the ventricle; therefore the electrical voltages produced by this portion of the myocardium will disappear. Instead of positive (R) waves over the infarcted area, Q waves will be recorded (either a QR or a QS complex).

To summarize: Abnormal Q waves are the characteristic markers of transmural infarction.* They signify the loss of positive electrical voltages caused by the death of heart muscle.

---

*As discussed in the next chapter, the equation of pathologic Q waves with transmural necrosis is an oversimplification. Not all transmural infarcts lead to Q waves, and not all Q wave infarcts correlate with transmural necrosis.

The new Q waves of an MI generally appear within the first day or so of the infarct. With an anterior wall infarction, they will be seen in one or more of leads V_1 to V_6, I, and aV_L (Fig 8-4). With an inferior wall MI, they will appear in leads II, III, and aV_F (Fig. 8-5).

LOCALIZATION OF INFARCTIONS

As mentioned, MIs are generally localized to a specific portion of the left ventricle, affecting either the anterior or the inferior wall. Anterior infarcts (Figs. 8-9 to 8-11) are sometimes considered as anteroseptal, strictly anterior, or anterolateral depending on the leads that show signs of the infarct.

Anterior Wall Infarctions

The characteristic feature of an anterior wall infarct is the *loss of normal R wave progression in the chest leads*. Recall that normally there is a progressive increase in the height of the R wave as you move from lead V_1 to lead V_6. An anterior infarct interrupts this progression, and the result is

pathologic Q waves in one or more of the chest leads.

Anteroseptal infarcts. Remember (from Chapter 4) that the ventricular septum is depolarized from left to right and that leads V_1 and V_2 show small positive r waves (septal r waves). Now consider the effect of damaging the septum. Obviously, there will be a loss of septal depolarization voltages; thus in leads V_1 and V_2 the r waves will be lost and an entirely negative (QS) complex will appear.

The septum is supplied with blood by the left anterior descending coronary artery, and septal infarction generally suggests that there has been an occlusion of this artery or one of its branches.

Strictly anterior infarcts. Normally leads V_3 and V_4 show RS- or Rs-type complexes. If the anterior wall of the left ventricle is infarcted, the positive R waves that reflect the voltages produced by this muscle area will be lost. Instead, Q waves (as part of QS or QR complexes) will be seen in leads V_3 and V_4. A strictly anterior infarct generally

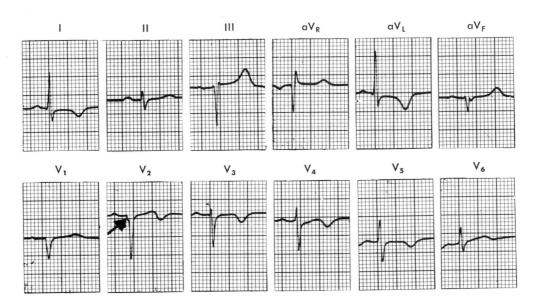

Fig. 8-9. Anterior wall infarction. Notice the QS complexes in leads V_1 and V_2, indicating anteroseptal infarction. There is also a characteristic notching (*arrow,* V_2) of the QS complex, often seen with infarcts. In addition, note the diffuse ischemic T wave inversions in leads I, aV_L, and V_2 to V_5, indicating generalized anterior wall ischemia.

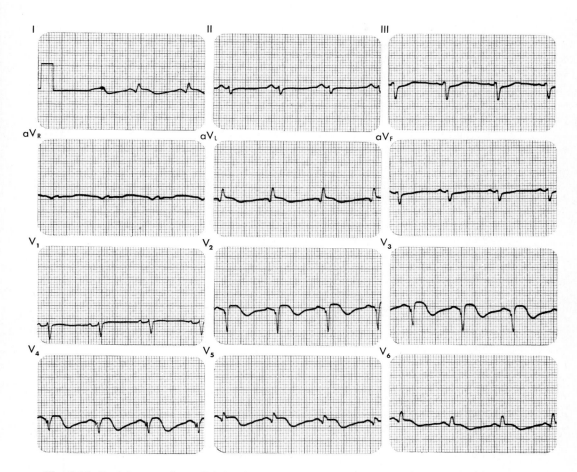

Fig. 8-10. Evolving anterior wall infarction. The patient sustained the infarct 1 week earlier. Notice the abnormal Q waves (leads I, aV_L, and V_2 to V_5) with slight ST segment elevations and deep T wave inversions. Left axis deviation resulting from left anterior hemiblock is present as well. (See Chapter 7.)

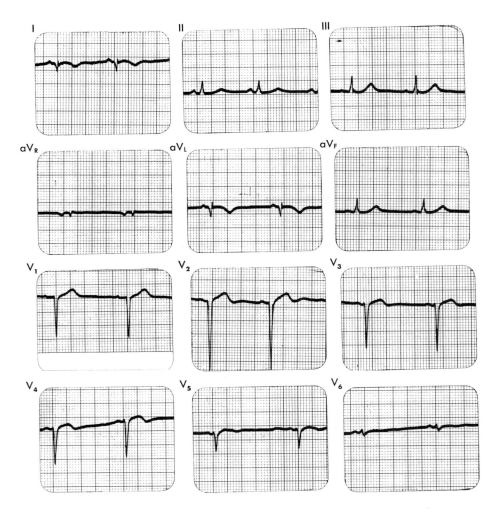

Fig. 8-11. Evolving anterior wall infarction. The infarct occurred 1 week earlier. Notice the poor R wave progression in leads V_1 to V_5 with Q waves in leads I and aV_L. T waves are slightly inverted in these leads. Right axis deviation in this case is the result of loss of lateral wall forces, with Q waves in I and aV_L.

results from occlusion of the left anterior descending coronary artery.

Anterolateral infarcts. An infarction of the lateral wall of the left ventricle produces changes in the more laterally situated chest leads (V_5 and V_6). With a lateral wall infarct abnormal Q waves, as part of QS or QR complexes, will appear in leads V_5 and V_6 (Fig. 7-7). The infarct is often caused by occlusion of the left circumflex coronary artery, but it may also result from occlusion of the left anterior descending coronary artery or a branch of the right coronary artery.

Differentiating anterior wall infarcts. The foregoing classification of anterior infarctions is not absolute. Often there is overlap. You can describe MIs by simply calling any infarct that shows ECG changes in one or more of leads I, aV_L, and V_1 to V_6 as "anterior" and then specifying which leads show Q waves and ST-T changes.

Inferior Wall Infarctions

Infarction of the inferior (diaphragmatic) portion of the left ventricle is indicated by changes in leads II, III, and aV_F (Figs. 8-12 to 8-14). These three leads, as shown in the frontal plane axis diagram, are oriented downward or inferiorly (Fig. 5-1). Thus they will record voltages from the inferior portion of the ventricle. An inferior wall infarct will produce abnormal Q waves in leads II, III, and aV_F. It is generally caused by occlusion of the right coronary artery, less commonly by a left circumflex coronary obstruction.

"Posterior" Infarctions

The posterior (back) surface of the left ventricle can also be infarcted. This may be difficult to diagnose because characteristic abnormal ST elevations may not appear in any of the 12 conventional leads. Instead, tall R waves and ST depressions may occur in leads V_1 and V_2 (reciprocal to the Q waves and ST segment elevations that would be recorded at the back of the heart). During the evolving phase of such infarcts, when deep T wave inversions appear in the posterior leads, the anterior chest leads will show reciprocally tall positive T waves (Fig. 8-15).

In most cases of posterior MI the infarct extends either to the lateral wall of the left ventricle, producing characteristic changes in lead V_6, or to the inferior wall of the left ventricle, producing characteristic changes in leads II, III, and aV_F (Fig. 8-15). Because of the overlap between *inferior* and

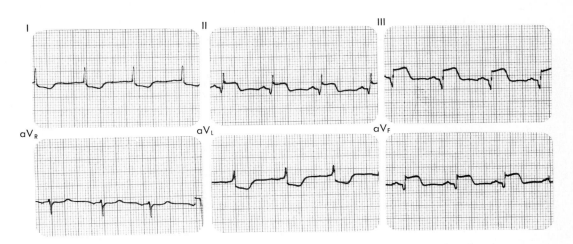

Fig. 8-12. Acute inferior wall infarction. Notice the ST elevations in leads II, III, and aV_F with reciprocal ST depressions in leads I and aV_L. Abnormal Q waves are also present in leads II, III, and aV_F.

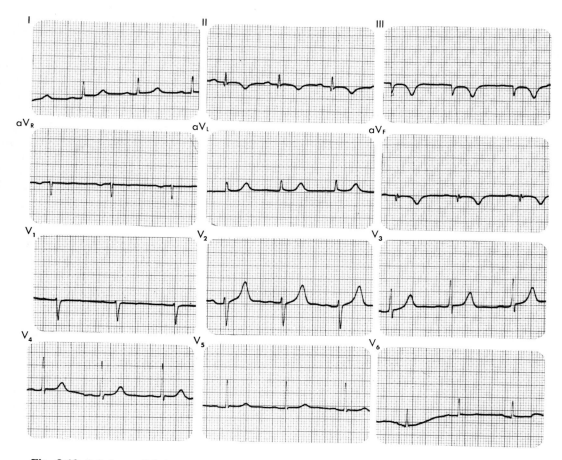

Fig. 8-13. Inferior wall infarct. This patient sustained a myocardial infarction 1 month previously. Notice the abnormal Q waves and symmetric T wave inversions in leads II, III, and aV$_F$. There is also T wave flattening in lead V$_6$. Q waves and ST-T changes after infarction may persist indefinitely or may resolve partially or completely.

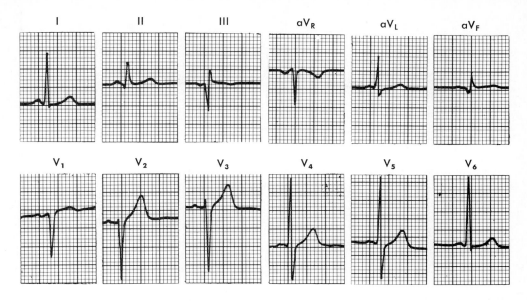

Fig. 8-14. Old inferior wall infarct. Notice the prominent Q waves in leads II, III, and aV$_F$ from a patient who sustained an MI 1 year previously. The ST-T changes have essentially reverted to normal.

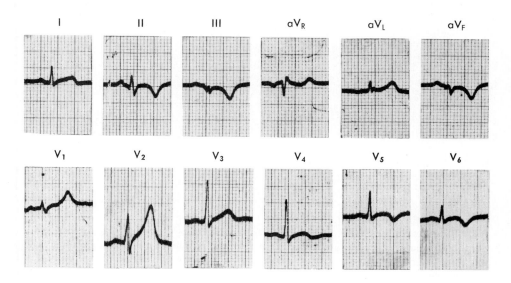

Fig. 8-15. Posterior infarction. Notice the tall R waves in V$_1$ and V$_2$. In addition, there is evidence of a prior inferior infarction (Q waves in II, III, aV$_F$) and probably a lateral infarction as well (T wave inversions in V$_4$ to V$_6$) Note also the reciprocally tall positive T waves in anterior precordial leads V$_1$ and V$_2$. (From Goldberger AL: Myocardial infarction: electrocardiographic differential diagnosis, ed 3, St Louis, 1984, The CV Mosby Co.)

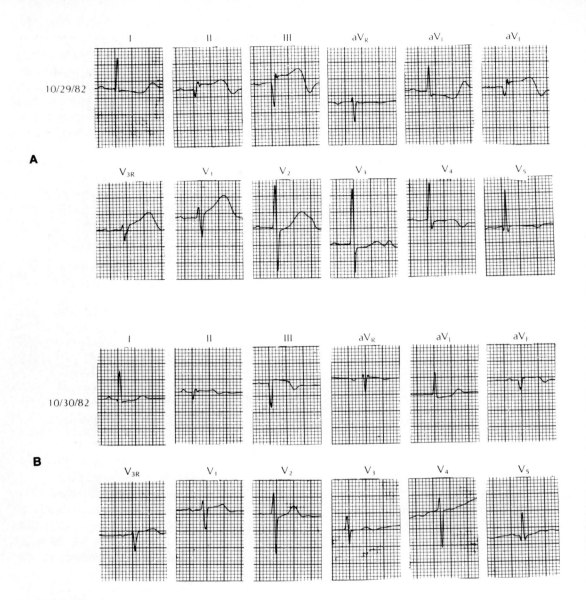

Fig. 8-16. Acute right ventricular infarction with inferior wall infarction. **A,** Q waves and ST segment elevations in leads II, III, and aV_F are accompanied by ST elevations in the right precordial leads (V_{3R} and V_1). ST-T changes in V_5 and V_6 are consistent with lateral wall ischemia. ST depression in I and aV_L is probably reciprocal to an inferior wall injury current. **B,** Follow-up tracing showing diminution of acute ST changes. The patient was hypotensive, and right-sided heart catheterization showed elevated right-sided heart filling pressures but relatively low pulmonary capillary wedge pressure. The patient responded favorably to volume expansion. (From Goldberger AL: Myocardial infarction: electrocardiographic differential diagnosis ed 3, St Louis, 1984, The CV Mosby Co.)

posterior infarcts the more general term "infero-posterior" can be used when the ECG shows changes consistent with either inferior or posterior infarction.

Right Ventricular (RV) Infarctions

A related topic is right ventricular (RV) infarction. Clinical and autopsy studies have shown that patients with an inferoposterior infarct not uncommonly have associated RV involvement. In one postmortem study, RV infarction was found in about one of four cases of inferoposterior MI but not in cases of anterior MI. Clinically patients with an RV infarct may have elevated central venous pressure (distended neck veins) because of the abnormally high diastolic filling pressures in the right side of the heart. If the RV damage is severe, hypotension and even cardiogenic shock may result. AV conduction disturbances are not uncommon in this setting. The presence of jugular venous distension in a patient with an acute inferoposterior MI should always suggest this diagnosis. In addition, many of these patients will have ST elevations in leads reflecting the right ventricle, such as V_1 and V_2 and V_{3R} to V_{5R} (p. 28, footnote), as shown in Fig. 8-16.

Recognition of RV infarction is of major clinical importance. Volume expansion may be critical in patients who are hypotensive and have a low or normal pulmonary capillary wedge pressure despite elevated central venous pressure.

SEQUENCE OF Q WAVES AND ST-T CHANGES WITH TRANSMURAL INFARCTIONS

Up to now we have discussed separately the ventricular depolarization (QRS) and repolarization (ST-T) changes produced by a transmural MI. As shown in the examples in Figs. 8-4 and 8-5, these changes occur simultaneously.

Ordinarily the earliest sign of transmural infarction is ST segment elevations (with reciprocal ST depressions). The ST elevations (current of injury pattern) usually persist for hours to days. During this same period Q waves will begin to appear in leads showing ST elevations. Following these changes, the ST segments start to return to the baseline; and the T waves become inverted during the evolving phase.

In the weeks or months following an infarct, what should you expect to happen to the Q waves and the ST-T changes just described? The answer is that you cannot make any certain predictions. In most cases the abnormal Q waves will persist for months, and even years, after the acute infarction. However, occasionally they will diminish in size and even disappear entirely. In some cases abnormal T wave inversions will persist indefinitely. In others there will be improvement but minor nonspecific ST-T abnormalities (such as slight T wave flattening) may persist (Figs. 8-4 and 8-5).

NORMAL AND ABNORMAL Q WAVES

One diagnostic problem frequently faced is deciding whether Q waves are abnormal. Not all Q waves are indicators of MI. For example, we normally expect to see a Q wave in lead aV_R. Furthermore, small "septal" q waves are normally seen in the left chest leads (V_4 to V_6) and in one or more of leads I, aV_L, II, III, and aV_F. Recall from Chapter 4 the significance of these septal q waves. The ventricular septum depolarizes from left to right. Left chest leads record this spread of voltages toward the right as a small negative deflection (q wave) as part of a qR complex, where the R wave represents the spread of left ventricular voltages toward the lead. When the electrical axis is horizontal, such qR complexes will be seen in leads I and aV_L. When the electrical axis is vertical, qR complexes will appear in leads II, III, and aV_F.

These normal septal q waves must be differentiated from the pathologic Q waves of infarction. Normal septal q waves are characteristically narrow and of low amplitude. As a rule septal q waves are less than 0.04 second in duration. A Q wave of 0.04 second or more in lead I, in all three inferior leads (II, III, aV_F), or in leads V_3 to V_6 is generally abnormal.

What about a Q wave of 0.04 second or more width in leads V_1 and V_2? A large QS complex can be seen as a normal variant in lead V_1 and rarely in leads V_1 and V_2. However, QS waves in these leads may be the only evidence of an anterior septal MI. An abnormal QS complex resulting from infarction will sometimes show a notch as it descends or it may be slurred instead of descending and rising abruptly (Fig. 8-9). Further criteria for differentiating normal from abnormal Q waves in these leads lie beyond the scope of this book.

What about a wide Q wave in lead aV_L or Q waves in leads III and aV_F, which can also occur normally? Again, the precise criteria to differentiate normal from abnormal Q waves in these leads lie beyond the scope of this book. However, the following can be taken as general rules:

1. An inferior wall MI should be diagnosed with certainty only when abnormal Q waves are seen in leads II, III, and aV_F. If prominent Q waves appear just in leads III and aV_F, then the likelihood of MI is increased by the presence of abnormal ST-T changes in all three inferior limb leads.
2. An anterior wall MI should not be diagnosed from lead aV_L alone. Look for abnormal Q waves and ST-T changes in the other anterior leads (I and V_1 to V_6).

Furthermore, just as not all Q waves are abnormal, so not all abnormal Q waves are a result of MI. For example, poor R wave progression in the chest leads, sometimes with actual QS complexes in the right to middle chest leads (for example, V_1 to V_3), may occur with left bundle branch block, left ventricular hypertrophy, and chronic lung disease in the absence of MI. Prominent noninfarctional Q waves are often a characteristic feature of idiopathic hypertrophic subaortic stenosis (IHSS) (Fig. 8-17). Noninfarctional Q waves also occur with dilated cardiomyopathy (Fig. 10-18). As mentioned before, normal people may sometimes have a QS wave in lead V_1 and rarely in leads V_1 and V_2. Prominent Q waves in the absence of MI are sometimes referred to as a *pseudoinfarct pattern*.*

VENTRICULAR ANEURYSM

After a large MI, in some patients a ventricular aneurysm will develop. An aneurysm is a severely

---

*See Goldberger AL: Myocardial infarction: electrocardiographic differential diagnosis, ed 3, St Louis, 1984, The CV Mosby Co.

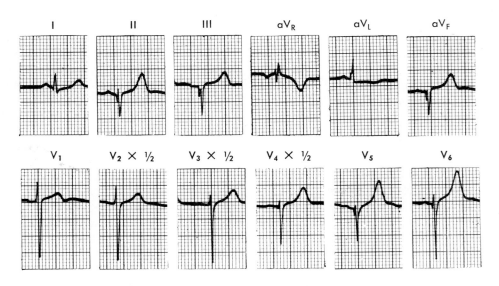

Fig. 8-17. Idiopathic hypertrophic subaortic stenosis (IHSS). Notice the prominent pseudoinfarctional Q waves, which are the result of septal hypertrophy. (From Goldberger AL: Myocardial infarction: electrocardiographic differential diagnosis, ed 3, St Louis, 1984, The CV Mosby Co.)

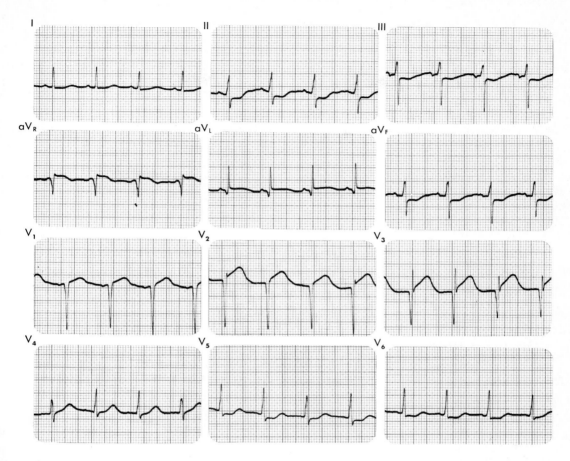

Fig. 8-18. Anterior wall aneurysm. The patient sustained an infarct several months prior to this ECG. Notice the prominent Q waves in leads V_1 to V_3 and aV_L with persistent ST elevations in these leads and with reciprocal ST depressions in the inferior leads (II, III, and aV_F). Persistent ST elevations more than 2 to 3 weeks after an infarct suggest ventricular aneurysm.

scarred portion of infarcted ventricular myocardium that does not contract normally. Instead, during ventricular systole the aneurysmic portion bulges outward while the rest of the ventricle is contracting. Ventricular aneurysms may occur on the anterior or inferior surface of the heart. The ECG may be helpful in making the diagnosis of ventricular aneurysm following an MI. Patients with ventricular aneurysms frequently have persistent ST segment elevations following the infarct. As mentioned earlier, the ST segment elevations seen with acute infarction generally resolve within several days. The persistence of ST segment elevations for several weeks or more is suggestive of a ventricular aneurysm (Fig. 8-18). However, the absence of persisting ST segment elevations does not rule out the possibility of an aneurysm.

Ventricular aneurysms are of clinical importance for several major reasons. They may lead to congestive heart failure. They may be associated with serious ventricular arrhythmias. A thrombus may form in an aneurysm and break off, resulting in stroke or some other embolic complication.

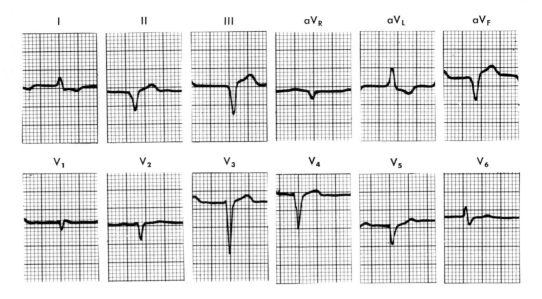

Fig. 8-19. Multiple infarcts. This ECG shows evidence of previous anterior wall and inferior wall MIs. Notice the poor R wave progression and QS complexes in chest leads V_1 to V_5, as well as the QS waves in leads II, III, and aV_F.

MULTIPLE INFARCTIONS

To this point we have discussed localized single infarcts. Not infrequently, however, patients may have two or more MIs at different times. For example, a new anterior wall infarct may develop in a patient with a previous inferior wall infarction. In such cases the ECG will initially show abnormal Q waves in leads II, III, and aV_F. During the anterior infarct new Q waves and ST-T changes will appear in the anterior leads. Fig. 8-19 is the ECG of a patient with multiple infarcts (anterior and inferior).

SILENT MI

Most patients with acute MI have symptoms. They may experience the classic syndrome of crushing substernal chest pain. In other cases the pain may be atypical (feeling like indigestion or upper back or jaw pain). However, in some cases the patient may experience few if any symptoms. Therefore it is not unusual to see abnormal Q waves on a patient's ECG that indicate a previous infarct, without any clinical history of a definite MI.

DIAGNOSIS OF MI IN THE PRESENCE OF BUNDLE BRANCH BLOCK

In some cases the diagnosis of infarction is made more difficult because the patient's baseline ECG will show a bundle branch block pattern or a bundle branch block may develop as a complication of the infarct. Then the ECG picture becomes more complex.

Right Bundle Branch Block with MI

The diagnosis of an MI can be made relatively easily in the presence of RBBB. Remember that RBBB affects primarily the terminal phase of ventricular depolarization, producing a wide R′ wave in the right chest leads and a wide S wave in the left chest leads. MI affects the initial phase of ventricular depolarization, producing abnormal Q waves. When RBBB and an infarct occur together, there will be a combination of these patterns: the QRS complex will be abnormally wide (0.12 sec or more) as a result of the bundle branch block, lead V_1 will show a terminal positive deflection, and lead V_6 will show a wide S wave; if the in-

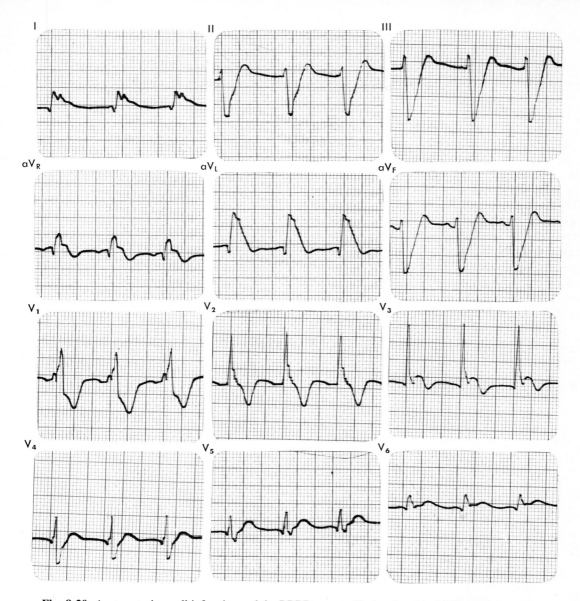

Fig. 8-20. Acute anterior wall infarction and the RBBB pattern. Notice the wide QRS complexes with an rSR′ wave in lead V_1 and a qRS pattern in V_5, indicating RBBB. There is, furthermore, a pattern of acute anterior wall infarction (Q waves and ST elevations in leads I and aV_L plus marked reciprocal ST depressions in II, III, and aV_F). Finally, notice the left axis deviations caused by the left anterior hemiblock. This combination (left anterior hemiblock and RBBB) is an example of bifascicular block and may herald complete heart block in patients with an acute anterior infarction.

farction is anterior, there will be a loss of R wave progression with abnormal Q waves in the anterior leads and characteristic ST-T changes; if it is in-

ferior, pathologic Q waves and ST-T changes will be seen in leads II, III, and aV_F. Fig. 8-20 shows RBBB and acute MI. (See also p. 315.)

Left Bundle Branch Block with MI

The diagnosis of LBBB in the presence of MI is considerably more complicated and confusing than that of RBBB. The reason is that LBBB interrupts both the early and the late phases of ventricular stimulation (Chapter 7). It also produces secondary ST-T changes. As a general rule LBBB will hide the diagnosis of an infarct. *Thus a patient with a chronic LBBB pattern in whom an acute MI develops may not show the characteristic changes of infarction described in this chapter.* Occasionally patients with LBBB will manifest primary ST-T changes indicative of ischemia or actual infarction. The secondary T wave inversions of uncomplicated LBBB are seen in leads V_4 to V_6 (with prominent R waves). The appearance of T wave inversions in leads V_1 to V_3 (with prominent S waves) is a primary abnormality that cannot be ascribed to the LBBB itself (Fig. 8-21).

The problem of diagnosing infarction with LBBB is further complicated by the fact that the LBBB pattern has several features that resemble those seen with infarction. An LBBB pattern can therefore mimic an infarct pattern. Recall (from Chapter 7) that LBBB typically shows poor R wave progression in the chest leads because of the reversed way the ventricular septum is activated: from right to left, the opposite of what happens normally. Consequently, with LBBB, there is a loss of the normal septal R waves in the right chest leads. This loss of normal R wave progression simulates the pattern seen with an anterior wall infarct.

Fig 7-5 shows an example of LBBB with poor R wave progression. Anterior wall infarction was not present. Notice that the ST segments in the right chest leads are elevated, resembling the pattern seen during the hyperacute or acute phase of an infarction. ST segment elevation in the right chest leads is also commonly seen with LBBB in the absence of infarction.

As a general rule a patient with an LBBB pattern should not be diagnosed as having suffered a myocardial infarction simply on the basis of poor R wave progression in the right chest leads or ST

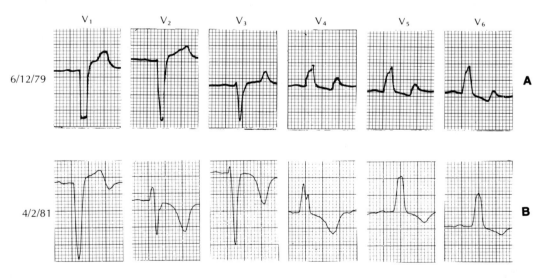

Fig. 8-21. A, Typical left bundle branch block pattern. Notice the poor R wave progression in the right precordial leads and the discordance of QRS and ST-T vectors reflected by ST elevations in the right precordial and ST depressions with T wave inversions in the left precordial leads. **B,** Subsequently the ECG from this patient showed development of primary T wave inversions in leads V_1 to V_3 caused by anterior ischemia and probable infarction. (From Goldberger AL: Myocardial infarction: electrocardiographic differential diagnosis, ed 3, St Louis, 1984, The CV Mosby Co.)

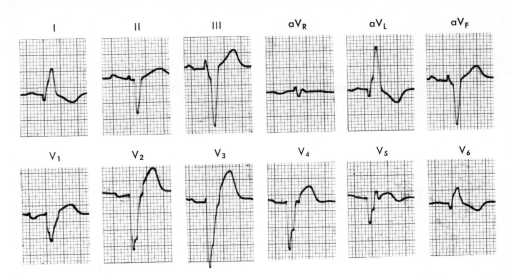

Fig. 8-22. Anterior wall infarction with LBBB. Notice the prominent Q waves in the left chest leads as part of QR complexes. See text. (From Goldberger AL: Myocardial infarction: electrocardiographic differential diagnosis, ed 3, St Louis, 1984, The CV Mosby Co.)

elevations in those leads. However, the presence of Q waves as part of QR complexes in the left chest leads (V_5 and V_6) with LBBB generally indicates an underlying MI (Fig. 8-22). In addition, the appearance of ST elevations in the left chest leads or in other leads with prominent R waves suggests ischemia (Fig. 8-22, *lead V_5*).

In the next chapter this discussion of the ECG with ischemia and infarction will continue, focusing on the *subendocardial* ischemia patterns.

REVIEW

Myocardial ischemia occurs when the blood supply to the myocardium is not adequate. *Myocardial infarction* (MI) refers to necrosis of the myocardium caused by severe ischemia.

Myocardial ischemia or infarction can affect the entire thickness of the ventricular muscle (*transmural* injury) or may be localized to just the inner layer of the ventricle (*subendocardial* ischemia or infarction). Transmural MI produces a typical sequence of ST-T changes and abnormal Q waves. The ST-T changes can be divided into two phases: (1) acute, marked by ST segment elevations (current of injury pattern) and sometimes tall positive T waves (hyperacute T waves), and (2) evolving, characterized by the appearance of deeply inverted T waves in leads that showed the hyperacute T waves and ST elevations. These ST-T changes occur during a period of hours or days and usually resolve over a period of weeks or months. During the first day or so after a transmural infarction, new abnormal Q waves will often appear in one or more leads.

When ST segment elevations persist for more than 2 or 3 weeks after an acute MI, this may signify that a ventricular aneurysm has developed. The abnormal Q waves tend to persist but may become smaller with time and, rarely, may even disappear.

Transmural MI can also be described in terms of its location. With an *anterior* infarction, ST segment elevations and abnormal Q waves occur in one or more of leads V_1 to V_6, I, and aV_L. (Reciprocal ST depressions may be seen in leads II, III, and aV_F.) With an *inferior* infarction, ST elevations and Q waves will appear in leads II, III, and aV_F and there may be reciprocal ST depressions in one or more of the anterior leads.

Right ventricular MI is a common complication of inferoposterior infarcts. In acute cases the ECG may also show elevated ST segments in the right chest leads.

The pathologic Q waves of infarction must be distinguished from normal Q waves. For example, small normal "septal" q waves as part of qR complexes may be seen in the left chest leads (V_4 to V_6), in leads II, III, and aV_F (with a vertical electrical axis), and in leads I and aV_L (with a horizontal axis). These septal q waves are normally less than 0.04 second in width.

A QS wave may be seen normally in lead V_1 and occasionally in leads V_1 and V_2. Q waves may also be seen as normal variants in leads aV_F, III, and aV_L.

Multiple MIs can occur, and the ECG will show old Q waves from the preceding infarct as well as new Q waves with ST-T changes from the current infarct.

When *right bundle branch block* complicates an acute MI, the diagnosis of both conditions is possible. The RBBB prolongs the QRS width, and lead V_1 shows a tall positive final deflection. In addition, abnormal Q waves and ST segment elevations resulting from the acute MI will be present in the chest leads (with an anterior MI) and in leads II, III, and aV_F (in inferior MI).

When *left bundle branch block* complicates an acute MI, it is often difficult to diagnose the MI because the LBBB may mask both the abnormal Q waves of the infarction and the ST segment elevations and T wave inversions of the ischemia. In addition, LBBB may produce QS waves in the right chest leads with ST segment elevations and poor R wave progression across the chest *without* MI. The presence of QR complexes in the left chest leads with LBBB is suggestive of underlying MI. T wave inversions in the right chest leads or ST segment elevations in the left chest leads or in leads with prominent R waves suggest ischemia with underlying LBBB.

Questions

See the end of Chapter 9.

9

Myocardial Ischemia and Infarction—II

SUBENDOCARDIAL ISCHEMIA AND INFARCT PATTERNS

Transmural myocardial infarction (MI) may be associated with abnormal Q waves and the typical progression of ST-T changes described in Chapter 8. In other cases (described in this chapter), however, myocardial ischemia with or without actual infarction may be limited to the *subendocardial* layer of the ventricle.

SUBENDOCARDIAL ISCHEMIA

How can subendocardial ischemia occur without transmural ischemia or infarction? The subendocardium is most distant from the coronary blood supply and closest to the high pressure of the ventricular cavity and therefore is particularly vulnerable to ischemia. It can become ischemic while the outer layer of the ventricle (epicardium) remains normally perfused with blood.

The most common ECG change with subendocardial ischemia is ST segment depression (shown in Fig. 9-1). It may be limited to the anterior leads (I, aV_L, and V_1 to V_6) or to the inferior leads (II, III, and aV_F), or it may be seen more diffusely in both groups of leads. As shown in Fig. 9-1, the ST depression with subendocardial ischemia has a characteristic squared-off shape. (ST segment elevations may be seen in lead aV_R.)

Recall from the previous chapter that acute transmural infarction produces ST segment elevation, a current of injury pattern. This results from epicar-

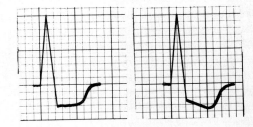

Fig. 9-1. Subendocardial ischemia may produce ST depressions.

dial injury. With pure subendocardial ischemia just the opposite occurs—ST segment depression (except in lead aV_R, which often shows ST elevation).

To summarize: Myocardial ischemia involving just the subendocardium produces ST segment depression while acute ischemia involving the epicardium produces ST elevation. This difference in the direction of the injury current vector is depicted in Fig. 9-2.

ECG Changes with Angina Pectoris

The term *"angina pectoris"* refers to transient attacks of chest discomfort caused by myocardial ischemia. Angina is a symptom of coronary artery disease. The classic attack of angina is experienced as a dull, burning, or boring substernal pressure or pain. It is typically precipitated by exertion, stress,

SUBENDOCARDIAL INJURY:
ST Depression

TRANSMURAL (EPICARDIAL) INJURY:
ST Elevation

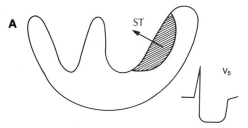
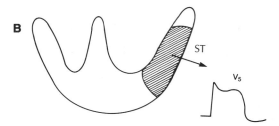

Fig. 9-2. Subendocardial versus epicardial injury currents. **A,** Acute subendocardial ischemia. The electrical forces *(arrow)* responsible for the ST segment are deviated toward the inner layer of the heart, causing ST depressions in lead V_5, which faces the outer surface of the heart. **B,** Acute epicardial ischemia as seen in a case of transmural MI. Electrical forces *(arrow)* responsible for the ST segment are deviated toward the outer layer of the heart, causing ST elevations in the overlying lead.

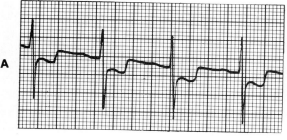
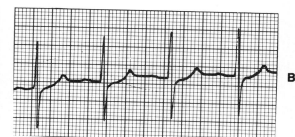

Fig. 9-3. This patient complained of chest pain while being examined. **A,** Notice the marked ST depressions in lead V_4. **B,** Five minutes later, after nitroglycerin, the ST segments have reverted to normal, with relief of the angina.

exposure to cold, and so on, and is relieved by rest and nitroglycerin.

Many patients with classic angina will have an ECG pattern of subendocardial ischemia (with ST depressions) during an attack. When the pain disappears, the ST segments generally return to the baseline.

Fig. 9-3 shows an example of ST depressions during a spontaneous episode of angina. Not all patients with angina will have ST depressions during chest pain. The presence of a normal ECG does not rule out underlying coronary artery disease.

However, the appearance of transient ST segment depression with chest pain is a strong indicator of myocardial ischemia.

Exercise Testing

Many patients with coronary artery disease will have a normal ECG while at rest; however, during exercise, ischemic changes may appear on their ECGs because of the extra oxygen requirements imposed on their heart by exertion. To assist in diagnosing coronary artery disease, the ECG can be recorded while the patient is being exercised

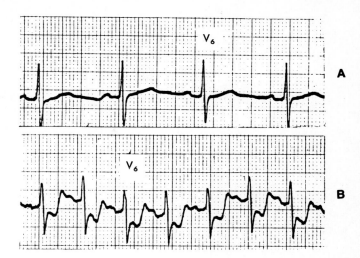

Fig. 9-4. Positive exercise test. **A,** Baseline rhythm strip from a patient with coronary artery disease. **B,** Notice the marked ST depressions with increased heart rate. (From Goldberger AL: Myocardial infarction: electrocardiographic differential diagnosis, ed 3, St Louis, 1984, The CV Mosby Co.)

under controlled conditions. Such *stress electrocardiography* is usually performed while the patient walks on a treadmill or pedals a bicycle. The test is stopped when the patient develops angina, fatigue, or diagnostic ST changes or when the heart rate reaches 85% to 90% of a maximum predetermined rate, predicted from the patient's age. (This is known as *submaximal testing.*)

Fig. 9-4, *A,* is the normal resting ECG of a patient. Fig. 9-4, *B,* shows marked ST segment depressions recorded while the patient was exercising. The appearance of ST depressions constitutes a positive (abnormal) result. Most cardiologists accept horizontal or downward ST depression of at least 1 mm or more, lasting at least 0.08 second, as a positive (abnormal) test result (Fig. 9-4, *B*). ST depression of less than 1 mm, or depression of only the J point, with a rapid upward sloping of the ST segment, is considered a negative (normal) test response (Fig. 9-5).

Exercise electrocardiography is often helpful in diagnosing coronary artery disease. However, like all tests, it may give both false-positive and false-negative results. For example, up to 10% of normal men and an even higher percentage of normal women will have false-positive exercise tests. False-positive tests also can be seen in patients taking digitalis and in those with hypokalemia, left ven-

tricular hypertrophy, ventricular conduction disturbances, or Wolff-Parkinson-White syndrome (p. 140). False-negative tests also can occur despite the presence of significant underlying coronary artery disease. *Therefore, a normal exercise test does not exclude coronary artery disease.*

To summarize: Subendocardial ischemia, such as occurs with typical angina pectoris (and as may sometimes be elicited with stress testing), often produces ST segment depressions in multiple leads.

Silent Myocardial Ischemia

A patient with coronary artery disease may have episodes of myocardial ischemia *without* angina; hence the term *"silent ischemia."* Silent ischemia is sometimes detected during exercise testing. The most useful way of assessing it is by ambulatory ECG (Holter) monitoring (Chapter 3). A 24-hour ECG monitoring of patients with coronary artery disease reveals a surprisingly high frequency of ST depressions *not* associated with angina. For further discussion of this important topic, readers are referred to the Bibliography. (See also p. 108.)

SUBENDOCARDIAL INFARCTION

If ischemia to the subendocardial region is severe enough, actual subendocardial infarction may occur. In such cases the ECG often shows persistent

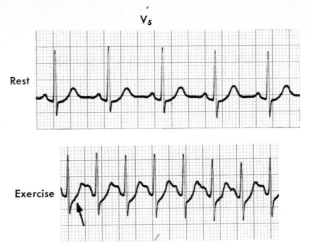

Fig. 9-5. Physiologic ST segment depression with exercise. Notice the J junction depression *(arrow)* with sharply upsloping ST segments. (From Goldberger AL: Myocardial infarction: electrocardiographic differential diagnosis, ed 3, St Louis, 1984, The CV Mosby Co.)

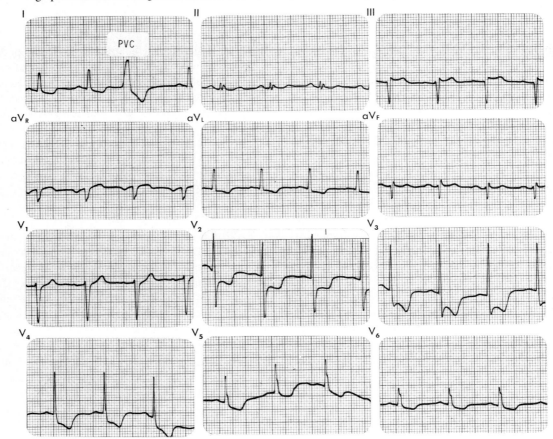

Fig. 9-6. Non–Q wave (''subendocardial'') infarction. This patient complained of severe chest pain. Subsequently cardiac enzymes were elevated. Notice the marked ST depressions, best seen in chest leads V_2 to V_5, consistent with subendocardial infarction. There is also a premature ventricular contraction *(PVC)* in lead I. Slight ST elevations are seen in lead aV_R and lead III.

ST depressions instead of the transient depressions seen with reversible subendocardial ischemia.

Fig. 9-6 shows an example of subendocardial infarction. Do Q waves appear with pure subendocardial infarction? The answer is that if only the subendocardium is infarcted abnormal Q waves usually do not appear. As a rule Q waves are seen only with transmural infarction. Subendocardial in-

farction generally affects ventricular repolarization (ST-T complex) and not depolarization (QRS complex); but exceptions may occur (pp. 121-122).

Another pattern sometimes seen in cases of *nontransmural* (non–Q wave) infarction is T wave inversions with or without ST segment depressions. Fig 9-7 shows a subendocardial infarction pattern with deep T wave inversions. (T wave inversions

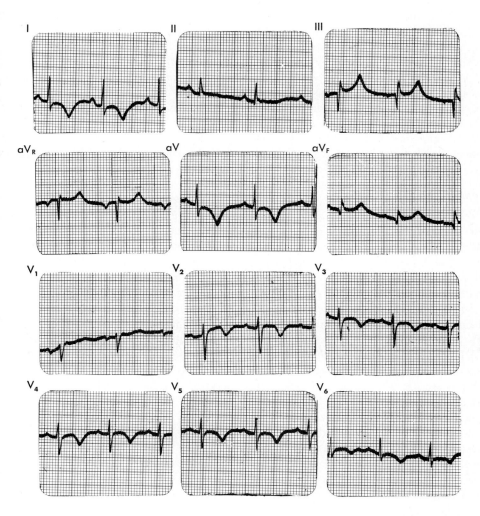

Fig. 9-7. Non–Q wave ("subendocardial") infarction. This patient complaining of chest pain had cardiac enzyme elevations. Notice the deep T wave inversions in leads I, aV$_L$, and V$_2$ to V$_6$. (Prominent Q waves in leads III and aV$_F$ represent an old inferior wall infarction.) Patients with acute infarcts may have deep ST segment depressions or T wave inversions without Q waves.

may also be seen in some cases of noninfarctional ischemia.)

To summarize: Subendocardial infarction can produce either (1) persistent ST depressions without Q waves or (2) T wave inversions without Q waves.

VARIETY OF ECG CHANGES SEEN WITH MYOCARDIAL ISCHEMIA

It should be apparent by now that myocardial ischemia can produce a wide variety of ECG changes. For example, transmural infarction (discussed earlier) causes abnormal Q waves as well as ST segment elevations followed by T wave inversions. Ventricular aneurysm may be associated with persistent ST segment elevations. Subendocardial ischemia (seen, for example, during an anginal attack or during a stress test) may produce transient ST depressions. Actual subendocardial infarction may lead to persistent ST depressions or to T wave inversions without Q waves.

ECG Changes Associated with Noninfarctional Ischemia

The foregoing paragraph does not mention all the possible ECG patterns seen with myocardial ischemia. We will briefly consider several others that may occur.

Myocardial ischemia does not always cause diagnostic ST-T changes. In some patients the ECG may remain entirely normal during episodes of ischemia. In others there may be only subtle changes in the ST-T complex. For example, you may see just a slight T wave flattening or minimal T wave inversions. These are *nonspecific ST-T changes*. (See also Chapter 10.)

Nonspecific ST-T changes may be abnormal, but they are not definite indicators of ischemia. They may be a sign of ischemic heart disease. However, they may also be caused by many other conditions, such as drug effects, hyperventilation, or electrolyte abnormalities. Therefore you should *not* make a definite diagnosis of myocardial ischemia solely on the basis of nonspecific ST-T changes.

To complete our discussion of noninfarctional ischemia, we will consider one other condition, *Prinzmetal's angina*. Recall that the ECG with classic or typical angina may show the pattern of subendocardial ischemia with ST segment depressions. However, a small but important group of patients will have an atypical form of angina (first reported by Dr. Myron Prinzmetal). Their angina is atypical because during episodes of chest pain they have ST segment elevations, a pattern described previously with acute transmural infarction. In these patients with Prinzmetal's angina the ST segment elevations are transient. Following the episode of chest pain the ST segments return to the baseline, without the characteristic evolving pattern of Q waves and T wave inversions seen with acute transmural MI. Thus Prinzmetal's angina is atypical because the ECG shows ST elevations rather than the ST depressions seen with typical angina.

Patients with Prinzmetal's angina are also atypical because their chest pain often occurs at rest or at night (in contrast to classic angina pectoris, which usually occurs with exertion or emotional stress). Prinzmetal's angina pattern is significant because it is a marker or coronary artery *spasm,* causing transient transmural ischemia. These episodes of spasm may occur in patients with otherwise normal coronary arteries. In other cases, spasm is associated with high-grade coronary obstruction (Fig. 9-8). Increasing evidence implicates cocaine as one cause of coronary spasm.

At this point we can summarize the diversity of ECG changes seen with ischemic heart disease—including Q waves, ST segment elevations or depressions, tall positive T waves or deep T wave inversions, nonspecific ST-T changes, and even a normal ECG (Fig. 9-9).

DIFFERENTIAL DIAGNOSIS OF ST ELEVATIONS AND ST DEPRESSIONS

ST elevations (current of injury pattern) are the earliest sign of acute transmural MI. Transient elevations, as mentioned, are also seen with Prinzmetal's angina. ST elevations persisting for several weeks after an acute MI may be a sign of a ventricular aneurysm.

However, not all ST segment elevations are in-

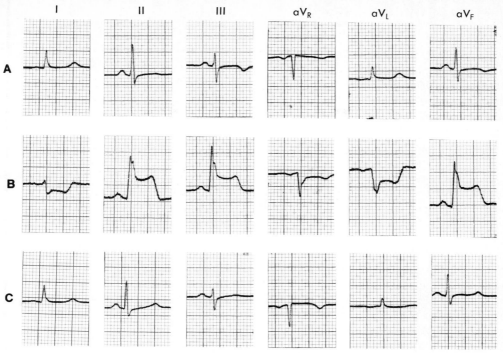

Fig. 9-8. Prinzmetal's (variant) angina with transient ST elevations. This patient, a 30-year-old man, had a history of exertional as well as rest angina. **A,** The baseline resting ECG shows nonspecific inferior lead ST-T changes. **B,** With chest pain, marked ST segment elevations occur in leads II, III, and aV_F and there are reciprocal ST depressions in leads I and aV_L. The rightward axis shift and slight widening of the QRS are consistent with left posterior hemiblock. **C,** Return of the ST segments to baseline after nitroglycerin administration. Cardiac catheterization in this case showed a severe right coronary obstruction with intermittent spasm producing total occlusion and transient ST elevations. (From Goldberger AL: Myocardial infarction: electrocardiographic differential diagnosis, ed 3, St Louis, 1984, The CV Mosby Co.)

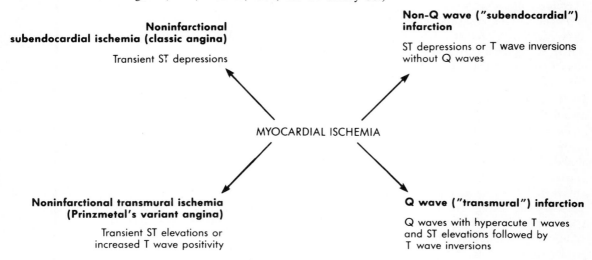

Fig. 9-9. Diversity of ECG changes with myocardial ischemia. T wave inversions may also occur with noninfarctional ischemia, and the ECG either be normal or show only nonspecific ST-T changes. (Adapted from Goldberger AL: Myocardial infarction: electrocardiographic differential diagnosis, ed 3, St Louis, 1984, The CV Mosby Co.)

dicators of ischemia. For example, *acute pericarditis* (p. 135) is associated with ST elevations. (The ECG changes with acute pericarditis are described in Chapter 10.) In other cases ST elevation may occur as a *normal variant* (Fig. 10-15). Many young adults have them, usually most prominent in the chest leads. This pattern of benign ST segment elevation is called the "early repolarization variant" (also described in Chapter 10). Finally, chronic ST elevations are often seen in leads V_1 and V_2 associated with the patterns of *left ventricular hypertrophy* and *left bundle branch block*.

Subendocardial ischemia with or without actual infarction is characterized by ST segment depression. However, not all the ST depressions you will see are indicative of subendocardial ischemia. For example, in Chapter 6 we discussed the left ventricular "strain" pattern often seen with *left ventricular hypertrophy*. As shown in Fig. 6-12, the ST segment may be slightly depressed with left ventricular strain. Another cause is an *acute transmural infarct*. Remember that acute anterior wall infarction may be associated with reciprocal ST depressions in one or more of leads II, III, and aV_F. Conversely, acute inferior wall infarction may be associated with reciprocal ST depressions in one or more of the anterior leads (I, aV_L, V_1 to V_6). Therefore, whenever you see ST depressions, it is important to look at all the leads and to evaluate these changes in context.

The ST segment may also be depressed by two other important factors (both described in Chapter 10). The first is *digitalis effect*. As shown in Fig. 10-1, digitalis may produce scooping of the ST-T complex with slight ST depression. The second factor is *hypokalemia*. As shown in Fig. 10-9, with a low serum potassium the ST segment may be slightly depressed. Prominent U waves may also appear. In some cases it may be difficult to sort out which factors are responsible for the ST depressions you are seeing. For example, a patient with left ventricular hypertrophy and "strain" may be taking digitalis and may also be having acute subendocardial ischemia.

DIFFERENTIAL DIAGNOSIS OF DEEP T WAVE INVERSIONS

Deep T wave inversions, as described previously, are seen during the evolving phase of transmural MI (Fig. 8-4, *B*) and also sometimes with non–Q wave (nontransmural or subendocardial) MI (Fig. 9-7). They are the result of a delay in regional repolarization produced by the ischemic injury.

However, just as not all ST segment elevations reflect ischemia, so not all deep T wave inversions are abnormal. For example, T wave inversions may be seen normally in leads with a *negative QRS complex* (such as aV_R). The T wave may be normally inverted in lead V_1 and sometimes in lead V_2 in adults. Furthermore, as mentioned earlier (p. 45, footnote), some adults have a persistent *juvenile T wave inversion pattern* with inverted T waves in the right and middle chest leads (V_1 to V_3).

Not all abnormal T wave inversions are caused by myocardial infarction. T wave inversions in the right chest leads may be caused by right ventricular strain (Fig. 10-16) and in the left chest leads by left ventricular strain (Fig. 6-10). Diffusely inverted T waves are seen during the evolving phase of pericarditis. Very deep widely splayed T wave inversions (with a long QT interval and sometimes prominent U waves) have been described in some patients with cerebrovascular accident, particularly subarachnoid hemorrhage (*CVA T wave pattern*) (Fig. 9-10). The cause of these marked repolarization changes with some types of cerebrovascular injury is not certain, but it probably reflects changes in the autonomic nervous system. As described in Chapter 7, secondary T wave inversions (resulting from abnormal depolarization) are seen in the right chest leads with RBBB and in the left chest leads with LBBB. Deep T wave inversions have also been reported following bouts of tachycardia (posttachycardia T wave syndrome) and after electronic ventricular pacing (post-pacemaker T wave pattern). Patients with the mitral valve prolapse syndrome may have inverted T waves in the inferolateral leads (II, III, aV_F, V_5, and V_6).

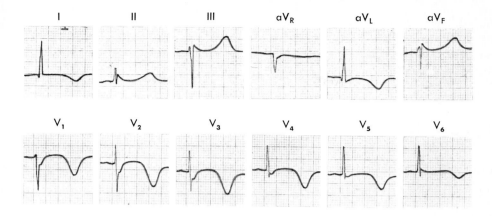

Fig. 9-10. Acute subarachnoid hemorrhage with giant T wave inversions. Subarachnoid hemorrhage may cause deeply inverted T waves, usually with markedly prolonged QT intervals, simulating the pattern seen in MI. (From Goldberger AL: Myocardial infarction: electrocardiographic differential diagnosis, ed 3, St Louis, 1984, The CV Mosby Co.)

This list of noninfarctional factors causing deep T wave inversions is by no means complete, but it should convey the point that *T wave inversions are not always indicative of myocardial ischemia*. For a more complete discussion of the differential diagnosis of the ST-T changes of myocardial infarction, readers are referred to the Bibliography.

COMPLICATIONS OF MI

Up to now we have considered just the diagnosis of MI from the ECG and also the differential diagnosis of these patterns. We will conclude with a brief review of the major complications of MI.

The complications can be divided into two groups: (1) mechanical and (2) electrical. The *mechanical* complications include heart failure, cardiogenic shock, left ventricular aneurysm, rupture of the heart, pericarditis, papillary muscle dysfunction, infarct extension and expansion, and embolism. (Diagnosis of these problems lies outside the scope of this book.) The *electrical* complications include the arrhythmias and conduction disturbances seen as a consequence of myocardial ischemia. MI can lead to virtually any arrhythmia. (The general subject of arrhythmias is discussed in Part II of this book.) The conduction disturbances include AV block (heart block) and intraventricular block (bundle branch block). (The conduction disturbances are discussed in Chapters 7 and 15.)

THE ECG IN MI: A CLINICAL PERSPECTIVE

One final note of caution should be made. The ECG is a reasonably sensitive, but hardly perfect, indicator of acute MI. Most patients with an acute MI will show the ECG changes described in Chapters 8 and 9. However, particularly during the early minutes or hours after an infarct, the ECG may be relatively nondiagnostic or even normal. Furthermore, as mentioned, an LBBB pattern may completely mask the changes of an acute infarct. Therefore the ECG must always be considered in clinical perspective and the diagnosis of myocardial ischemia or infarction not be dismissed simply because the ECG does not show the classic changes.

It should also be emphasized that the distinction between transmural and subendocardial (nontransmural) MIs on the basis of the ECG findings is an oversimplification. In some cases extensive infarction may occur without Q waves while in others nontransmural injury may occur with Q waves. Furthermore, current evidence suggests that "subendocardial'' infarction may have as ominous a long-term prognosis as ''transmural'' infarction. For these reasons a number of authorities have suggested that electrocardiographers abandon the terms ''transmural'' and ''subendocardial'' and instead use ''Q wave'' and ''non–Q wave'' when describing an infarction.

REVIEW

Subendocardial ischemia generally produces ST segment depressions, which may appear only in the anterior leads (I, aV_L, and V_1 to V_6) or only in the inferior leads (II, III, and aV_F) or may appear diffusely in both groups of leads. (Lead aV_R often shows ST segment elevation.)

These ischemic ST segment depressions may be seen during attacks of typical angina pectoris. Similar ST segment depressions may develop during exercise (with or without chest pain) in people with ischemic heart disease. Recording the ECG during exercise (stress electrocardiography) is a method of determining the presence of ischemic heart disease. ST segment depression of 1 mm or more, lasting 0.08 second or more, is generally considered a *positive* (abnormal) response. However, *false-negative* (normal) results can occur in patients with ischemic heart disease and *false-positive* results can occur in normal people.

Ischemic ST segment changes may also be detected during ambulatory ECG (Holter) monitoring. Analysis of these records has shown that many episodes of myocardial ischemia are not associated with angina pectoris (''silent ischemia'').

With *subendocardial (non–Q wave) infarction* the ECG may show persistent ST segment depressions. Another pattern sometimes seen with subendocardial (nontransmural) infarction is deep T wave inversions with or without ST segment depressions. Abnormal Q waves *do not* usually occur with subendocardial infarction.

Prinzmetal's angina occurs in patients with transient ST segment elevations, suggestive of epicardial or transmural ischemia, during attacks of angina. These patients often have atypical chest pain, which occurs at rest or at night, in contrast to classic angina, which is typically exertional and is associated with ST segment depressions. Prinzmetal's (variant) angina pattern is generally a marker of coronary artery spasm with or without underlying coronary obstructions.

The ST segment elevations of acute transmural MI can be simulated by the ST elevations of Prinzmetal's angina as well as by the normal variant ST elevations seen in some healthy people (''early repolarization pattern'') and by the ST elevations of acute pericarditis.

The abnormal ST depressions of subendocardial ischemia or infarction may be simulated by the pattern of left ventricular strain, digitalis effect (Chapter 10), or hypokalemia (Chapter 10).

T wave inversions can be a sign of ischemia or infarction but may also occur in a variety of other settings (including normal variant, ventricular hypertrophy [''strain'' pattern], pericarditis, subarachnoid hemorrhage, and secondary ST-T changes from bundle branch block).

Questions—Chapters 8 and 9

1. Answer these questions about the ECG below:
   a. What is the approximate heart rate?
   b. Are there any ST segment elevations?
   c. Are there any abnormal Q waves?
   d. What is the diagnosis?

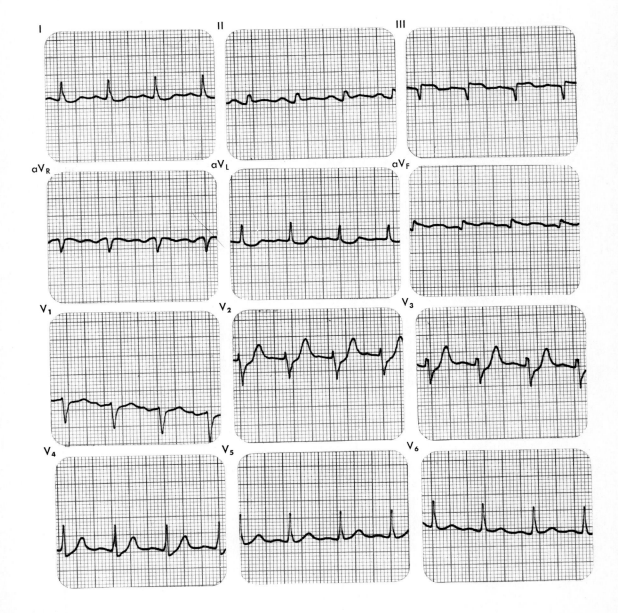

2. Answer these questions about the following ECG:
    a. What is the approximate mean QRS axis?
    b. Is the R wave progression in the chest leads normal?
    c. Are the T waves normal?
    d. What is the diagnosis?

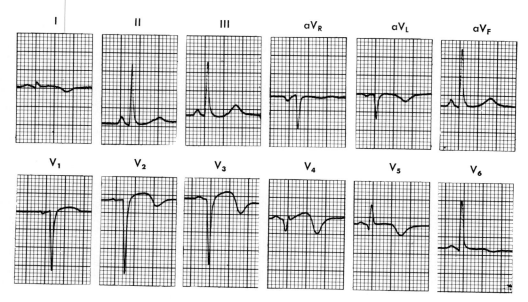

3. With an acute *transmural anterior* wall infarction, the ST segments in leads II, III, and aV_F are likely to be _____.

4. Persistent ST elevations several weeks or more after an infarct may be a sign of _____
    _____.

5. A patient with severe chest pain has persistent diffuse ST segment depressions with abnormal elevations of cardiac enzymes. The most likely diagnosis is
    a. Prinzmetal's angina
    b. Non–Q wave (subendocardial) infarction
    c. Hyperacute infarction
    d. Angina pectoris

6. What ECG abnormality is shown and of what symptom might this patient have been complaining?

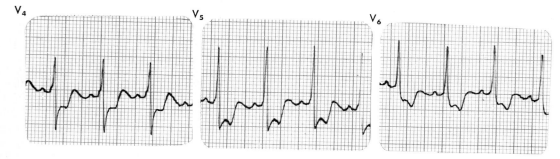

7. Does this ECG tracing show evidence of a previous MI?

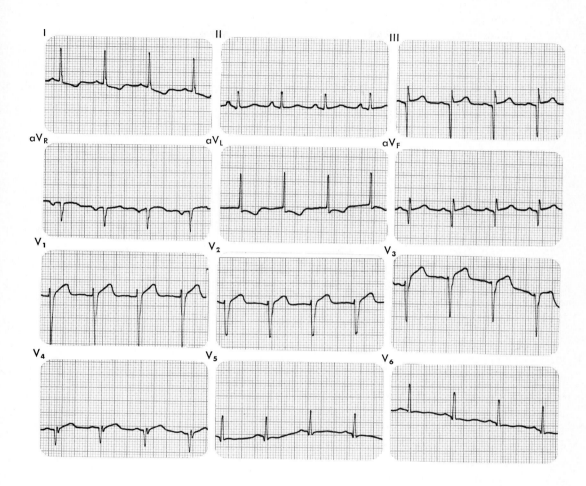

Answers

1. a. 100 beats/min.
   b. Yes. Leads II, III, and aV_F (with reciprocal ST depressions in leads V_2 to V_4, I, and aV_L).
   c. Yes. Best seen in leads III and aV_F.
   d. Acute inferior wall infarction.
2. a. About $+90°$. (Between $80°$ and $90°$ is acceptable.)
   b. No.
   c. No. Notice the inverted T waves in leads V_2 to V_6, I, and aV_L.
   d. (Evolving) anterior wall infarction.
3. Reciprocally depressed.
4. Ventricular aneurysm.
5. b.
6. Marked ST segment depressions. This patient had severe ischemic chest pain with a non–Q wave "subendocardial" infarct.
7. Yes. There is evidence of anterior wall infarction, with loss of R wave progression in the chest leads. There is also evidence of inferior wall infarction, with large Q waves in leads III and aV_F. In addition, note the tall R wave in lead aV_L (14 mm) with a "strain" pattern in leads I and aV_L. This patient had a history of hypertension, producing left ventricular hypertrophy.

10

Miscellaneous ECG Patterns

This chapter presents an electrocardiographic potpourri—a discussion a number of ECG patterns that have not been covered in detail to this point. We will briefly discuss drug effects, electrolyte disturbances, pericardial disease, early repolarization, pulmonary embolism, Wolff-Parkinson-White syndrome, and several other miscellaneous ECG patterns.

DRUG EFFECTS

Numerous drugs can affect the ECG. Generally the changes produced are slight and nonspecific. However, several commonly used drugs produce distinctive ECG changes. We will consider the patterns seen with digitalis, quinidine and related agents, and the psychotropics.

Digitalis is used to treat heart failure and certain arrhythmias and is a most frequently employed drug. One of its effects is to shorten repolarization time in the ventricles. This shortens the QT interval. Digitalis also often produces a characteristic scooping of the ST-T complex, as shown in Figs. 10-1 and 10-2, called *digitalis effect*. Notice that when digitalis effect occurs the ST segment and T wave are fused together and it is impossible to tell where one ends and the other begins. Digitalis effect can be seen in any patient taking therapeutic or toxic doses of a digitalis preparation (for example, digoxin or digitoxin). Digitalis *effect* must be distinguished from digitalis *toxicity* (Chapter 16), which involves arrhythmias, conduction disturbances, and systemic side effects produced by excessive amounts of digitalis.

Quinidine, procainamide, and disopyramide are antiarrhythmic drugs with similar properties. They may be useful in the therapy of ventricular or atrial arrhythmias. In contrast to digitalis, they prolong ventricular repolarization. Therefore they may prolong the QT interval and flatten the T wave. In toxic doses they may also prolong ventricular depolarization, leading to a widening of the QRS complexes. Occasionally these agents will produce prominent U waves resembling those seen with hypokalemia (p. 133).

Quinidine, a drug used to treat atrial or ventricular arrhythmias, may in selected cases actually cause fainting or even sudden death as a result of ventricular tachycardia *(quinidine syncope)*. This paradoxical effect is most likely to occur with very long QT intervals and prominent U waves (Fig.

DIGITALIS EFFECT

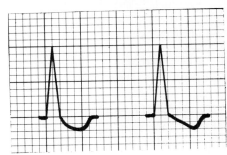

Fig. 10-1. Notice the characteristic scooping of the ST-T complex produced by digitalis. Not all patients taking digitalis exhibit these changes, however.

DIGITALIS EFFECT

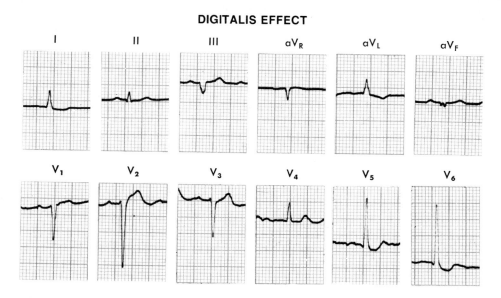

Fig. 10-2. Notice the characteristic scooping of the ST-T complex, best seen in leads V_5 and V_6. Low voltage is also present, with a total QRS amplitude of 5 mm or less in all six extremity leads.

QUINIDINE EFFECTS AND EARLY TOXICITY

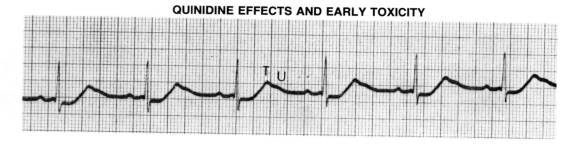

Fig. 10-3. Lead V_6. Quinidine blood level 2.9 μg/ml (therapeutic range). Notice the prolonged repolarization with prominent U waves, similar to the pattern of hypokalemia. Some patients in whom quinidine causes marked repolarization prolongation (often with large U waves) may be at increased risk of ventricular tachycardia (torsade de pointes, Chapter 14). This patient did, in fact, subsequently develop torsade de pointes. (From Goldberger E: Textbook of clinical cardiology, St Louis, 1982, The CV Mosby Co.)

10-3). The dispersion of repolarization in such cases may allow for "reentrant" (p. 143) ventricular arrhythmias, in particular, *torsade de pointes,* a potentially lethal complication that can occur in patients taking therapeutic doses. (See also Chapter 14.)

Psychotropic drugs (for example, the phenothi-azines and tricyclic antidepressants) can markedly alter the ECG and, in toxic doses, induce a fatal ventricular tachyarrhythmia or asystole. They may also prolong the QRS, causing a bundle branch block–like pattern, or lengthen repolarization (long Q-T-U intervals), predisposing to torsade de pointes (p. 191). Fig. 10-4 presents the typical findings, in

TRICYCLIC OVERDOSE

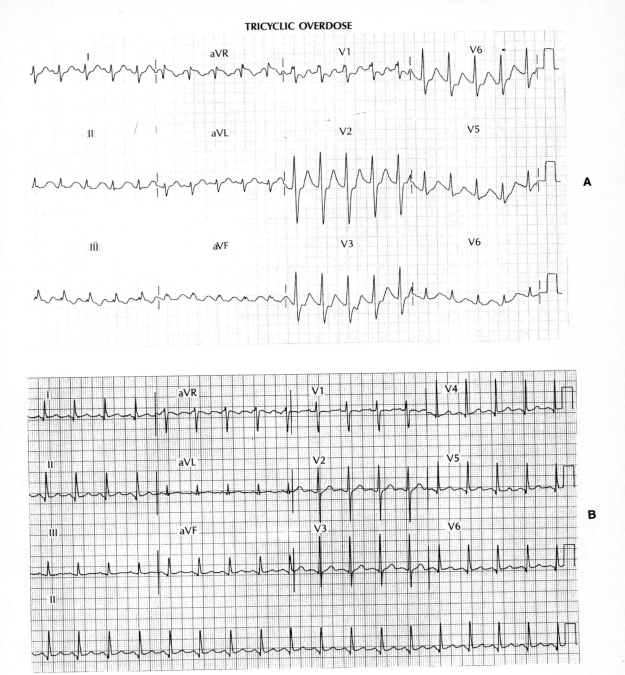

Fig. 10-4. A, The ECG from a patient with tricyclic antidepressant overdose shows three major findings: sinus tachycardia (from anticholinergic and adrenergic effects), prolongation of the QRS (from slowed conduction), and prolongation of the QT (from delayed repolarization). **B,** A repeat ECG 4 days later shows persistent sinus tachycardia but normalization of the QRS and QT.

EFFECTS OF HYPERKALEMIA

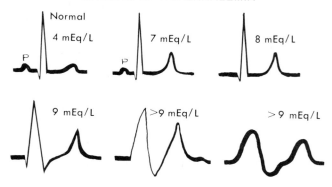

Fig. 10-5. The earliest change with hyperkalemia is peaking (''tenting'') of the T wave. With progressive increases in serum potassium, the QRS complexes widen, P waves disappear, and, finally, a ''sine-wave'' pattern leads to asystole (Fig. 10-8). These changes do not necessarily occur with a specific serum K^+ level. For example, some patients can have a normal ECG with a K^+ of 7 mEq/L whereas others will have cardiac arrest at 9 mEq/L or less.

this case from a young adult who took an overdose of tricyclic antidepressant. Notice the prolonged QRS and QT intervals, along with a sinus tachycardia.

ELECTROLYTE DISTURBANCES

Abnormal serum concentrations of potassium and calcium can produce marked effects on the ECG. Hyperkalemia can, in fact, be lethal because of its cardiac toxicity.

Hyperkalemia

Hyperkalemia produces a distinctive sequence of ECG changes affecting both depolarization (QRS) and repolarization (ST-T). The normal serum potassium concentration is between 3.5 and 5.0 mEq/L. The first change seen with abnormal elevation of the serum potassium concentration is narrowing and peaking of the T wave. As shown in Figs. 10-5 and 10-6, the T wave with hyperkalemia has a characteristic ''tented'' shape and may be-

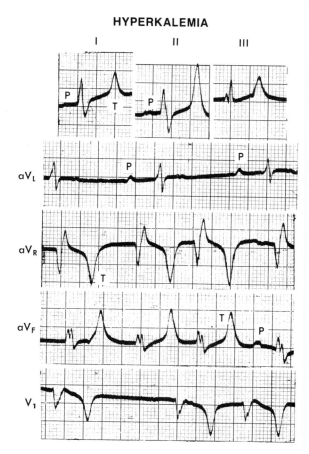

HYPERKALEMIA

Fig. 10-6. Notice the peaked T waves, widened QRS complexes, and prolonged PR intervals. Intermittently a junctional rhythm is present with no P waves.

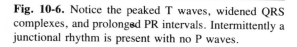

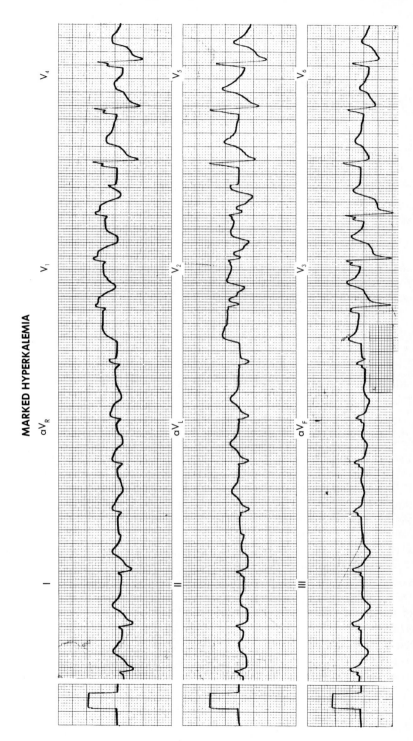

Fig. 10-7. In this patient the K$^+$ concentration was 8.5 mEq/L. Notice the absence of P waves and the bizarre wide QRS complexes.

SEVERE POTASSIUM TOXICITY
LEAD I

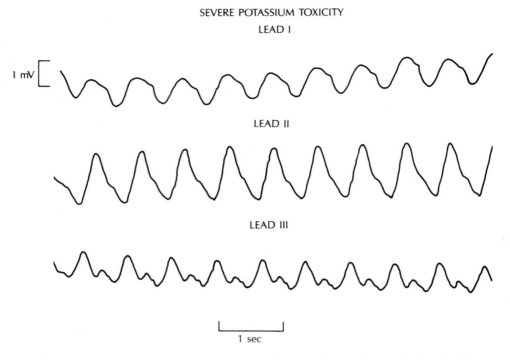

Fig. 10-8. Marked elevations of the serum potassium may slow cardiac conduction, leading to a "sine-wave" pattern and ultimately to cardiac arrest. Compare with Fig. 10-5.

come quite tall. With further elevation of the serum potassium, the PR interval becomes prolonged and the P waves become smaller and may disappear entirely. Continued elevations produce an intra-ventricular conduction delay, with widening of the QRS (Fig. 10-7). As the concentration rises fur-ther, the QRS continues to widen, leading to a large undulating ("sine-wave") pattern (Fig. 10-8) and eventual asystole. The sequence of changes seen on the ECG with progressive hyperkalemia is out-lined in Fig. 10-5. Because hyperkalemia may be fatal, recognition of the earliest signs of T wave peaking may prove lifesaving (Fig. 10-6). Hyper-kalemia can be seen in several clinical settings. The most common is kidney failure, in which there is reduced excretion of potassium.

Hypokalemia

Hypokalemia also produces distinctive changes in the ST-T complex. The most common pattern

seen is ST segment depression with prominent U waves and prolonged repolarization* (Figs. 10-9 and 10-10). With hypokalemia the U waves typi-cally become enlarged and may even exceed the height of the T waves. Hypokalemia can be caused by several factors. The most common are (1) uri-nary potassium losses resulting from diuretic ther-apy and (2) potassium losses associated with metabolic alkalosis from vomiting or gastric suc-tion.

Hypercalcemia and Hypocalcemia

Hypercalcemia shortens, and hypocalcemia lengthens, ventricular repolarization (Fig. 10-11).
Hypercalcemia causes shortening of the QT in-

---

*Technically the QT interval with hypokalemia may remain normal while repolarization is prolonged (as shown by the prom-inent U waves). However, the T wave and U wave often merge, so the QT interval cannot always be accurately measured.

HYPOKALEMIA

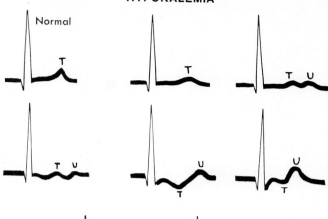

Fig. 10-9. Variable ECG patterns may be seen with hypokalemia, ranging from slight T wave flattening to the appearance of prominent U waves, sometimes with ST depressions or T wave inversions. These patterns are not directly related to the specific level of serum potassium.

HYPOKALEMIA

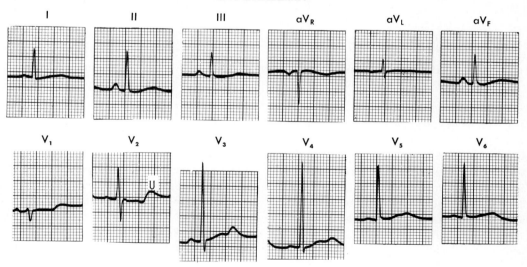

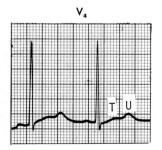

Fig. 10-10. The serum K^+ was 2.2 mEq/L. Notice the prominent U waves.

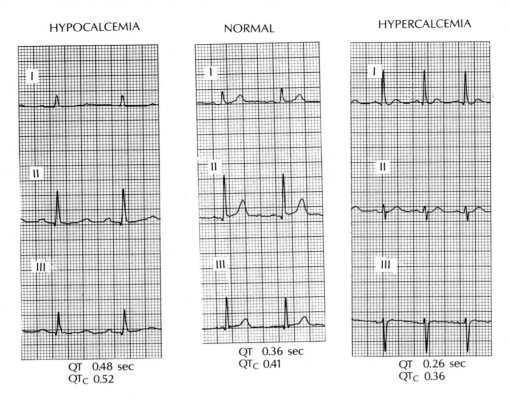

Fig. 10-11. Hypocalcemia prolongs the QT interval by stretching out the ST segment. Hypercalcemia curtails the QT by shortening the ST segment.

terval. It may be life threatening at high levels and lead to coma and death. A short QT interval in a comatose patient is sometimes the first clue to the diagnosis of hypercalcemia. Hypercalcemia may be caused by numerous factors, including malignant tumors (especially breast and lung), multiple myeloma, hyperparathyroidism, and excessive amounts of vitamin D.

Hypocalcemia lengthens or prolongs the QT interval. Common causes include intestinal malabsorption, pancreatitis, kidney failure, and hypoparathyroidism.

PERICARDITIS AND PERICARDIAL EFFUSION

Pericarditis (inflammation of the pericardium) may be caused by a number of factors—including viral or bacterial infection, metastatic tumors, collagen vascular diseases, myocardial infarction, and uremia.

As mentioned in Chapter 8, the ECG patterns

of pericarditis resemble those seen with acute myocardial infarction. The early phase of acute pericarditis is characterized by ST segment elevations. This is a current of injury pattern resulting from the inflammation of the heart's surface (epicardium) that often accompanies pericardial inflammation. Fig. 10-12 shows an example of the ST segment elevations with acute pericarditis. The major difference between these and the ones occurring with myocardial infarction is their distribution. The ST segment elevations with acute myocardial infarction are characteristically limited to either the anterior leads or the inferior leads because of the localized area of the infarct. The pericardium envelops the heart, and the ST-T changes occurring with pericarditis are therefore more generalized. ST elevations may be seen in both anterior and inferior leads. For example, in Fig. 10-12 notice the elevations in leads I, II, aV_L, aV_F, and V_2 to V_6.

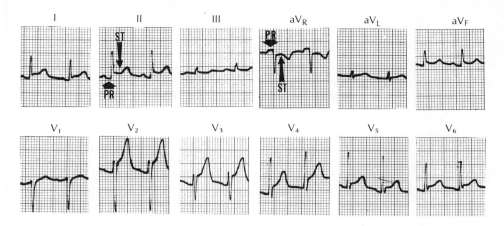

Fig. 10-12. Acute pericarditis causing diffuse ST segment elevations in leads I, II, aV$_F$, and V$_2$ to V$_6$, with reciprocal ST depression in aV$_R$. By contrast, an atrial current of injury causes PR segment elevation in lead aV$_R$ with reciprocal PR depression in the left chest leads and lead II. (From Goldberger AL: Myocardial infarction: electrocardiographic differential diagnosis, ed 3, St Louis, 1984, The CV Mosby Co.)

Not only does acute pericarditis affect ventricular repolarization (the ST segment), it also affects repolarization of the atria, which starts during the PR segment (end of the P wave to beginning of the QRS). In particular, pericardial inflammation often causes an atrial current of injury, reflected by elevation of the PR in lead aV$_R$ and depression of the PR in other limb leads and the left chest leads (V$_5$ and V$_6$). Thus with acute pericarditis the PR and ST segments typically point in opposite directions—the PR being elevated (often by only 1 mm or so) in aV$_R$, the ST being usually slightly depressed in that lead. Other leads may show PR depression and ST elevation.*

Fig. 10-12 illustrates these subtle but often helpful repolarization changes seen with acute pericarditis. The presence of PR changes may be a useful clue in the differential diagnosis of ST segment elevation, suggesting acute pericarditis as the cause.

The ST elevations seen with acute pericarditis are sometimes followed (after a variable time) by T wave inversions (Fig. 10-13). This sequence of elevations and inversions is the same as that described with myocardial infarction. In some cases the T wave inversions caused by pericarditis will resolve completely with time and the ECG will return to normal. In other cases they may persist for long periods.

We have concentrated on the similarity between the ECG patterns of acute pericarditis and acute myocardial infarction because both may produce ST segment elevations followed by T wave inversions. However, the ST-T changes with pericarditis, as noted, tend to be more diffuse than the localized changes of myocardial infarction. Another major difference is that pericarditis does not produce abnormal Q waves, such as those seen with transmural infarction. With transmural MI the abnormal Q waves occur because of the death of heart muscle and the consequent loss of positive depolarization voltages. (See Chapter 8.) Pericarditis, on the other hand, generally causes only a superficial inflammation and does not produce transmural myocardial necrosis. Thus abnormal Q waves never result from pericarditis alone.

Pericardial effusion refers to an abnormal accumulation of fluid in the pericardial sac. In most cases this fluid accumulates as the result of peri-

---

*This constitutes an exception to the earlier statement (p. 18) that repolarization of the atria generally is not recorded on the ECG.

PERICARDITIS, EVOLVING PATTERN

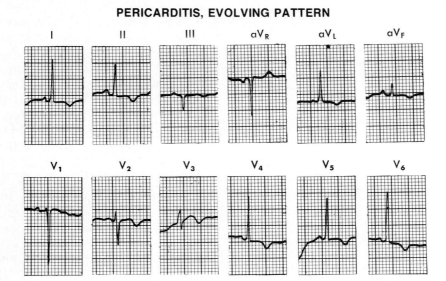

Fig. 10-13. Notice the diffuse T wave inversions in leads I, II, III, aV_L, aV_F, and V_2 to V_6.

carditis. In some cases, however, such as myxedema (hypothyroidism) or rupture of the heart, pericardial effusion may occur in the absence of pericarditis. The major clinical significance of pericardial effusion is the danger of cardiac tamponade, in which the fluid actually "chokes off" the heart, leading to a drop in blood pressure and sometimes to cardiac arrest. (See Chapter 17.)

The most common ECG sign of pericardial effusion (with or without actual tamponade) is low voltage of the QRS complexes. In such cases the low voltage is probably due to short-circuiting of cardiac voltages by the fluid surrounding the heart.

In our discussion of hypertrophy patterns (Chapter 6), the criteria for high voltage were mentioned. *Low voltage* is said to be present when the total amplitude of the QRS complexes in each of the six limb leads is 5 mm (0.5 mV) or less.* Fig. 10-2 shows an example of low voltage.

Following is a list of the major factors that can lead to low voltage complexes:

1. Obesity
2. Emphysema
3. Pericardial effusion
4. Hypothyroidism
5. Diffuse myocardial injury (for example, extensive myocardial infarction or myocardial fibrosis)
6. Infiltration of the heart muscle (for example, amyloidosis)
7. Normal variant

Obesity can cause low voltage because of the fat tissue that lies between the heart and the chest wall. In patients with emphysema there is increased inflation of the lungs. This extra air acts to insulate the heart. Of the causes of low voltage listed, obesity and emphysema are among the most common. However, when you see low voltage (particularly with sinus tachycardia), pericardial effusion should always be high on your list because it can lead to fatal tamponade (p. 191).

Myxedema (hypothyroidism), as noted, may cause a pericardial effusion without actual peri-

*Low voltage in the limb leads may or may not be accompanied by low voltage in the chest leads (defined as a total QRS amplitude of 10 mm or less in V_1 to V_6).

**ELECTRICAL ALTERNANS IN
PERICARDIAL TAMPONADE**

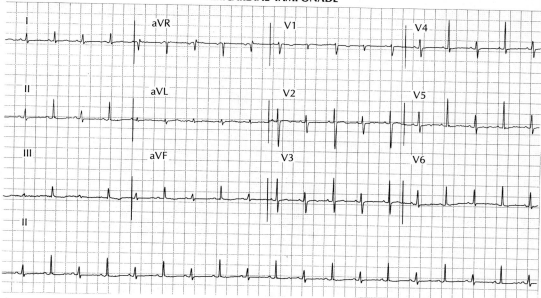

Fig. 10-14. In patients with pericardial effusion and cardiac tamponade, electrical alternans may develop. Notice the beat-to-beat alternation in the P-QRS-T axis caused by swinging of the heart in a large pericardial effusion. Relatively low QRS voltage and sinus tachycardia are also present.

carditis. Hypothyroidism also generally causes sinus bradycardia (Chapter 11). Therefore the combination of low voltage and sinus bradycardia should suggest the possible diagnosis of myxedema.

Electrical alternans is another pattern that can occur with pericardial effusion and tamponade (Fig. 10-14). It is characterized by a beat-to-beat shift in the QRS axis associated with mechanical swinging of the heart to-and-fro in a large accumulation of fluid. It is virtually pathognomonic of cardiac tamponade, although *not* every patient with tamponade will manifest this pattern.

To summarize: Pericarditis causes a diffuse current of injury pattern with ST segment elevations in the anterior and inferior leads, followed by T wave inversions in these leads. Abnormal Q waves, however, are not seen with pericarditis alone. Pericardial effusion is one of the causes of low voltage on the ECG.

EARLY REPOLARIZATION VARIANT

Recall, from Chapter 4, that the normal ST segment is isoelectric, riding along the baseline and gradually rising into the T wave (see Fig. 2-10). Although slight deviations (generally of less than 1 mm) may be seen in normal people, more marked ST elevations may signify an abnormal condition (such as myocardial infarction, Prinzmetal's angina, ventricular aneurysm, or pericarditis).

In Fig. 10-15, from a *normal* young adult, notice the marked elevation of the ST segments. This is a benign variant known as the *early repolarization pattern*. With early repolarization the ST segments in the chest leads may rise to 3 mm above the baseline. Although most common in young people, such elevations can also occur in older persons, simulating the pattern seen with acute pericarditis or MI. However, they are stable and do not undergo the evolutionary sequence seen with acute pericar-

EARLY REPOLARIZATION

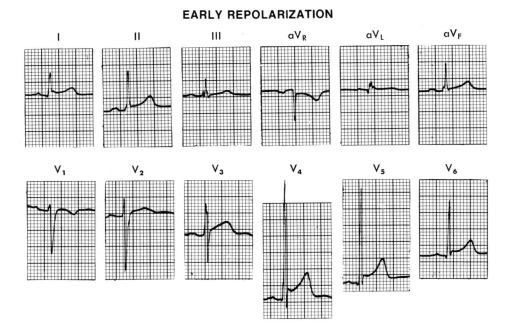

Fig. 10-15. ST segment elevation, usually most marked in the chest leads, is sometimes seen as a normal variant. This "early repolarization" pattern may be confused with ST segment elevations of acute myocardial infarction or pericarditis.

ACUTE PULMONARY EMBOLISM

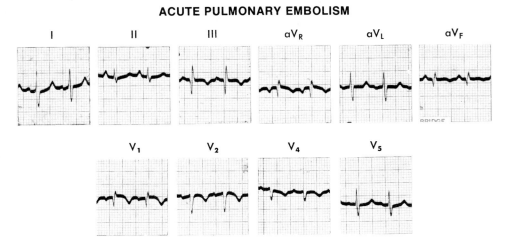

Fig. 10-16. Several features occasionally seen with pulmonary embolism are sinus tachycardia, S waves in lead I with Q waves and T wave inversions in lead III ($S_IQ_{III}T_{III}$ pattern), and poor R wave progression with T wave inversions (right ventricular "strain") in chest leads V_1 to V_4 resulting from acute right ventricular overload.

ditis; and they are not associated with reciprocal ST depressions (except in lead aV_R), contrary to what is observed with acute MI.

PULMONARY EMBOLISM

The ECG is not a sensitive test for pulmonary embolism. In some cases the obstruction produced by an embolus in the pulmonary artery system can lead to ECG changes, but generally there is no single pattern that is always diagnostic. The following may all be seen (Fig. 10-16):

1. An RBBB pattern (wide rSR' in lead V_1)
2. A right ventricular "strain" pattern (inverted T waves in leads V_1 to V_4)
3. The so-called $S_IQ_{III}T_{III}$ pattern (an S wave in lead I and a new Q wave in lead III with T wave inversion in that lead) (This pattern, which may simulate that produced by acute inferior wall MI, is probably due to acute right ventricular dilation.)

4. Shifting of the QRS axis to the right
5. ST segment depressions indicative of subendocardial ischemia
6. Sinus tachycardia (Other arrhythmias also occur, such as ventricular ectopy and atrial fibrillation.)

The appearance of these changes, particularly in combination, is suggestive but not diagnostic of pulmonary embolism. Many patients with massive pulmonary emboli will have only minor, relatively nonspecific, changes on their ECG. Thus both the diagnostic sensitivity and the specificity of the ECG with pulmonary embolism are limited. Fig. 10-16 shows a classic example of the changes seen with pulmonary embolism.

CHRONIC LUNG DISEASE (EMPHYSEMA)

Patients with chronic lung disease from emphysema often have a relatively characteristic combination of ECG findings (Fig. 10-17)—including

CHRONIC LUNG DISEASE

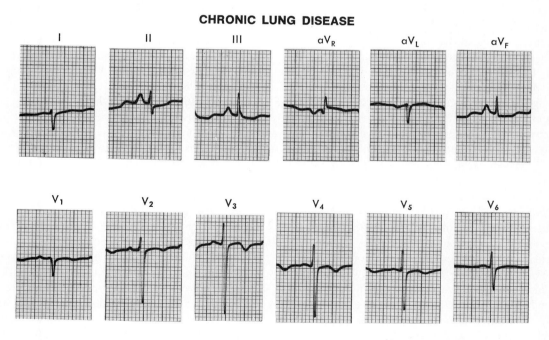

Fig. 10-17. Notice the characteristic relatively low voltages in the limb leads, right axis deviation, P pulmonale, and poor R wave progression. T wave inversions (V_1 to V_5) are due to right ventricular "strain."

(1) low voltage, (2) poor R wave progression in the chest leads, and (3) a vertical or rightward QRS axis in the frontal plane. Excessive pulmonary air trapping causes the low voltage. The poor R wave progression results, in part, from the downward displacement of the diaphragm; thus the chest leads are actually placed *relatively* higher than usual. In addition, right ventricular dilation may contribute to the delayed chest lead transition zone. Finally, the anatomically vertical position of the heart in the chest of a patient with emphysema, and sometimes right ventricular enlargement, causes the mean QRS axis to be vertical or even rightward (greater than + 100°). P pulmonale (Fig. 10-17) may also be present.

CONGESTIVE HEART FAILURE

Congestive heart failure (CHF) is a complex syndrome that may result from multiple causes—including ischemic heart disease, systemic hypertension, valvular heart disease, and cardiomyopathy. The ECG may provide helpful clues to a specific diagnosis in some of these patients. For example, prominent Q waves and typical ST-T changes suggest underlying ischemic heart disease. Left ventricular hypertrophy patterns (Chapter 6) may be seen with hypertensive heart disease, aortic valve disease (stenosis or regurgitation), or mitral regurgitation. The combination of left atrial enlargement (or atrial fibrillation) and signs of right ventricular hypertrophy should suggest mitral stenosis (Fig. 19-1). Left bundle branch block (Chapter 7) may be seen with congestive heart failure caused by ischemic heart disease, valvular abnormalities, hypertension, or cardiomyopathy.

In some patients marked enlargement and decreased function of the left (and often the right) ventricle occur without coronary artery disease, hypertension, or significant valvular lesions. The term *"dilated (congestive) cardiomyopathy"* is applied in such cases. Dilated cardiomyopathy can be idiopathic or associated with chronic excessive alcohol ingestion (alcoholic cardiomyopathy), viral infection, or some other etiology.

Patients with dilated cardiomyopathy from any cause may have a distinctive ECG pattern (the *ECG-CHF* triad) characterized by

1. Relatively low limb lead voltages (such that the QRS in each of the six limb leads $\leq$ 8 mm in amplitude)
2. Relatively prominent precordial lead QRS voltages (such that the sum of the S wave in either lead V_1 or lead V_2 plus the R wave in V_5 or $V_6 \geq$ 35 mm)
3. Poor R wave progression defined by a QS- or rS-type complex in leads V_1 to V_4

When this triad is present (Fig. 10-18), it strongly suggests underlying cardiomyopathy but does not indicate a specific etiology. It may occur not only with primary dilated cardiomyopathy but also with severe heart disease due to previous infarcts or significant valvular dysfunction. Furthermore, it is of only modest sensitivity; that is, its absence does not exclude underlying cardiomyopathy.

WOLFF-PARKINSON-WHITE SYNDROME

The Wolff-Parkinson-White (WPW) syndrome is an unusual and distinctive ECG abnormality caused by preexcitation of the ventricles. Normally the electrical stimulus passes to the ventricles from the atria via the AV junction. The physiologic lag of conduction through the AV junction results in the normal PR interval of 0.12 to 0.2 second. Imagine the consequences of having an accessory conduction pathway between the atria and ventricles that would *bypass* the AV junction and *preexcite* the ventricles. This is exactly what occurs with the WPW syndrome: an accessory conduction fiber (the bundle of Kent) connects the atria and ventricles, bypassing the AV junction (Fig. 10-19).

Preexcitation of the ventricles with the WPW syndrome produces the following three characteristic changes on the ECG (Fig. 10-20):

1. The QRS is widened, giving the superficial appearance of a bundle branch block pattern. The wide QRS is caused not by a delay in ventricular depolarization but by early stimulation of the ventricles. (The QRS will be widened to the degree that the PR is shortened.)

ECG-CHF TRIAD

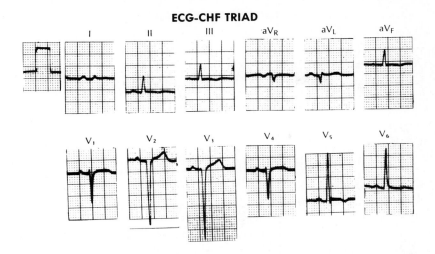

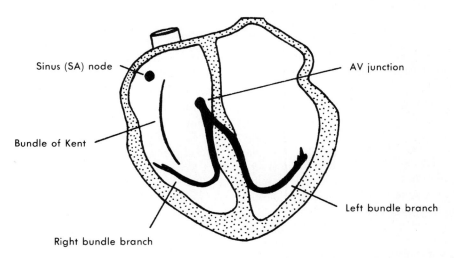

Fig. 10-18. Severe idiopathic dilated cardiomyopathy in a 29-year-old man. Poor precordial R wave progression simulates anterior wall infarction. The triad of relatively low limb lead QRS voltages, prominent precordial QRS voltages, and poor R wave progression in the chest leads is highly specific for dilated cardiomyopathy. (From Goldberger AL: Myocardial infarction: electrocardiographic differential diagnosis, ed 3, St Louis, 1984, The CV Mosby Co.)

Fig. 10-19. Anatomy of the preexcitation syndrome (Wolff-Parkinson-White) pattern. In a small percentage of the population an accessory fiber (bundle of Kent) connects the atria and ventricles. The consequences of this extra conduction path are discussed in the text.

WOLFF-PARKINSON-WHITE PATTERN

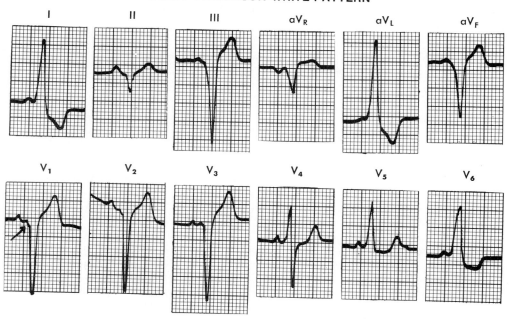

Fig. 10-20. Notice the characteristic triad of the WPW (type B) pattern: wide QRS complexes, short PR intervals, and a delta wave (*arrow* in lead V₁). The Q waves in leads II, III, and aV_F result from abnormal ventricular conduction rather than from inferior myocardial infarction.

2. The PR is shortened (often but not always <0.12 sec) because of ventricular preexcitation.

3. There is slurring, or notching, of the upstroke of the QRS complex. This is called a *delta* wave.

Fig. 10-20 shows the WPW pattern, with its classic triad of a widened QRS, a short PR interval, and a delta wave. It superficially resembles a bundle branch block pattern because of the widened QRS complexes. Depending on which area of the ventricles is preexcited first, the ECG will show a pattern resembling that of either a right bundle branch block with tall R waves in the right chest leads (type A pattern) or a left bundle branch block with a predominantly negative QS in lead V₁ (type B pattern).

The significance of the WPW syndrome is two-fold: First, patients with this pattern are prone to atrial arrhythmias, especially paroxysmal atrial tachycardia and sometimes atrial fibrillation. Second, the ECG of these patients is often mistaken as indicating a bundle branch block or myocardial infarction (Fig. 10-20).

The WPW syndrome predisposes to paroxysmal atrial tachycardia in particular because of the accessory conduction pathway. For example, an impulse traveling down the AV junction may recycle up the bundle of Kent and then back down the AV junction, and so on.* This type of reentry mech-

*When paroxysmal atrial tachycardia develops in a patient with the WPW syndrome, the QRS complex generally becomes narrow. The wide QRS seen with WPW and a normal sinus rhythm occurs because the stimulus travels concomitantly down the bundle of Kent and down the AV junction, resulting in a *fusion* beat. When atrial tachycardia occurs, the impulse usually travels down the AV junction and back up the bundle of Kent in a retrograde fashion, resulting in a loss of the delta wave.

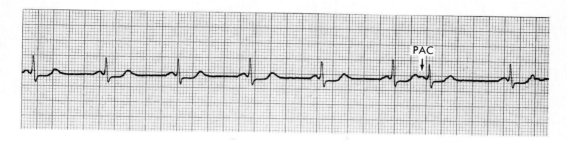

Fig. 10-21. Possible Lown-Ganong-Levine (LGL) type of preexcitation with short PR intervals (0.12 sec). In addition, notice the single premature atrial contraction.

anism *(circus movement)* can account for various tachycardias.

Another type of preexcitation variant, the Lown-Ganong-Levine (LGL) pattern, is caused by a bypass tract (James fiber) that connects the atria and AV junction. Bypassing the AV node results in a short PR interval (less than 0.12 sec). However, the QRS width is not prolonged because ventricular activation occurs normally. Therefore the LGL pattern (Fig. 10-21) consists of a normal-width QRS with a short PR and no delta wave; the WPW consists of a wide QRS with a short PR and a delta wave. Patients with the LGL pattern may also have ''reentrant'' paroxysmal atrial tachycardia (PAT) or paroxysmal atrial fibrillation or flutter.*

DIFFERENTIAL DIAGNOSIS OF WIDE QRS COMPLEXES

Discussion of the WPW syndrome allows us now to review all the major ECG patterns that produce a widened QRS complex. This list includes four major categories:

1. Bundle branch blocks, including the classic RBBB or LBBB patterns
2. ''Toxic'' conduction delays caused by some extrinsic factor, such as hyperkalemia or drugs (quinidine and related antiarrhyth-

mics, phenothiazines, tricyclic antidepressants)
3. Beats arising in the ventricles, which may be premature ventricular contractions (PVCs, p. 180), ventricular escape beats (p. 214), or pacemaker beats (p. 85)
4. Wolff-Parkinson-White type preexcitation

Differentiation among these possibilities is usually easy. Right and left bundle branch blocks were described in Chapter 7. Hyperkalemia produces widening of the QRS complex often with loss of P waves. Widening of the QRS in any patient taking an antiarrhythmic or psychotropic should always suggest possible drug toxicity. Pacemakers generally produce an LBBB pattern with a pacemaker spike before each QRS. The WPW syndrome is recognized by the combination of a short PR interval and a wide QRS, usually with a delta wave.

ST-T CHANGES: SPECIFIC AND NONSPECIFIC

The concluding topic of Part I of this book is a review of the major factors causing ST-T (repolarization) changes. The term *''nonspecific ST-T change,''* defined earlier (Chapter 9), is commonly used in clinical electrocardiography. Many factors, such as drugs, ischemia, electrolyte imbalances, infections, and pulmonary disease, can affect the ECG. As mentioned earlier, the repolarization phase (ST-T complex) is particularly sensitive to such effects and can show a variety of nonspecific

---

*Not all persons with a short PR interval and normal QRS will have LGL preexcitation, however. A short PR may be seen as a normal variant *without* a bypass tract. Therefore care must be taken not to ''overread'' an ECG on which the only noteworthy finding is a short PR.

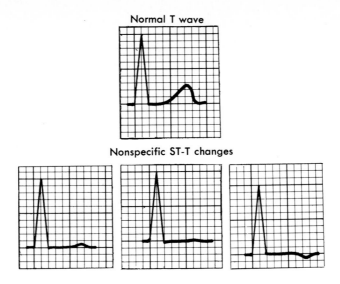

Fig. 10-22. Flattening of the T wave *(left* and *middle)* or slight T wave inversion *(right)* is an abnormal but relatively nonspecific change that may be caused by numerous factors.

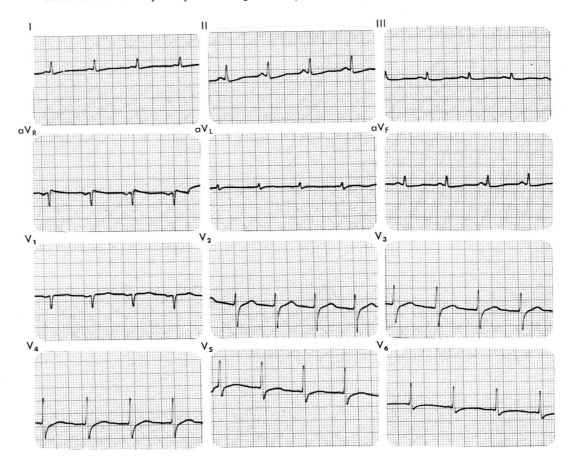

Fig. 10-23. Nonspecific ST-T changes. Notice the diffuse T wave flattening.

changes as a result of multiple factors (Figs. 10-22 and 10-23). These changes include slight ST depressions, T wave flattening, and slight T wave inversions (diagrammed in Fig. 10-22).

In contrast to these nonspecific ST-T changes, there are certain fairly specific changes associated with particular conditions (such as the tall tented T waves of hyperkalemia). Some of these relatively specific ST-T changes are shown in Fig. 10-24. However, even such apparently specific changes can be misleading. For example, ST elevation is characteristic of acute transmural myocardial infarction, yet ST elevations are also seen in Prinzmetal's angina and ventricular aneurysms as well as in pericarditis and benign (normal) early repolarization. Similarly, deep T wave inversions are most characteristic of ischemia but may occur in other conditions as well (p. 120).

To summarize: Repolarization abnormalities (ST-T changes) can be grouped into two general categories: First are the nonspecific ST-T changes, which include slight ST segment deviation and flattening or inversion of the T wave. These are not diagnostic of any particular condition but must always be interpreted in clinical context. Second are the relatively specific ST-T changes that are more strongly, but not always definitively, diagnostic of some particular underlying cause (for example, hyperkalemia or myocardial ischemia).

PEDIATRIC ELECTROCARDIOGRAPHY

The normal ECG patterns seen in children differ considerably from those seen in adults (Chapter 4). The topic of pediatric electrocardiography falls outside the scope of this book, but a few critical points of difference between pediatric and adult ECGs will be mentioned briefly. The normal ECG of the newborn and infant resembles the pattern seen in right ventricular hypertrophy, with tall R waves in the right chest leads and right axis deviation. During the first decade of life the T waves in the right to middle chest leads are normally inverted. This pattern sometimes persists into adolescence and adulthood and is called the *juvenile* T wave variant. As mentioned in Chapter 6, children and young adults may also have tall voltage in the chest leads as a normal variant.

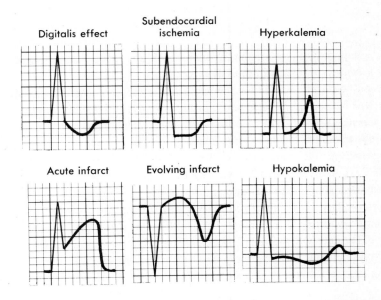

Fig. 10-24. Relatively specific ST-T changes. Notice that they are not absolutely specific for the abnormalities shown.

REVIEW

The ECG can be influenced by numerous factors.

Many *drugs* affect it. *Digitalis effect* refers to the characteristic scooped-out depression of the ST segment produced by therapeutic doses of digitalis. *(Digitalis toxicity* refers to the arrhythmias and conduction disturbances produced by excessive doses of digitalis.) *Quinidine, procainamide,* and *disopyramide* as well as the *psychotropic* drugs can prolong the QT interval and, in toxic doses, widen the QRS complex. These drugs may also cause a potentially lethal type of ventricular tachycardia called *torsade de pointes* (Chapter 14). Patients likely to develop this complication often show prolonged QT intervals and large U waves.

Electrolyte disturbances can also affect the ECG. *Hyperkalemia* produces a sequence of changes. First, there is narrowing and peaking (tenting) of the T wave. Further elevation of the serum potassium concentration leads to PR prolongation and then to loss of P waves and to QRS widening, followed by eventual ventricular fibrillation and asystole. *Hypokalemia* may produce ST depressions and prominent U waves. The QT interval becomes prolonged. (In some cases you are actually measuring the QU and not the QT interval, because it may be impossible to tell where the T wave ends and the U wave begins.) *Hypercalcemia* may shorten the QT interval, and *hypocalcemia* may prolong it.

Pericarditis produces diffuse ST segment elevations, usually in one or more of the chest leads and also in leads I, aV_L, II, and aV_F. PR segment elevation in lead aV_R with PR depression in other leads may be caused by an atrial current of injury. Abnormal Q waves do not develop. The ST segment elevations may be followed by T wave inversions after a variable period.

Pericardial effusion often produces *low voltage* of the QRS complex (QRS amplitude of 5 mm or less in all six extremity leads). Low voltage is not specific for pericardial effusion but may also occur with obesity, emphysema, and diffuse myocardial injury or infiltration or as a normal variant.

Pericardial effusion complicated by *cardiac tamponade* is usually associated with sinus tachycardia and low voltage complexes. Some of these patients will also have *electrical alternans*, a pattern characterized by a beat-to-beat shift in the QRS axis.

Normally the ST segment is isoelectric. However, in some normal people, young adult males in particular, there will be normal ST segment elevations *(early repolarization variant)*, usually best seen in the chest leads (up to 3 mm of elevation). The pattern may simulate that of acute MI or pericarditis but does not show the successive changes that usually occur with those pathologies.

Pulmonary embolism may produce any of the following patterns: (1) acute RBBB, (2) right ventricular strain T wave inversions, (3) $S_I Q_{III} T_{III}$, (4) right axis shift, (5) ST depressions resulting from subendocardial ischemia, and (6) various arrhythmias.

The *WPW pattern* shows (1) a short PR interval (usually but not always <0.12 sec), (2) a wide QRS complex, and (3) slurring or notching of the initial part of the QRS complex. This slurring is called a *delta* wave. Patients with the WPW pattern are particularly prone to attacks of supraventricular tachycardias (paroxysmal atrial tachycardia or rapid atrial fibrillation). Another form of preexcitation, the Lown-Ganong-Levine pattern, is characterized by a short PR interval and a normal QRS.

The differential diagnosis of ECG patterns with a wide QRS complex includes four major possibilities: (1) right or left bundle branch block, (2) toxic conduction delays caused by hyperkalemia or certain drugs, (3) beats arising in the ventricles, such as PVCs or pacemaker beats, and (4) WPW preexcitation.

Questions

1. The following factors may all affect ventricular repolarization (ST-T complex). Put an "L" next to those that may prolong ventricular repolarization (lengthen the QT interval). Put an "S" next to those that may shorten the QT interval.

    Digitalis
    Quinidine
    Procainamide
    Hypokalemia
    Hypocalcemia
    Hypercalcemia

2. Put an "X" next to those factors that can widen the QRS complex.

    Hypokalemia
    Hyperkalemia
    Wolff-Parkinson-White syndrome
    Digitalis effect
    Quinidine toxicity
    Right bundle branch block

3. Which of the following factors can produce ST segment elevations?

    Hypokalemia
    Early repolarization pattern
    Digitalis effect
    Ventricular aneurysm
    Hypocalcemia
    Left ventricular strain
    Pericarditis

4. Match ECGs *A, B,* and *C* with the following causes:
   Digitalis effect
   Hyperkalemia
   Hypokalemia

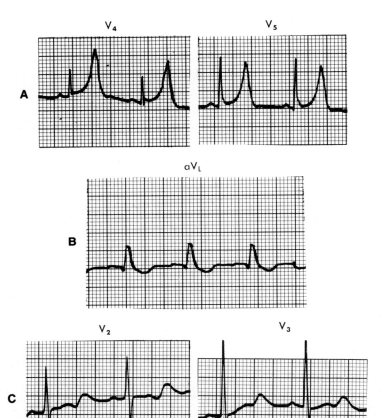

5. What caused the wide QRS in the following ECG?
   a. Right bundle branch block
   b. Quinidine toxicity
   c. Posterolateral infarction
   d. Wolff-Parkinson-White pattern
   e. Hyperkalemia

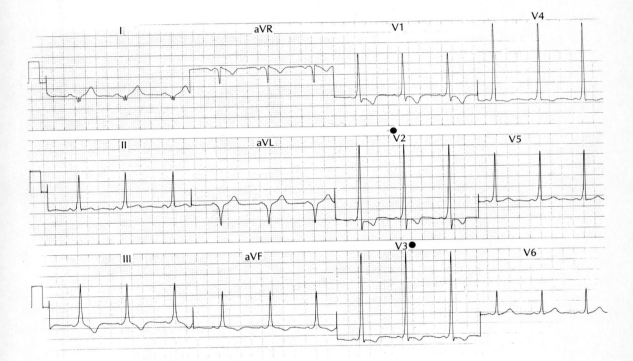

Answers

1. Digitalis (S); quinidine (L); procainamide (L); hypokalemia (L); hypocalcemia (L); hypercalcemia (S).

2. Hyperkalemia (X); Wolff-Parkinson-White syndrome (X); quinidine toxicity (X); right bundle branch block (X).

3. Early repolarization variant; ventricular aneurysm; pericarditis.

4. Digitalis effect, *B;* hyperkalemia, *A;* hypokalemia, *C.*

5. d. Notice the diagnostic triad of a wide QRS, short PR interval, and delta wave (slurred initial portion of the QRS). Compare this with Fig. 10-20, which also shows the Wolff-Parkinson-White pattern. The present example, however, mimics a right bundle branch block and thus is sometimes called the *type A* WPW pattern. The pattern in Fig. 10-20 mimics that of LBBB and is sometimes called the *type B* pattern. WPW patterns are also at times mistaken for hypertrophy (tall R waves) or infarction (*pseudoinfarction* Q waves).

II

CARDIAC RHYTHM DISTURBANCES

11

Sinus Rhythms

NORMAL SINUS RHYTHM

The diagnosis of normal sinus rhythm (NSR) was described in Chapter 3. When the sinus (SA) node is pacing the heart, atrial depolarization spreads from right to left and downward toward the AV junction. An arrow representing the depolarization wave will point downward and toward the left. Therefore, with normal sinus rhythm, the P wave is negative in lead aV_R and reciprocally positive in lead II (Fig. 4-3).

Do not be confused by the polarity of the P wave in other leads. With normal sinus rhythm the P wave may be upright, negative, or biphasic in one or more of the extremity leads. When diagnosing normal sinus rhythm, pay particular attention to the polarity of the P wave in lead aV_R and lead II. The diagnosis of normal sinus rhythm requires examining lead aV_R and finding a negative P wave preceding each QRS complex. Each sinus beat will also produce a positive P wave preceding the QRS complex in lead II (Fig. 11-1).

By convention, *normal sinus rhythm* is defined as sinus rhythm with a heart rate between 60 and 100 beats/min. Sinus rhythm with a heart rate of less than 60 beats/min is called *sinus bradycardia;* one with a heart rate greater than 100 beats/min is *sinus tachycardia.*

REGULATION OF THE HEART RATE

The heart, like the other organs of the body, has a special nerve supply from the autonomic nervous

NORMAL SINUS RHYTHM

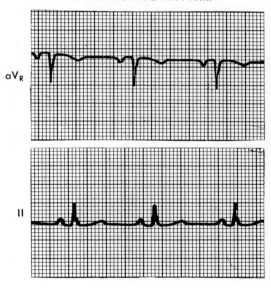

Fig. 11-1. Each QRS complex is preceded by a P wave that is negative in lead aV_R and positive in lead II.

system, which controls involuntary muscle action. The autonomic nerve supply to the heart (and, in particular, the SA node and AV junction) consists of two opposing groups of fibers: the sympathetic nerves and the parasympathetic nerves. Sympathetic stimulation produces an increased heart rate and also increases the strength of myocardial contraction. The parasympathetic nervous supply to the heart is from the vagus nerve. Vagal stimulation

153

produces a slowing of the heart rate as well as a slowing of conduction through the AV junction. In this way the autonomic nervous system exerts a counterbalancing control of the heart rate. The sympathetic nervous system acts as a cardiac accelerator while the parasympathetic (vagal) system produces a braking effect. For example, when you become excited or upset, increased sympathetic stimuli (and diminished parasympathetic tone) result in an increased heart rate and increased contractility, producing the familiar sensation of a pounding heart (palpitations).

SINUS TACHYCARDIA

Sinus tachycardia *is simply sinus rhythm with a heart rate exceeding 100 beats/min.* Generally in adults the heart rate with sinus tachycardia is between 100 and 180 beats/min.

Fig. 11-2 shows an example of sinus tachycardia. Each QRS complex is preceded by a P wave. Notice that the P waves are positive in lead II. With sinus tachycardia at very fast rates, the P wave may merge with the preceding T wave and become difficult to distinguish.

Sinus tachycardia is an arrhythmia, but not necessarily an abnormal rhythm. For example, most normal persons develop a sinus tachycardia during exercise or excitement. In general, a sinus tachycardia will be seen with any condition that produces an *increase* in sympathetic tone or a *decrease* in vagal tone.

The following conditions are commonly associated with sinus tachycardia:

1. Anxiety, emotion, and exertion
2. Drugs (such as epinephrine, ephedrine, tricyclic antidepressants, isoproterenol, and cocaine) that increase sympathetic tone
3. Drugs (such as atropine) that block vagal tone
4. Fever
5. Congestive heart failure (Sinus tachycardia caused by increased sympathetic tone is generally seen with pulmonary edema.)
6. Pulmonary embolism (Sinus tachycardia is the most common arrhythmia seen with acute pulmonary embolism [Chapter 10].)
7. Acute myocardial infarction, which may produce virtually any arrhythmia (Sinus tachycardia persisting after an acute infarct is generally a bad prognostic sign and implies extensive heart damage.)
8. Hyperthyroidism (Sinus tachycardia occurring at rest is a common finding.)
9. Hypotension and shock associated with myocardial infarction, sepsis, or blood loss
10. Alcohol withdrawal

Treatment of sinus tachycardia must be directed at the underlying cause (for example, infection, hyperthyroidism, congestive heart failure). Patients with a sinus tachycardia may complain of palpitations.

Sinus tachycardia is our first example of a supraventricular tachycardia (SVT). A *supraventricular tachycardia* is a tachycardia in which the pacemaker is located in either the atria or the AV junction, *above* the ventricles. In subsequent chapters we will consider other types of SVTs, such as paroxysmal atrial tachycardia (PAT), atrial flutter, and atrial fibrillation.

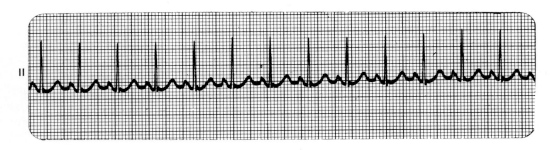

Fig. 11-2. Sinus tachycardia.

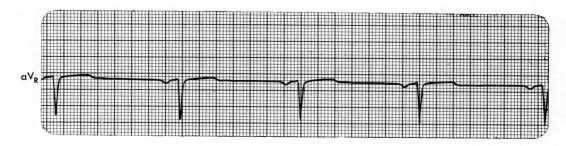

Fig. 11-3. Sinus bradycardia.

SINUS BRADYCARDIA

With sinus bradycardia, sinus rhythm is present and the heart rate is less than 60 beats/min (Fig. 11-3).

Sinus bradycardia is usually caused by a relative increase in vagal tone or a decrease in sympathetic tone that slows the pacemaker rate of the SA node. Sinus bradycardia commonly occurs in the following conditions:

1. As a normal variant (Many normal people have a resting pulse rate of less than 60 beats/min, and trained athletes may have a pulse rate as low as 35 beats/min.)
2. Drugs that increase vagal tone, such as digitalis or edrophonium, or that decrease sympathetic tone, such as the beta blockers (In addition, calcium channel–blocking drugs such as diltiazem hydrochloride and verapamil may cause marked sinus bradycardia.)
3. Hypothyroidism (This is generally associated with a sinus bradycardia, just as hyperthyroidism produces a resting sinus tachycardia.)
4. "Sick sinus syndrome" (Some patients, particularly elderly ones, will have marked sinus bradycardia without obvious cause, probably from degenerative disease of the sinus node. This "sick sinus syndrome" is discussed further at the end of this chapter and in Chapter 18. See also Fig. 11-6.)
5. Sleep apnea syndrome
6. Carotid sinus syndrome

Most people with sinus bradycardia have no symptoms. If the heart rate is very slow (in the 40s), light-headedness and even syncope may occur. In such cases a drug such as atropine, which blocks vagal tone, may be needed acutely to increase the heart rate. In cases of chronic sinus bradycardia causing symptoms (for example, in the *sick sinus syndrome*) an electronic pacemaker may be needed.

SINUS ARRHYTHMIA

Even in healthy persons the sinus node does not pace the heart at a perfectly regular rate. There is normally a slight beat-to-beat variation in sinus rate. Sometimes, as shown in Figs. 11-4 and 11-5, when this variability in sinus rate is more accentuated, the term *"sinus arrhythmia"* is used. Sinus arrhythmia therefore is sinus rhythm with an apparently irregular rate.

The most common cause of sinus arrhythmia is respiration. With inspiration the heart rate normally increases slightly; with expiration it slows slightly. This respiratory, or *phasic,* sinus arrhythmia is caused by slight changes in vagal tone occurring during the different phases of respiration (Fig. 11-4).

Occasionally a *nonphasic* sinus arrhythmia occurs, and the heart rate varies from beat to beat without relation to the respiratory cycle (Fig. 11-5).

Phasic sinus arrhythmia is a normal finding, particularly in children or young adults. A nonphasic sinus arrhythmia, while not strictly normal, does not have any special pathologic or therapeutic significance.

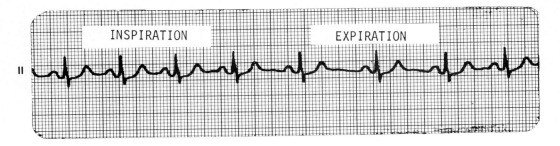

Fig. 11-4. Phasic sinus arrhythmia. Normally there is a slight increase in the heart rate with inspiration and a slight decrease with expiration.

MONITOR LEAD

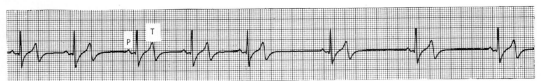

Fig. 11-5. Nonphasic sinus arrhythmia. The monitor lead shows a markedly irregular rhythm. Each QRS complex is preceded by a P wave, with a constant PR interval. This arrhythmia resulted from acute myocarditis. (Notice that the T waves are biphasic.)

SINUS ARREST AND ESCAPE BEATS

Up to this point we have considered normal sinus rhythm, sinus tachycardia, sinus bradycardia, and sinus arrhythmia. Suppose for some reason the sinus node fails to function for one or more beats. Such failure to pace is called *sinoatrial block (SA block)*. It may occur intermittently, with simply a missing beat (no P wave or QRS complex) at occasional intervals, or it may be more extreme. An example of the latter is *sinus pause* or *arrest* (Fig. 11-6), in which the sinus node fails to function altogether for a prolonged period. This type of block will lead to cardiac arrest with asystole unless the sinus node regains function or some other pacemaker (escape pacemaker) takes over. Fortunately, other parts of the cardiac conduction system are capable of producing electrical stimuli and functioning as an escape pacemaker in these circumstances. Escape beats may come from the atria, the AV junction, or the ventricles.

Fig. 11-7 shows a junctional escape beat. (The characteristics of escape beats are described in Chapter 12.)

SA block and sinus arrest can be caused by numerous factors, including hypoxia, myocardial ischemia or infarction, hyperkalemia, digitalis toxicity, and toxic reactions to other drugs such as the beta blockers and calcium-channel blockers (diltiazem, verapamil). In elderly people the sinus node may undergo degenerative changes and fail to function effectively. Then periods of SA block and even sinus arrest can occur, leading at times to light-headedness and syncope. The term *"sick sinus syndrome"* refers to this type of sinus node dysfunction (Figs. 11-6 and 18-13).

To summarize: The term *"arrhythmia"* refers to any heart rhythm other than strictly normal sinus rhythm. Sinus bradycardia, sinus tachycardia, sinus arrhythmia, and SA block are all arrhythmias. However, sinus bradycardia in a resting person,

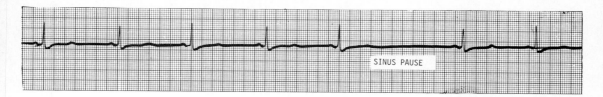

Fig. 11-6. Sinus pause in a patient with sick sinus syndrome. The monitor lead shows sinus bradycardia with a long (about 2.4 second) pause.

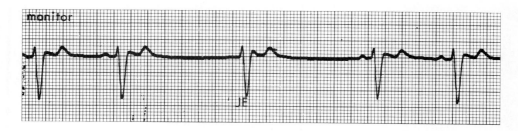

Fig. 11-7. Junctional escape beat (*JE*). The monitor strip shows a sinus pause with each escape beat.

sinus tachycardia with exercise, or phasic sinus arrhythmia with respiratory changes in heart rate may be normal. In other settings, such as hypothyroidism or pulmonary emboli, sinus bradycardia or sinus tachycardia respectively may be important diagnostic clues.

The next few chapters describe other common arrhythmias in which the cardiac pacemaker is located *outside* the sinus node—in the atria, AV junction, or ventricles.

REVIEW

With *normal sinus rhythm* (NSR) each heartbeat originates in the sinus node. The P wave is always negative in lead aV_R and positive in lead II. The rate is between 60 and 100 beats/min.

With *sinus tachycardia* the heart rate is greater than 100 beats/min while with *sinus bradycardia* it is less than 60 beats/min. There are multiple causes of sinus bradycardia and sinus tachycardia, and both arrhythmias may occur normally.

With *sinus arrhythmia* there is variability of the sinus rate from beat to beat, and it may be either phasic with respiration or nonphasic. *SA block* describes failure of the sinus node to function for one or more beats. *Sinus arrest,* leading to fatal asystole, may occur unless NSR resumes or unless *escape beats* from other foci in the atria, AV junction, or ventricles take over. SA block and sinus arrest may be seen particularly in elderly people as a consequence of the *sick sinus syndrome.* Digitalis toxicity or toxic reactions to other drugs (beta blockers, calcium blockers) must always be excluded in anyone with marked sinus bradycardia, SA block, or sinus arrest.

Questions

1. Is normal sinus rhythm present?

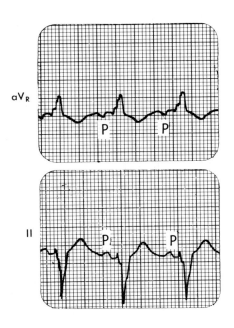

2. Is normal sinus rhythm present?

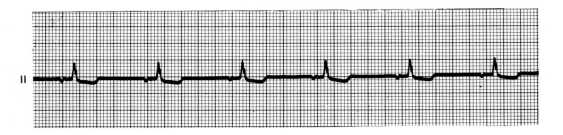

Answers

1. Yes. The P waves are negative in lead aV_R and positive in lead II. Don't be confused by the unusual QRS complexes (positive in lead aV_R and negative in lead II) produced by the abnormal axis deviation. Diagnosis of normal sinus rhythm depends only on the P waves.

2. No. Each QRS complex is preceded by a P wave. However, notice that the P waves are *negative* in lead II. These retrograde P waves were produced in this case by a junctional (or ectopic atrial) rhythm.

12

Supraventricular Arrhythmias—I

PREMATURE ATRIAL CONTRACTIONS, PAROXYSMAL ATRIAL TACHYCARDIA, AV JUNCTIONAL RHYTHMS

The intrinsic pacemaker of the heart is the sinus (SA) node, and normally it initiates each heartbeat. However, pacemaker stimuli can arise from other parts of the heart—the atria, the AV junction, or the ventricles. The terms *"ectopy," "ectopic pacemaker,"* and *"ectopic beat"* are used to describe these non-sinus beats. Ectopic beats are often premature; that is, they come before the next sinus beat is due. Thus we may find premature atrial contractions (PACs), premature AV junctional contractions (PJCs), and premature ventricular contractions (PVCs). Ectopic beats can also come after a pause in the normal rhythm, as in the case of AV junctional or ventricular *escape* beats. Ectopic beats originating in the AV junction (node) or atria are referred to as *supraventricular* (that is, coming from *above* the ventricles).

In this chapter and the next, ectopic atrial and AV junctional (supraventricular) rhythms are described. Chapter 14 deals with ventricular ectopy.

PREMATURE ATRIAL CONTRACTIONS

Premature atrial contractions (PACs)* are ectopic beats arising from somewhere in either the left or the right atrium but not in the sinus node. The atria therefore are depolarized from an ectopic site. Following atrial stimulation, the stimulus may spread normally through the AV junction into the ventricles. For this reason, ventricular depolarization (the QRS) is generally not affected by PACs.

PACs have the following major features (Fig. 12-1):

1. The beat is premature, occurring before the next normal beat is due. This is in contrast to escape beats (p. 157), which come after a pause in the normal rhythm.

2. The PAC is often, but not always, preceded by a visible P wave that usually has a slightly different shape and/or slightly different PR interval from the P wave seen with normal sinus beats. The PR interval of the PAC may be either longer or shorter than the PR interval of the normal beats.

3. Following the PAC there is generally a slight pause before the normal sinus beat resumes.

4. Occasionally, no clear P wave will be seen preceding the PAC (Fig. 12-2). In some of these cases the P wave may be "buried" in the T wave of the preceding beat.

5. The QRS complex of the PAC is usually identical or very similar to the QRS complex of the preceding beats. Remember that with

---

*The terms *"premature atrial contractions," "premature atrial beats," "premature atrial depolarizations,"* and *"atrial extrasystoles"* are used synonymously.

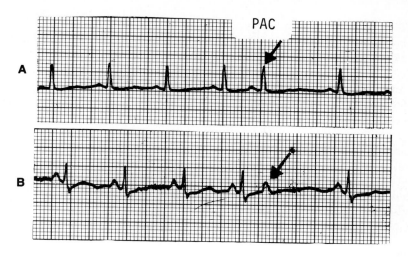

Fig. 12-1. Premature atrial contractions. Notice, **A,** the PAC after the fourth sinus beat and, **B,** the blocked PAC also after the fourth sinus beat. The premature P wave falls on the T wave of the preceding beat and is not followed by a QRS complex because the AV node is still in a refractory state.

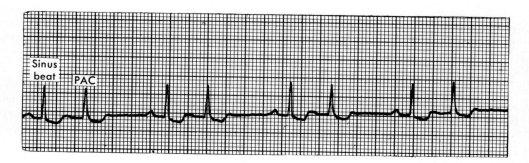

Fig. 12-2. Atrial bigeminy. Every other beat is a premature atrial contraction.

PACs the atrial pacemaker is in an ectopic location but the ventricles are depolarized in a normal way. This contrasts with premature ventricular contractions (PVCs), discussed in Chapter 14, in which the QRS complex is abnormally wide because of abnormal depolarization of the ventricles. Occasionally PACs will result in aberrant ventricular conduction so the QRS is wider than normal. Differentiation of such PACs "with aberration" from premature ventricular contrac-

tions may be difficult. (See Chapter 18.)

Sometimes, when the PAC is very premature, the stimulus will reach the AV junction shortly after it has already been stimulated by the preceding normal beat. Because the AV junction, like all other conduction tissue, requires time to recover its capacity to conduct impulses, this premature atrial stimulus may reach the junction when it is still *refractory*. In such cases the PAC may not be conducted to the ventricles and no QRS complex will appear. This situation will result in a *blocked*

PAC. The ECG (Fig. 12-1, *B*) will show a premature P wave *not* followed by a QRS complex. Following the blocked P wave, there is a slight pause before the next normal beat resumes. The blocked PAC, therefore, produces a slight irregularity of the heartbeat. If you do not search carefully for these blocked PACs you will overlook them.

PACs may occur frequently (for example, five or more times/min) or sporadically. Two PACs occurring consecutively are referred to as "paired PACs." Sometimes, as shown in Fig. 12-2, each sinus beat is followed by a PAC. (This pattern is referred to as *atrial bigeminy*.)

Clinical Significance

PACs are very common. They may occur both in persons with normal hearts and in persons with organic heart disease. Finding PACs, therefore, does not imply that the person has cardiac disease. In normal subjects PACs may be seen with emotional stress, with excessive coffee drinking, or as a result of sympathomimetic drugs (epinephrine, isoproterenol, theophylline). PACs may produce palpitations—the patient may complain of feeling a skipped beat or an irregular pulse. PACs may also be seen with any type of heart disease. Frequent PACs are sometimes the forerunner of atrial fibrillation (Chapter 13) or paroxysmal atrial tachycardia.

PAROXYSMAL ATRIAL TACHYCARDIA

Paroxysmal atrial tachycardia (PAT) is the second tachyarrhythmia we shall discuss. The first was sinus tachycardia (Chapter 10). *PAT is simply a run of three or more consecutive PACs.* As described later in this chapter (pp. 167-168), most of the cases of so-called PAT are actually related to a *reentrant*-type mechanism involving the AV junction. Hence the terms *"PAT"* and *"AV junctional* or *nodal tachycardia"* are sometimes used synonymously. Another term often used is *"paroxysmal supraventricular tachycardia"* (PSVT).

In some cases the run of PAT will be brief and self-limited. In others it may be sustained for hours, days, or even weeks. Figs. 12-3 to 12-5 show several examples.

PAT has the following characteristics:

1. The heart rate is generally between 140 and 250 beats/min. Recall that with sinus tachycardia the heart rate in adults does not generally exceed 160 to 180 beats/min.
2. The rate is usually extremely regular. Each beat falls exactly on time, and the RR intervals between beats do not generally show any variability. This also contrasts with sinus tachycardia, in which there is generally some slight but discernible beat-to-beat variability.
3. P waves may or may not be visible. When seen, they are generally different from the P

PAROXYSMAL ATRIAL TACHYCARDIA (PAT)

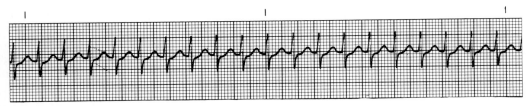

Fig. 12-3. This strip shows PAT (a run of more than three PACs). The rate is about 167 beats/min. Notice the marked regularity of the rhythm. No P waves are visible. This type of PAT is probably due to a rapidly circulating impulse in the AV junction and is also sometimes referred to as an AV nodal (junctional) reentrant tachycardia or paroxysmal supraventricular tachycardia (PSVT). (See text.)

PAROXYSMAL ATRIAL TACHYCARDIA

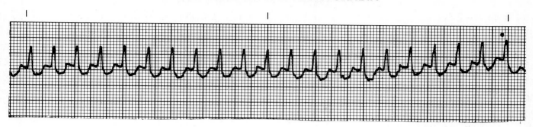

Fig. 12-4. PAT with a rate of about 200 beats/min.

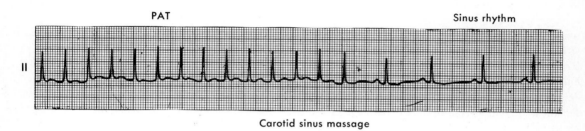

PAT   Sinus rhythm

II

Carotid sinus massage

Fig. 12-5. Paroxysmal atrial tachycardia treated with carotid sinus massage. The first 14 beats in this rhythm strip show PAT with a rate of about 150 beats/min. Carotid sinus massage resulted in abrupt termination of the tachycardia, with the appearance of normal sinus rhythm.

waves in a patient with normal sinus rhythm. The PR interval may be the same as, greater than, or less than the patient's usual PR interval.

4. The QRS complexes are usually of normal width, since intraventricular conduction is generally normal. (A wide QRS will be seen if the patient has an underlying bundle branch block or if the PAT induces a "rate-related" bundle branch block.)

Clinical Significance

PAT may be seen both in normal persons and in those with organic heart disease. It, therefore, does not necessarily imply that the patient has any significant cardiac abnormality. For example, healthy adults can have attacks of PAT that may break spontaneously or that occasionally require

special treatment. PAT may also occur with heart disease of any type. One special condition associated with PAT is *ventricular preexcitation*, seen in the Wolff-Parkinson-White or Lown-Ganong-Levine syndrome (Chapter 10).

Patients with PAT usually complain of lightheadedness or palpitations. Occasionally PAT produces syncope. A run of PAT in a patient with limited cardiac reserve may precipitate angina pectoris or congestive heart failure.

Treatment

Many times PAT will resolve spontaneously or after the patient is sedated. There are several methods of direct therapy. A number of these involve increasing the amount of *vagal tone* on the heart. Recall that the vagus nerve exerts a braking effect on the heart, slowing stimulus formation and conduction in the sinus node and the AV junction. Patients with PAT have an excessive number of stimuli traveling through the AV junction. Therefore, one approach to treating PAT is to increase vagal tone. There are several ways of doing this. The patient may try *Valsalva's maneuver* (straining and bearing down as if to have a bowel movement). *Carotid sinus massage* may also terminate an attack of PAT by increasing vagal tone (Fig. 12-5).

Numerous drugs can also be used to treat PAT. Verapamil, a calcium blocker, is highly effective. Digitalis acts by increasing vagal tone at the AV junction. Edrophonium also increases vagal tone. Propranolol and other beta blockers (for example, metoprolol or esmolol) decrease sympathetic stimulation. Phenylephrine, an intravenous vasoconstrictor, raises the blood pressure rapidly, causing a reflex increase in vagal tone similar to what occurs with carotid sinus massage. Quinidine or procainamide may be useful. Intravenous adenosine, the latest drug approved for treatment of PAT, also slows conduction through the AV junction.

It is essential to be familiar with the adverse effects and contraindications of any drug prior to its use. The clinical pharmacology of antiarrhythmic agents is discussed in many texts (see Bibliography). In general, most patients will respond to one of the aforementioned drugs. Often therapy is effective within minutes. Occasionally PAT requires more immediate therapy. Younger patients and those without significant underlying cardiovascular disease may tolerate heart rates up to 250 beats/min with complaints only of palpitations or light-headedness. However, in patients with limited cardiac reserve, heart rates above 160 beats/min (or even less) may have disastrous consequences. In these persons, myocardial ischemia or even infarction may develop. They may also have congestive heart failure or hypotension. In such emergency circumstances, when PAT is associated with angina, congestive heart failure, or hypotension and when initial therapy with vagal maneuvers and rapidly acting drugs fails, electrical cardioversion may be required.

Electrical cardioversion is the use of a direct current (DC) shock to treat certain tachyarrhythmias. The shock is administered with special paddles placed on the chest wall. In treating some arrhythmias, such as ventricular flutter or ventricular fibrillation, an *unsynchronized* DC shock is given. In treating PAT and other supraventricular arrhythmias, such as atrial fibrillation and atrial flutter, it is essential to give a *synchronized* DC shock. The shock is synchronized so it does not occur during the *vulnerable period* of ventricular repolarization (simultaneous with the apex of the T wave). It has been noted that DC shocks given to the heart during the vulnerable period may produce ventricular fibrillation. *Therefore, in treating PAT, a synchronized DC shock must be given.* The details of electrical cardioversion lie outside the scope of this book.

AV JUNCTIONAL RHYTHMS

With PACs the ectopic pacemaker is located somewhere in the atria outside the sinus node. Under certain circumstances, the AV junction may also function as an ectopic pacemaker, producing an AV junctional rhythm. In older textbooks, the term "AV nodal" or "nodal" rhythm is used to refer to AV junctional rhythm. The terms *"AV junctional," "junctional," "AV nodal,"* and *"nodal"* are all essentially synonymous.

In Chapter 4 the basic mechanism of AV junctional rhythms and the pattern seen with AV junctional escape beats were described. When the AV junction is the cardiac pacemaker, the atria are stimulated in a *retrograde* fashion, from bottom to top. An arrow representing the spread of atrial depolarization with junctional rhythm will point upward, just opposite the direction of atrial depolarization when normal sinus rhythm is present (Fig. 4-3). This retrograde stimulation of the atria will produce a positive P wave in lead aV_R and a negative P wave in lead II (Fig. 4-5). With AV junctional rhythm the ventricles will be depolarized normally (unless a bundle branch block is present), resulting in a narrow QRS complex.

In some cases of AV junctional rhythm the atria will be stimulated before the ventricles. In other cases the stimulus may reach the ventricles first. Finally, in still other cases the atria and the ventricles will be stimulated simultaneously. If the atria are stimulated first, the P wave will precede the QRS complex. (A retrograde P wave preceding the QRS may also occur with some ectopic atrial beats. However, the distinction between ectopic atrial and AV junctional beats is usually not of clinical importance.) If the ventricles are first to be stimulated, the QRS will precede the P wave. If atrial and ventricular depolarizations are simultaneous, the P wave will be "buried" in the QRS and not be seen.

To summarize: AV junctional beats can be recognized on the ECG by one of the following three patterns (Fig 12-6):

1. Retrograde P waves (positive in lead aV_R, negative in lead II) preceding the QRS complexes
2. Retrograde P waves following the QRS complexes
3. Absent P waves (buried in the QRS), so the baseline between QRS complexes is flat

AV junctional rhythms can be considered in two general classes—slow escape rhythms and tachycardias—depending on the rate. The *slow* junctional escape rhythms are less than 60 beats/min. The junctional *tachycardias* have rates between 100 and 250 beats/min.

AV Junctional Escape Rhythms

AV junctional escape beats were mentioned in the section on sinus arrest (p. 156). An AV junctional escape beat (Fig. 11-7) is simply a beat that comes after a pause when the normal sinus pacemaker fails to function. The AV junctional escape beat therefore is a "safety beat." Following this escape beat, the normal sinus pacemaker may resume function. However, if it does not, a slow AV junctional escape rhythm may continue. An AV junctional escape rhythm is a consecutive run of AV junctional beats. The heart rate is usually slow, between 30 and 60 beats/min.

Fig. 12-7 shows an example of an AV junctional escape rhythm. It is not surprising that the basic

AV JUNCTIONAL BEATS

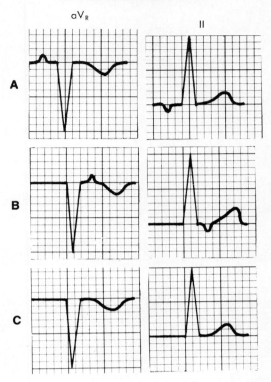

Fig. 12-6. AV junctional beats produce P waves that point upward in lead aV_R and downward in lead II—just the opposite of what is seen in sinus rhythm. The P wave may precede the QRS complex, **A,** follow it, **B,** or occur simultaneously with it, **C.** In the last instance no P wave will be visible.

rate of the AV junction is slower than that of the sinus node. If the AV junction had a faster inherent rate, it would compete with the sinus node for control of the heartbeat.

AV junctional escape rhythm can be seen in a number of clinical settings—digitalis toxicity (Chapter 16), toxic reactions to beta blockers or calcium-channel blockers (diltiazem, verapamil), acute myocardial infarction, hypoxemia, hyperkalemia. Treatment depends on the cause (for example, stopping the digitalis and oxygenating the patient). If the heart rate becomes excessively slow

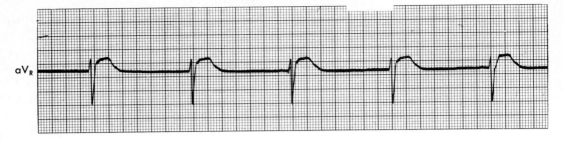

Fig. 12-7. This strip shows a slow junctional escape rhythm at 43 beats/min with no visible P waves.

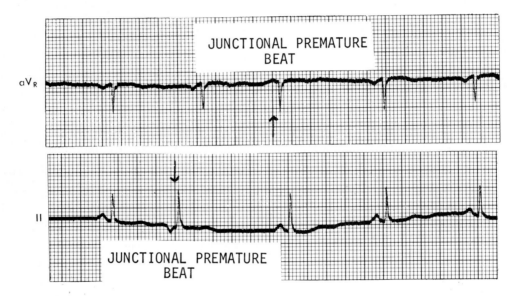

Fig. 12-8. Notice the retrograde P waves (positive in lead aV_R, negative in lead II) on the ECG of a patient with junctional premature beats. The P wave polarity is the reverse of what is seen with normal sinus rhythm.

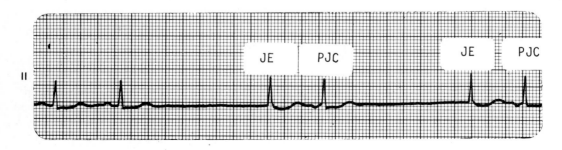

Fig. 12-9. The junctional escape beat (*JE*) comes after a pause and is followed by a premature junctional contraction (*PJC*). Notice the retrograde (inverted) P wave preceding the PJC in lead II.

with an AV junctional rhythm, then drugs such as atropine (a vagal blocker) or isoproterenol (a sympathomimetic stimulant) may be used acutely to increase the heart rate.

AV Junctional Tachycardias

As mentioned, the AV junction can also be the site of ectopic stimuli producing premature AV junctional contractions (PJCs) and junctional tachycardia.

PJCs are simply premature beats formed in the AV junction. They resemble premature atrial contractions (PACs), except that the P waves, when seen, will be retrograde with a PJC (Figs. 12-8 and 12-9). If no P wave is seen before the premature beat, then there may be no way of telling if it is a PAC (with the P wave lost in the preceding T wave) or a PJC (with the P wave buried in the QRS). The distinction is purely academic. PACs and PJCs have the same clinical significance, and treatment is the same.

An AV junctional tachycardia, analogous to PAT, is simply a run of three or more consecutive PJCs (Figs. 12-10 and 12-11). AV junctional tachycardia and most cases of PAT can be considered clinically as a single entity. They have the same clinical significance and treatment. Current evidence indicates that most cases of PAT are actually due to

JUNCTIONAL TACHYCARDIA

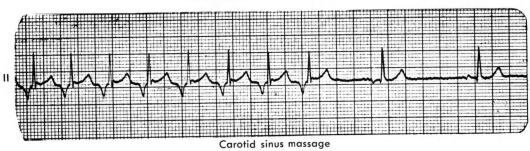

Carotid sinus massage

Fig. 12-10. Notice the retrograde P waves preceding the QRS complexes in this lead II strip from a patient with paroxysmal junctional tachycardia.

JUNCTIONAL TACHYCARDIA

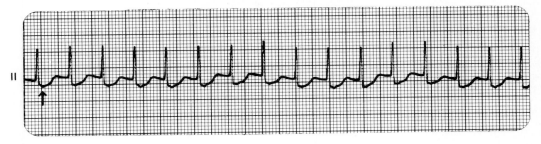

Fig. 12-11. The heart rate is about 150 beats/min. This lead II strip shows retrograde P waves (*arrow*) that are barely visible and are buried in the ST-T complexes.

reentry* involving the AV junction. The terms *"AV junctional"* and *"AV nodal"* are sometimes used synonymously in connection with these reentrant tachycardias. A minority of cases of atrial tachycardia are due to an "automatic" atrial focus firing at a rapid rate.

More detailed discussions of the diagnosis and therapy of *reentrant* versus *automatic* supraventricular tachycardias are given in selected Bibliographic references.

The differential diagnosis of PAT and AV junctional tachycardia from other tachyarrhythmias is described in Chapter 18.

*The term *"reentry"* is used by cardiologists to describe a rapidly circulating electrical wave that may arise in virtually any part of the heart and cause a tachycardia. For example, reentry can lead to the types of supraventricular tachycardia described in this chapter or be the mechanism of a ventricular tachycardia (described in Chapter 14). Review of Chapter 10 at this point for a brief discussion of reentry with the Wolff-Parkinson-White preexcitation syndrome is suggested. The terminology might seem a bit confusing, but it is necessary only to remember that the following terms have been used to describe the same arrhythmia: *"AV nodal reentrant tachycardia," "AV junctional tachycardia,"* and *"paroxysmal supraventricular tachycardia"* (PSVT). Remember also that the condition still commonly goes by its older designation "paroxysmal atrial tachycardia" (PAT).

REVIEW

Stimuli that pace the heart can arise not only in the sinus node but in other cardiac tissues as well—the atria, AV junction, or ventricles.

The terms *"ectopy," "ectopic pacemaker,"* and *"ectopic contraction* or *beat"* are used to describe these stimuli. There are two major categories of ectopic beats:

1. *Premature* (extra beats that come before the next normal beat is expected; examples are PACs, PJCs, and PVCs)
2. *Escape* (usually AV junctional or ventricular beats that are *not* premature but come after a pause in the normal rhythm)

PACs show the following:

1. Usually there is a slightly different-shaped P wave with a slightly longer or shorter PR interval than in the preceding complexes. Sometimes the P wave of the PAC will be hidden in the T wave of the preceding normal beat.
3. Occasionally the atrial stimulus cannot penetrate the AV junction. In such cases of *blocking* the premature P wave will *not* be followed by a QRS complex.

PAT is a run of three or more consecutive PACs. It shows the following features:

1. The heart rate is generally between 140 and 250 beats/minute.
2. The rhythm is usually extremely regular.
3. P waves may or may not be visible, and the shape of the P wave and length of the PR interval may differ from the patient's usual pattern.

AV junctional rhythm shows the following features:

1. The P wave, when seen, is negative in lead II and positive in lead aV_R, just the reverse of the pattern seen with normal sinus rhythm. These are called *retrograde* P waves.
2. The retrograde P wave may precede or follow the QRS complex.
3. In some cases the retrograde P wave will be buried within the QRS complex. If this occurs, the baseline between QRS complexes remains completely flat.

AV junctional rhythms are categorized as junctional escape rhythms and junctional tachycardias. An

AV junctional escape rhythm is a run of AV junctional beats with a slow rate, generally between 40 and 60 beats/minute. AV junctional tachycardia, by contrast, is a run of three or more consecutive PJCs. It has the same clinical significance as PAT.

Questions

True or false (1 to 4):
1. PAT is sinus rhythm with a rate of 140 to 250 beats/minute.
2. PAT is invariably a sign of serious organic heart disease.
3. PAT is usually extremely regular.
4. PAT is defined as a run of three or more consecutive PACs.
5. Why might the patient whose rhythm strip is shown below complain of occasional palpitations?

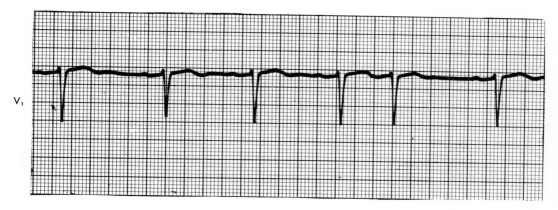

6. What is the beat marked **X**?

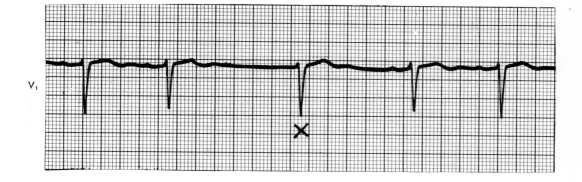

7. a. What is the approximate heart rate?
   b. What arrhythmia is present?

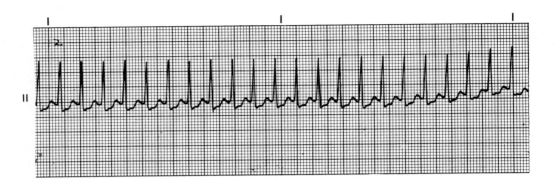

Answers

1. False. PAT is an *ectopic* rhythm with the pacemaker *outside* the sinus node.
2. False. PAT frequently occurs in structurally normal hearts.
3. True.
4. True.
5. Palpitations might have been caused by occasional PACs. Notice that the fifth beat here is a PAC (or possibly a PJC, since the P wave of the premature beat is not seen).
6. Junctional escape beat. Notice that the beat comes after a pause in normal rhythm and is not preceded by a P wave.
7. a. Approximately 210 beats/min. (Count the number of QRS cycles in 6 sec and multiply by 10.)
   b. PAT. As noted on p. 162 and on p. 168 (footnote), this type of PAT is sometimes referred to as paroxysmal supraventricular tachycardia (PSVT) and is likely due to a reentrant mechanism involving the AV node (junction). This type of PSVT may also occur with a bypass tract (p. 42, footnote).

13

Supraventricular Arrhythmias—II

ATRIAL FLUTTER AND ATRIAL FIBRILLATION

Atrial flutter and atrial fibrillation (Fig. 13-1) are two distinct but related tachyarrhythmias. Like paroxysmal atrial tachycardia (PAT), they are *ectopic*. In other words, with all three the atria are being stimulated *not* from the sinus node but from an ectopic site or sites. With PAT the atria are stimulated at a rate generally between 140 and 250 beats/min. With atrial flutter the atrial rate is even faster, generally between 250 and 350 beats/min. Finally, with atrial fibrillation the atrial depolarization rate is between 400 and 600 beats/min. Thus it can be seen that all three conditions are part of a continuum in which the atrial stimulation rate is increasing.

With both atrial flutter and atrial fibrillation there are no true P waves on the ECG. Instead we see characteristic flutter (F) waves and fibrillation (f) waves. Notice the pronounced *sawtooth* shape of the F waves in Fig. 13-1.

ATRIAL FLUTTER

With atrial flutter the stimulation rate is about 300 per minute (Fig. 13-2). What happens to the ventricles during this rapid bombardment of the atria? The answer is that with atrial flutter (and atrial fibrillation) the ventricular (QRS) rate varies depending on the ability of the AV junction to transmit stimuli from the atria to the ventricles. If the ventricles respond to each flutter wave, then the ventricular rate will be around 300 beats per minute. Most commonly the ventricular rate with atrial flutter is about 150, 100, or 75 beats per minute. Atrial flutter with a ventricular response of 150 beats/min is called 2:1 flutter because the ratio of the atrial rate (300) to the ventricular rate (150) is 2 to 1. Atrial flutter with a ventricular rate of 100 beats/min is 3:1, and with 75 beats/min usually 4:1. As mentioned, atrial flutter with a ventricular rate equal to the atrial rate, 300 beats/min, or 1:1 flutter is very rare. Characteristically patients with atrial flutter will increase or decrease their ventricular rate by stepwise fractions of the atrial rate (Fig. 13-1). Thus a patient may change abruptly from atrial flutter with a ventricular response of 75 to 100 beats/min, to 150 beats/min, or even to 300 beats/min. In some patients the ventricular response with atrial flutter will be more variable.

Clinical Significance

Atrial flutter is rarely seen in people with normal hearts. This is in contrast to atrial fibrillation (described later), which may occur transiently in normal individuals. Atrial flutter is not specific for any particular type of heart disease but occurs, for example, in patients with valvular heart disease, acute myocardial infarction, chronic ischemic heart disease, cardiomyopathy, hypertensive heart disease, lung disease, and pulmonary emboli as well as after cardiac surgery.

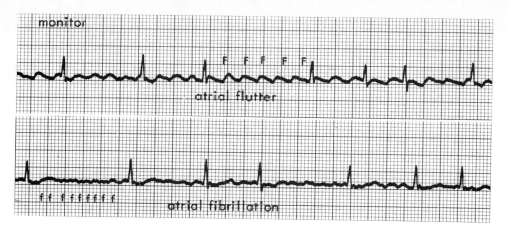

Fig. 13-1. Atrial flutter and fibrillation. Notice the sawtooth waves with atrial flutter (*F*) and the irregular fibrillatory waves with atrial fibrillation (*f*).

ATRIAL FLUTTER

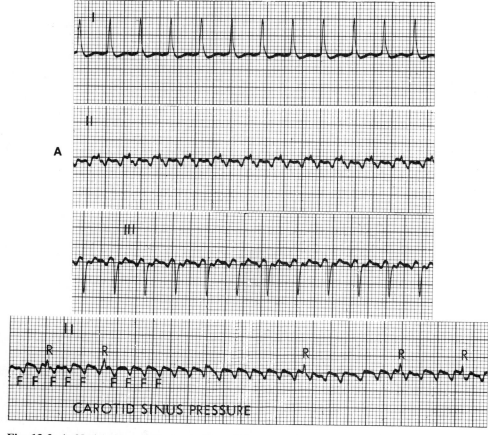

Fig. 13-2. A, Notice the variable appearance of flutter waves in different leads. In lead I the waves are barely apparent while in leads II and III the classic "sawtooth" waves appear. The ventricular rate is about 160 beats/min, and the flutter rate is about 320 beats/min; thus 2:1 conduction is present. **B,** Carotid sinus massage produces marked slowing of the ventricular rate by increasing vagal tone.

Treatment

Treatment of atrial flutter depends on the clinical condition. In some patients atrial flutter will revert spontaneously to normal sinus rhythm. In others who are hypoxic, treatment with oxygen may help restore normal sinus rhythm.

Patients in atrial flutter are frequently treated with digitalis. Digitalis has two major effects on atrial flutter. It *slows conduction through the AV junction,* thereby slowing the ventricular rate, and it *tends to increase the rate of atrial depolarization.* Increasing the atrial rate may convert atrial flutter to atrial fibrillation. Thus digoxin administered to a patient in atrial flutter may convert the patient to atrial fibrillation with a slower and more stable ventricular rate. Rarely patients may convert to normal sinus rhythm from atrial flutter following digitalization. In other cases, a second drug (such as quinidine) is added to help convert atrial flutter to normal sinus rhythm. Quinidine is an antiarrhythmic drug that is useful in treating both atrial flutter and atrial fibrillation. In selected cases either verapamil or diltiazem, calcium channel blockers, or a beta blocker such as propranolol may be used orally or intravenously to slow the ventricular response during atrial flutter.

In many patients atrial flutter will persist despite pharmacologic therapy with digitalis and quinidine. Fortunately, atrial flutter is one of the arrhythmias most easily treated with *electrical cardioversion.* As described in Chapter 12, a synchronized DC shock is given with the patient properly anesthetized. Of all the atrial arrhythmias, atrial flutter is probably the easiest to cardiovert electrically.

Another way of treating atrial flutter is with very rapid pacing of the atria by means of a temporary pacing wire (known as *overdrive* pacing). The details of this therapy, however, lie outside the scope of this book.

To summarize: Atrial flutter is a tachyarrhythmia in which the atria are stimulated (depolarized) usually at a rate of 250 to 350 beats/min, with a ventricular response that is often some fraction of the atrial rate ($1/2$, $1/4$, etc.). Atrial flutter may be treated with special drugs (digitalis, quinidine), synchronized DC shock, or rapid atrial pacing.

ATRIAL FIBRILLATION

With atrial fibrillation, one of the most commonly seen arrhythmias, the atria are stimulated (depolarized) at a very rapid rate, up to 600 times/min. This fibrillatory activity produces a characteristically irregular wavy pattern in place of the normal P waves. The irregular waves, seen in Fig. 13-3, are called *fibrillatory* or *f waves.* In some cases the f waves are relatively coarse (Fig. 13-4). In others a fine fibrillation is seen (Fig. 13-5). Atrial fibrillation, therefore, is characterized by rapid oscillatory depolarization of the atria, producing irregular undulations of the ECG baseline without true P waves.

Because of the rapid atrial depolarization rate, the AV junction in patients with atrial fibrillation is being bombarded by innumerable stimuli from the atria. If every stimulus (each f wave) penetrated the AV junction, the ventricles would beat at a rate of up to 600 times/min, with obvious consequences to the patient. Fortunately, the AV junction is refractory to most of these impulses and allows only

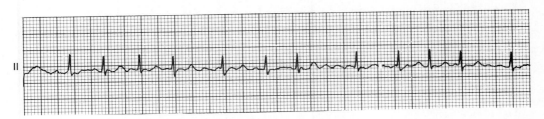

Fig. 13-3. Rapid undulation of the baseline because of fibrillatory (f) waves. There are no true P waves, and the ventricular rate is irregular.

ATRIAL FIBRILLATION WITH RAPID RESPONSE

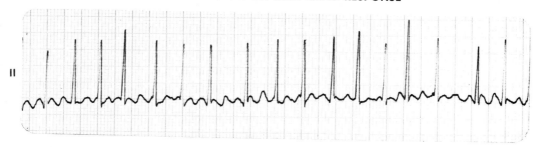

Fig. 13-4. Coarse atrial fibrillatory waves with a rapid ventricular response. This patient had hyperthyroidism. (The commonly used term "rapid atrial fibrillation" is actually a misnomer since "rapid" refers to the ventricular rate rather than the atrial rate. The same is true for "slow atrial fibrillation.")

ATRIAL FIBRILLATION

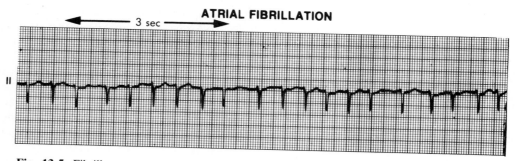

Fig. 13-5. Fibrillatory waves may be hard to find. In this tachyarrhythmia no atrial waves are evident. The ventricular rate is about 140 beats/min and irregular. Although no clear fibrillatory waves are visible here, the rhythm is nevertheless atrial fibrillation.

ATRIAL FIBRILLATION

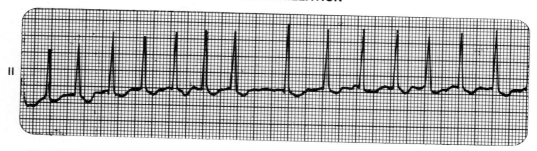

Fig. 13-6. A very irregular ventricular rate is present here. Although no clear P waves can be seen, this rhythm (like the one in Fig. 13-5) is nevertheless atrial fibrillation with a rapid ventricular response.

a fraction to reach the ventricles. In patients with a normal AV junction in whom atrial fibrillation suddenly develops, the ventricular rate is generally 110 to 180 beats/min. Fig. 13-5 shows an example of atrial fibrillation with a ventricular rate of about 140 beats/min. Characteristically, the ventricular rate with atrial fibrillation is haphazardly irregular because the AV junction is being stimulated in an apparently random fashion by the rapidly fibrillating atria.

To summarize: There are two ECG characteristics of atrial fibrillation. First, you will see the irregular wavy baseline produced by the rapid f waves. Second, the ventricular (QRS) rate is usually quite irregular. When the ventricular rate is very fast (Fig. 13-6), it may be difficult to distinguish the f waves. However, in such cases the diagnosis of atrial fibrillation can be made by finding a very irregular ventricular rate in the absence of definite P waves.

General Clinical Aspects

In some patients atrial fibrillation occurs *paroxysmally* and may last for only minutes, hours, or days. In others it is *chronic* and may persist for months or years.

Atrial fibrillation can occur both in normal persons and in patients with a variety of cardiac diseases. Paroxysmal atrial fibrillation is occasionally associated with emotional stress or excessive alcohol consumption in otherwise healthy people. In such cases it often spontaneously reverts to normal sinus rhythm or is converted easily with digitalis alone.

Atrial fibrillation is also one of the most common arrhythmias seen in patients with organic heart disease. Common pathologic causes include coronary artery disease, hypertensive heart disease, and valvular heart disease. Patients with coronary artery disease may go into paroxysmal atrial fibrillation in the course of an acute myocardial infarction. However, usually the fibrillation develops as a consequence of *chronic* ischemic myocardial disease, presumably resulting in atrial dilation or fibrosis. Patients with hypertensive heart disease typically have left ventricular and left atrial enlargement as a result of years of sustained high blood pressure.

Atrial fibrillation is also commonly caused by valvular heart disease, particularly when there is mitral valve involvement. For example, severe mitral stenosis or mitral regurgitation will produce atrial enlargement, predisposing to atrial arrhythmias.

Atrial fibrillation also occurs in other conditions. For example, patients with thyrotoxicosis (hyperthyroidism) may go into atrial fibrillation (Fig. 13-5). Atrial fibrillation (or flutter) is not uncommon following cardiac surgery. It may also occur with chronic pericarditis, pulmonary emboli, cardiomyopathies, and other forms of heart disease.

Clinical Consequences

What happens physiologically when atrial fibrillation develops? Normally, after the P wave, the atria contract and pump blood into the ventricles. With atrial fibrillation, normal atrial depolarization is lost and the atria fibrillate (quiver) instead of contracting synchronously. In these circumstances the normal atrial "kick" is lost, and the result is decreased cardiac output (since ventricular filling is decreased) and sometimes thromboembolization.

Decreased cardiac output. Hemodynamically the most significant effect of atrial fibrillation is decreased cardiac output, which will be especially marked in patients with underlying cardiac impairment and in elderly people, who appear to be more dependent on atrial contraction for filling of the ventricles. In addition, the amount of this decreased output will depend on the ventricular rate with atrial fibrillation. The faster the rate, the more decreased the cardiac output will be. Thus the patient in atrial fibrillation at a rate of 180 beats/min is more likely to be hypotensive or in congestive heart failure than would be the case with a rate of 100 beats/min. In patients with coronary artery disease this rapid ventricular rate can cause myocardial ischemia and even infarction (Chapter 8).

To summarize: Decreased cardiac output with atrial fibrillation reflects two major factors: (1) the loss of normal atrial contractility (atrial kick) and (2) the rapid ventricular rate. The drop in cardiac output with atrial fibrillation (as with any tachyarrhythmia) can produce one (or more) of the following three clinical problems: congestive heart failure, hypotension (even shock), and myocardial ischemia. Initial clinical assessment of the patient in atrial fibrillation must focus on these three areas. Is the patient showing signs of severe congestive failure (difficulty breathing, rales in the chest)? Is the patient's blood pressure low? Is there evidence of myocardial ischemia with anginal chest pain and/or ECG signs of acute ischemia or actual infarction (ST segment depressions or elevations)? *Patients in atrial fibrillation associated with pulmonary edema, hypotension, or acute myocardial ischemia require emergency therapy.*

Atrial thrombi and embolization. The second problem, resulting from the stagnation of blood, is the tendency in some patients for atrial thrombi to develop and dislodge into the arterial circulation, causing peripheral embolism. The thrombi can produce a cerebrovascular accident, occlusion of the blood supply to the legs, and other complications.

Not all patients with chronic atrial fibrillation will have atrial thrombi. The problem seems most common in patients with rheumatic mitral valve disease or cardiomyopathy. Therefore any patient with these disorders who has chronic atrial fibrillation will generally require long-term anticoagulation. The indications for long-term anticoagulation in other patients with chronic (or recurrent paroxysmal) atrial fibrillation are controversial and currently under investigation.

The risk that an atrial thrombus will break off and embolize is also increased when a patient in atrial fibrillation is converted to normal sinus rhythm. The sudden resumption of normal atrial contractions can dislodge part of the atrial clot. For this reason patients with chronic atrial fibrillation are generally anticoagulated for several weeks prior to and following cardioversion.

Treatment

We will not discuss the details of treating atrial fibrillation but instead will focus more broadly on the general clinical approach to patients with this arrhythmia. There are two ways of treating atrial fibrillation. The first is *pharmacologically,* with drugs like digitalis and quinidine. The second is with *electrical cardioversion,* the same as that described for PAT and atrial flutter. Treatment with

drugs generally takes hours or days to convert atrial fibrillation to sinus rhythm. Treatment with electrical cardioversion has an immediate effect. However, patients in chronic atrial fibrillation (present for months or years) may not convert to normal sinus rhythm with any therapy. This is particularly true in cases of chronic rheumatic heart disease with extremely dilated atria that are not capable of normal depolarization. Furthermore, the patient with a very large left atrium or with long-standing atrial fibrillation will often revert to atrial fibrillation eventually, even if electrical cardioversion was initially successful.

There are two major clinical questions to ask in approaching patients with atrial fibrillation. First, is the arrhythmia causing a significant decrease in cardiac output, as indicated by myocardial ischemia, hypotension, or congestive heart failure? Second, is the atrial fibrillation paroxysmal or chronic? As a general rule, patients in paroxysmal atrial fibrillation that is producing myocardial ischemia, shock, or pulmonary edema should be considered candidates for electrical cardioversion if they do not respond promptly to drug therapy. The longer the rapid heart rate persists, the greater will be the chance of irreversible myocardial damage.

In most cases atrial fibrillation does not require immediate electrical cardioversion. Drug therapy alone can be used initially to control the arrhythmia. The mainstay of treating atrial fibrillation with a rapid ventricular response is digitalis. Digitalis acts by slowing conduction of stimuli through the AV junction. In atrial fibrillation, as noted, the junction is being bombarded by stimuli from the atria, which are fibrillating 400 to 600 times/min. The prime clinical concern in patients with atrial fibrillation is to slow the ventricular rate. In patients with atrial fibrillation and a rapid ventricular rate, digitalis given intravenously (or even orally) can generally slow the ventricular rate below 100 beats/min in a matter of hours. Some patients with paroxysmal atrial fibrillation may actually convert to normal sinus rhythm after being given just digitalis. In other cases it is necessary to add a second drug, such as quinidine, to try to restore normal atrial depolarization.

The usual sequence in treating atrial fibrillation

pharmacologically is to slow the ventricular response with digitalis, which blocks the AV junction. If sinus rhythm is not restored after the patient has been digitalized, then quinidine or a related drug* can be started. Quinidine alone may sometimes increase conduction through the AV junction (because of its vagolytic effect). Therefore it should never be given to a patient in atrial fibrillation unless the ventricular rate has first been slowed (usually to less than 100 beats/min) with digitalis or another drug. As in the case of atrial flutter, verapamil, diltiazem, or a beta blocker can also be used in selected patients to help control the ventricular response to atrial fibrillation.

General Approach to the Patient

At the same time that you are starting to treat any patient with atrial fibrillation, you should be thinking of possible causes of this arrhythmia. Search for evidence of coronary artery disease, hypertensive heart disease, cardiomyopathy, valvular disease, or pericardial disease. A blood test of thyroid function should be obtained in a patient with unexplained atrial fibrillation, since thyrotoxicosis

---

*Procainamide and disopyramide have electrophysiologic actions similar to those of quinidine. Newer antiarrhythmics are also available and are currently being evaluated.

is a treatable cause of this arrhythmia. Remember that some patients, including young adults, may go into paroxysmal atrial fibrillation without underlying heart disease. The term *"lone atrial fibrillation"* is sometimes used to describe the condition in which chronic atrial fibrillation develops in such a patient.

Atrial Fibrillation and Other Arrhythmias

Atrial fibrillation may occur with other arrhythmias and conduction disturbances, just as you can have sinus rhythm with PVCs, AV heart block, and so on. Fig. 13-7 shows an example of atrial fibrillation with PVCs. Atrial fibrillation can also occur with complete heart block (Fig. 13-8), and in such cases there is a very slow and regular ventricular response. In any patient with atrial fibrillation and a very slow ventricular rate, always think of possible digitalis toxicity (Chapter 16).

Atrial fibrillation with the Wolff-Parkinson-White syndrome is discussed on p. 226.

Occasionally, it will be difficult to decide whether atrial fibrillation or atrial flutter is present (p. 238). The coarse atrial fibrillatory waves may resemble flutter waves (Fig. 19-3). In some of these cases the arrhythmia is referred to as flutter-fibrillation and has the same clinical significance and treatment as atrial fibrillation.

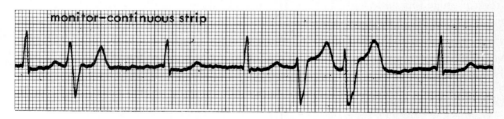

Fig. 13-7. Atrial fibrillation with PVCs.

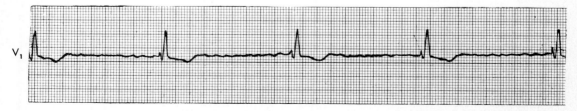

Fig. 13-8. Atrial fibrillation with complete heart block. The ventricular rate is very slow and regular because of the complete AV block.

REVIEW

Paroxysmal atrial tachycardia (PAT), *atrial flutter,* and *atrial fibrillation* are three supraventricular tachycardias that can be considered as parts of a continuum.

The *atrial* rate of *PAT* is generally 140 to 250 beats/min, that of atrial flutter 250 to 350 beats/min, and that of atrial fibrillation 400 to 600 beats/min.

Atrial flutter shows the following:

1. Characteristic sawtooth flutter waves instead of P waves
2. A variable ventricular rate (for example, one QRS complex with every fourth flutter wave, 4:1 flutter; one QRS with every two flutter waves, 2:1 flutter, and the ventricular rate half the atrial rate; or the rare 1:1 flutter, in which the ventricles contract about 300 times a minute)

Atrial flutter rarely occurs in normal hearts but is most often seen in patients with valvular heart disease, ischemic heart disease, lung disease, cardiomyopathy, or pulmonary emboli, and after cardiac surgery. It may be treated with a synchronized DC shock (cardioversion), with drug therapy, or with rapid atrial pacing.

Atrial fibrillation shows the following:

1. Rapid irregular undulations of the baseline (fibrillatory waves) instead of P waves
2. A ventricular rate that is usually grossly irregular (when the patient is given digitalis, the ventricular rate will slow)

In some cases atrial fibrillation occurs chronically. In others it is paroxysmal. Occasionally it is seen in normal people. Common causes are coronary artery disease, hypertensive heart disease, and rheumatic valvular disease. It may also occur with hyperthyroidism, cardiomyopathy, cardiac surgery, pulmonary emboli, and chronic pericarditis. It may be seen with other arrhythmias such as ventricular ectopy or complete heart block. With an extremely slow ventricular rate (50 beats/min or less) it may signify digitalis toxicity.

Paroxysmal atrial fibrillation can be converted to normal sinus rhythm with DC cardioversion or by means of drugs (digitalis, quinidine, or a related agent).

Questions

1. Answer the following questions about the rhythm strip below:
   a. What is the atrial rate?
   b. What is the ventricular rate?
   c. What is this arrhythmia?

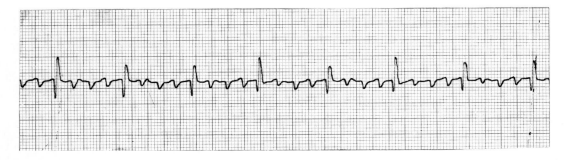

2. Answer the following questions about this rhythm strip:
   a. What is the *average* heart rate?
   b. What is the rhythm?

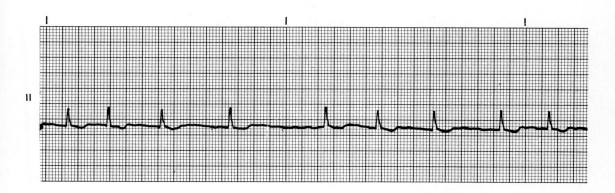

3. The atrial rate with atrial flutter is *(faster, slower)* than the atrial rate with atrial fibrillation.
4. The atrial rate with atrial flutter is *(faster, slower)* than the atrial rate with PAT.
5. The ventricular rate with atrial fibrillation is always greater than 100 beats/min (true or false).

Answers

1. a. About 300 beats/min.
   b. About 75 beats/min.
   c. Atrial flutter with 4:1 AV conduction.
2. a. About 70 beats/min. (Count the number of RR cycles in 6 sec and multiply by 10.)
   b. Atrial fibrillation.
3. Slower.
4. Faster.
5. False.

14

Ventricular Arrhythmias

The three preceding chapters have focused on *supra*ventricular arrhythmias—rhythm disturbances arising in the sinus node, the atria, or the AV junction (node), with normal ventricular depolarization. Now we will discuss another major ECG topic, the ventricular arrhythmias. Ectopic (nonsinus) beats frequently arise in the ventricles themselves, producing premature ventricular contractions, ventricular tachycardia, and sometimes ventricular fibrillation.

PREMATURE VENTRICULAR CONTRACTIONS

Premature ventricular contractions (PVCs)* are premature beats arising in the ventricles, analogous to premature atrial contractions (PACs) and premature junctional contractions (PJCs), which are *supra*ventricular premature beats. Recall that with PACs and PJCs the QRS complex is usually of normal width because the stimulus spreads normally through the bundle branches into the ventricles. With PVCs, on the other hand, the premature beat arises in either the right or the left ventricle. Therefore the ventricles will not be stimulated simultaneously, and the stimulus will spread through the ventricles in an aberrant direction. Thus the QRS complex will be wide with PVCs just as it is with a bundle branch block pattern. Figs. 14-1 to 14-3 show examples.

*In the ECG literature the terms "ventricular premature beat," "ventricular premature depolarization," and "ventricular extrasystole" are also used.

PVCs have two major characteristics:
1. They are premature and occur before the next normal beat is expected.
2. They are aberrant in appearance. The QRS is abnormally wide (usually 0.12 sec or more). The T wave and the QRS usually point in opposite directions.

Features

There are several features of PVCs that are of clinical importance.

Frequency. The frequency of PVCs refers to how many PVCs are seen per minute or per other unit of time. The frequency may range from one isolated PVC to many. As we will discuss, the difference between an occasional PVC and multiple PVCs may be the difference between no treatment and emergency therapy.

PVCs may occur in various combinations. For example, two PVCs occurring consecutively (Fig. 14-4) are referred to as a *pair*, or *couplet*. Three PVCs in a row are, by definition, *ventricular tachycardia*, discussed later in this chapter (Fig. 14-5). Sometimes, as shown in Fig. 14-6, *A*, PVCs occur so frequently that each normal beat is followed by a PVC. This produces a distinctive repetitive grouping of one normal beat–one PVC, with the sequence repeated several times. Such a pattern is called *ventricular bigeminy*. The sequence of two normal beats with a PVC is *ventricular trigeminy* (Fig. 14-6).

Coupling interval. The term "coupling inter-

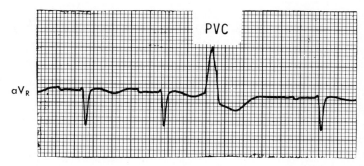

Fig. 14-1. A premature ventricular contraction is recognized because it comes before the next normal beat is expected and has a wide aberrant shape. (Also notice the long PR interval in the normal sinus beats, indicating first-degree AV block.)

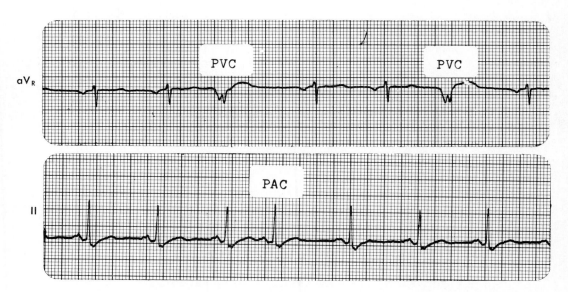

Fig. 14-2. Notice the wide aberrant shapes of premature ventricular contractions compared to the more narrow ones of PACs.

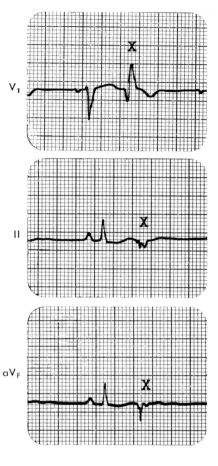

Fig. 14-3. Notice that the same premature ventricular contraction (**X**) recorded simultaneously in three different leads shows different shapes. Compare this with Fig. 14-9, illustrating multiform PVCs that show different shapes in the same lead.

Monitor lead

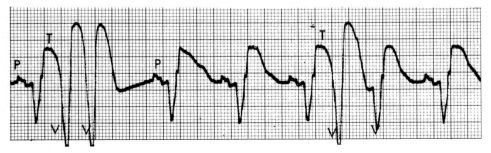

Fig. 14-4. Two premature ventricular contractions (**V**) are termed "paired PVCs" or a "couplet." These also show the R on T phenomenon. (See text and Fig. 14-10.)

VENTRICULAR TACHYCARDIA

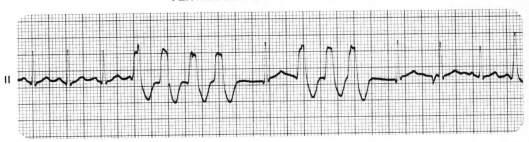

Fig. 14-5. Notice the two short bursts of ventricular tachycardia, defined as three or more consecutive PVCs.

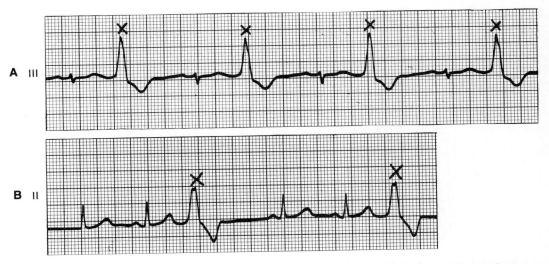

Fig. 14-6. Ventricular premature contractions. **A,** Ventricular bigeminy. Each normal sinus beat is followed by a PVC (marked **X**). **B,** Ventricular trigeminy. After every two sinus beats a PVC occurs.

val'' is frequently used and refers to the interval between the PVC and the preceding normal beat. In many cases, when there are multiple PVCs, there is *fixed coupling,* the coupling interval being approximately the same for each PVC (Fig. 14-6). At other times PVCs may show a *variable coupling interval.* Clinically, fixed and variably coupled PVCs are generally treated in the same fashion.

Compensatory pause. As you may have noticed, PACs and PVCs are usually followed by a pause before the next normal beat. The pause may be longer than the pause following a PAC, but there are exceptions. A fully compensatory pause (Fig. 14-7) indicates that the interval between the normal QRS complexes immediately before and immediately after the PVC is exactly twice the basic RR interval. A fully compensatory pause is more characteristic of PVCs than of PACs. Sometimes a PVC will fall almost exactly between two normal beats, and in such cases is said to be *interpolated* (Fig. 14-8).

FULLY COMPENSATORY PAUSE

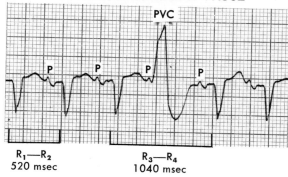

Fig. 14-7. Some PVCs cause a fully conpensatory pause—the interval between the two sinus beats that surround the PVC (R_3 and R_4 in this case) being exactly two times the normal interval between sinus beats (R_1 and R_2). Notice that the P waves come on time, except that the third P wave is interrupted by the PVC and therefore does not conduct normally through the AV junction. The next (fourth) P wave also comes on time. The fact that the sinus node is continuing to pace despite the PVC results in the fully compensatory pause.

INTERPOLATED PVC

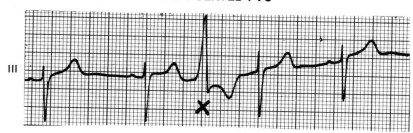

Fig. 14-8. Sometimes a PVC (marked X here) will fall between two normal beats, in which case it is *interpolated*.

Uniform and multiform PVCs. Premature beats arising from an ectopic focus in the ventricles may be *uniform* or *multiform*. These terms are used to describe the appearance of PVCs in a lead. Uniform PVCs, as the name implies, have the same appearance in any lead and arise from the same focus (Fig. 14-6). (They will, of course, have different shapes in different leads, just as any normal beat can.) By contrast, multiform PVCs have different morphologies in the same lead (Fig. 14-9). Multiform PVCs often, but not always, arise from different foci. Uniform PVCs are uni*focal* whereas multi*form* PVCs are not necessarily multi*focal*. Uniform PVCs may occur in healthy people or in persons with underlying organic heart disease. Multiform PVCs usually indicate organic heart disease.

R on T phenomenon. The "R on T" or "PVC on T" phenomenon refers to PVCs that are timed so they fall near the peak* of the T wave of the preceding normal beat (Fig. 14-10). PVCs falling on the T wave in this way are significant because

---

*Or at the nadir of a negative T wave.

MULTIFORM PVCs

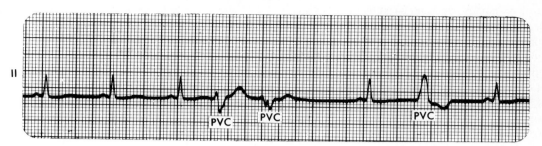

Fig. 14-9. Multiform PVCs here have different shapes in the same lead. (Compare with Fig. 14-3.)

R ON T PHENOMENON

Monitor lead

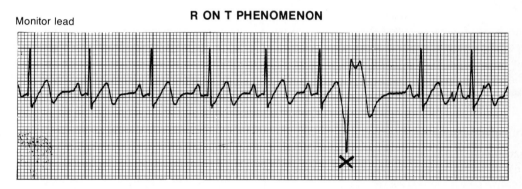

Fig. 14-10. A PVC (marked X) falling near the peak of the T wave of the preceding beat may predispose to ventricular tachycardia or ventricular fibrillation. PVCs exhibiting this R on T (PVC on T) timing should be treated, particularly when they occur in the setting of acute MI.

they may precipitate ventricular tachycardia or ventricular fibrillation, particularly in the course of acute myocardial infarction. Recall from our discussion of synchronized DC cardioversion (p. 164) that the peak of the T wave is a time during which an external stimulus is especially likely to produce ventricular tachycardia or fibrillation. However, ventricular tachycardia and ventricular fibrillation commonly occur without a preceding "R on T" beat, and not every "R on T" beat will precipitate a ventricular tachyarrhythmia.

Clinical Significance

PVCs are among the most commonly seen arrhythmias. They may occur both in normal people and in patients with serious organic heart disease. They may be a stable and benign finding, or the precursor of cardiac arrest and sudden death from ventricular fibrillation. Clearly, the physician needs certain ground rules to help decide which PVCs require treatment and which do not. A few general principles will be discussed here.

As mentioned, PVCs are not uncommon in normal people in all age groups. Young adults, for example, may have them because of anxiety or excessive caffeine intake. Certain drugs, such as epinephrine, isoproterenol, and aminophylline (all used in asthmatics), can provoke PVCs in normal hearts. Nevertheless, finding frequent PVCs should always prompt a careful search for underlying cardiac disease (heart murmurs, abnormal echocardiographic findings, etc.) and a careful drug history. Occasional unifocal PVCs in an otherwise healthy person are not usually a source of concern. PVCs are common in subjects with mitral valve prolapse and may also be seen with virtually any type of heart disease. For example, patients with valvular heart disease, hypertensive heart disease, or ischemic heart disease with or without myocardial infarction may have them. PVCs are the most common arrhythmia seen with acute myocardial infarction and may be a precursor of ventricular tachycardia and ventricular fibrillation.

PVCs, as noted, can be caused by the toxic effects on the heart of numerous drugs (such as epinephrine, isoproterenol, and aminophylline, which are cardiac stimulants). Ventricular ectopy is also an important sign of digitalis toxicity (discussed in Chapter 16). PVCs may be seen with electrolyte disturbances, such as hypokalemia or hypomagnesemia, and in patients with lung disease or hypoxemia from any cause.

Treatment

Treatment of PVCs depends on several considerations. In every case a search should be made for possibly reversible causes. Elimination of caffeine, certain drugs, and anxiety may be effective therapy in patients with occasional PVCs. Judicious administration of oxygen to hypoxemic patients or treatment of anemia, hypokalemia, or hypomagnesemia may be sufficient in appropriate cases. Withholding digitalis and checking the serum digoxin level are mandatory in any patient who develops PVCs while taking digitalis.

PVCs occurring during *acute* myocardial infarction are of particular concern because of the increased risk of ventricular tachycardia and ventricular fibrillation in this setting. As a general rule, patients with frequent PVCs (greater than five per minute), paired PVCs (two in a row), multifocal PVCs, or PVCs showing an R on T phenomenon should be treated immediately with an intravenous drug such as lidocaine or procainamide. Some cardiologists believe that even a single PVC occurring in a patient with an acute MI should

be similarly treated. In addition, some cardiologists recommend prophylactic administration of lidocaine to certain patients with acute MI because ventricular fibrillation may occur without any "warning" arrhythmia.

Drug Therapy

The use of antiarrhythmic drugs in patients with frequent PVCs, including short runs of ventricular tachycardia, who do not have acute myocardial infarction or ischemia is controversial and a matter of active investigation. As noted, PVCs may be seen in otherwise healthy people. Even in patients with underlying asymptomatic heart disease, there is no evidence that suppression of frequent isolated PVCs or short runs of ventricular tachycardia with drugs improves survival. Perhaps most important is the fact that drugs (such as quinidine, procainamide, disopyramide, mexiletine, tocainide, encainide, and flecainide) used to treat PVCs all have important and sometimes life-threatening side effects. Furthermore, not only do these drugs sometimes fail to suppress the ventricular ectopy, they also may actually make the situation worse by paradoxically increasing the severity of the ectopy (*proarrhythmic effect*). In some patients treatment with "antiarrhythmic" drugs can actually provoke a possibly fatal ventricular tachyarrhythmia.

For more complete discussion of these complex therapeutic issues the reader is referred to the Bibliography. It should be emphasized again that whenever you are confronted by a patient with frequent PVCs it is always important to search for potentially reversible causes (in particular, hypokalemia, hypomagnesemia, and certain drugs). Correcting metabolic problems or drug effects may obviate the need to treat the patient with additional, potentially toxic, medications.

VENTRICULAR TACHYCARDIA

PVCs are important primarily because they may be a precursor of sustained ventricular tachycardia and ventricular fibrillation, which are life-threatening arrhythmias. *Ventricular tachycardia is, by definition, simply a run of three or more consec-*

utive PVCs. Examples are shown in Figs. 14-5 and 14-11 to 14-13. Ventricular tachycardia may occur as a single isolated burst, may recur paroxysmally, or may persist for a long run. The heart rate is generally between 100 and 200 beats/min but may be faster.

Sustained ventricular tachycardia (lasting more than 30 sec) is a life-threatening arrhythmia for two major reasons. First, most patients are not able to maintain an adequate blood pressure at very rapid ventricular rates and quickly become hypotensive. Second, the condition may degenerate into ventricular fibrillation (Fig. 14-14).

Very rapid ventricular tachycardia with a sine-wave appearance is sometimes referred to as *ventricular flutter* and often leads to ventricular fibrillation (Fig. 14-15).

Treatment

There are two aspects to the treatment of ventricular tachyarrhythmias. The first is preventive. Treatment of malignant PVCs in patients with acute MI may be prophylactic against future bouts of ventricular tachycardia or particularly ventricular fibrillation. The second is suppressive. Patients with acute MI who are having frequent PVCs or intermittent runs of ventricular tachycardia generally require emergency administration of an intravenous antiarrhythmic drug, such as lidocaine, to attempt to suppress the ventricular ectopy.

Occasionally you will be required to treat a patient having a sustained run of very rapid ventricular tachycardia who is becoming hypotensive and losing consciousness. In such cases you can try giving the patient a sharp punch to the midsternum

PAROXYSMAL VENTRICULAR TACHYCARDIA

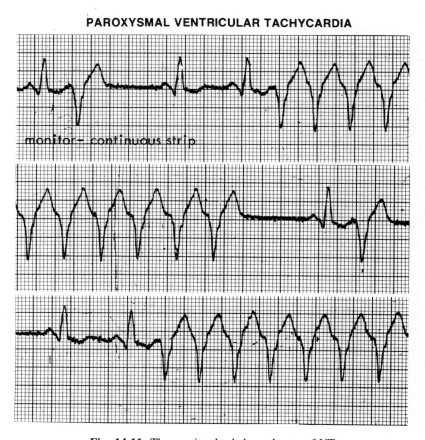

Fig. 14-11. The monitor lead shows bursts of VT.

SUSTAINED VENTRICULAR TACHYCARDIA TERMINATED BY DC SHOCK

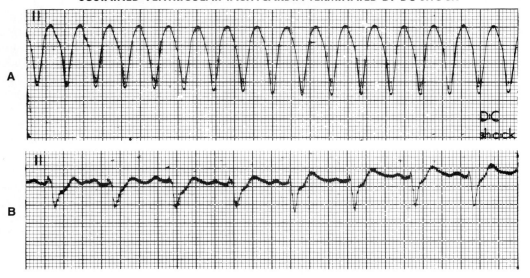

Fig. 14-12. A, Long run of VT. **B,** Normal sinus rhythm restored after direct current cardioversion.

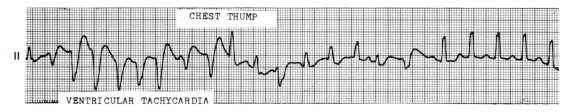

Fig. 14-13. VT terminated by a thump on the chest (''thump version'').

VENTRICULAR FIBRILLATION

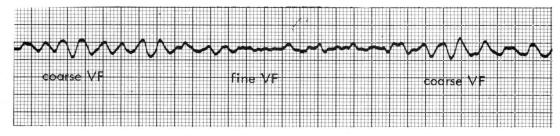

Fig. 14-14. VF may produce both coarse and fine waves. Immediate defibrillation should be performed.

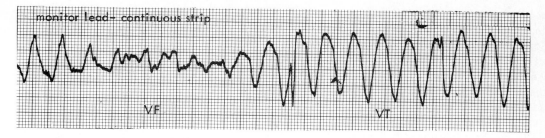

Fig. 14-15. Ventricular fibrillation (*VF*) and rapid ventricular tachycardia (*VT*) occurring together. This type of VT is sometimes referred to as ventricular flutter.

with your clenched fist. This treatment, termed *"thump version"* (Fig. 14-13) (p. 213, footnote), may restore a normal heart rhythm by itself in a case of ventricular tachycardia. While thump version is being tried, the electrical cardioverter should be charged up; if the thump does not restore normal rhythm, the patient must be given a DC shock. Immediately preceding or following electrical cardioversion, the patient should be started on intravenous medication to suppress further ectopy and the cause of the ventricular tachycardia should be carefully sought.

Causes

The etiologic factors of ventricular tachycardia are the same as those discussed earlier with PVCs. The same list of reversible causes of PVCs also applies in evaluating patients with ventricular tachycardia.

Sustained ventricular tachycardia, which may lead to syncope or sudden death, rarely occurs in patients without demonstrable heart disease. Most patients with this type of high-grade ventricular ectopy have some underlying structural cardiac abnormality, most commonly prior MI or some type of cardiomyopathy. Only some of these patients can be successfully managed with antiarrhythmic drug therapy. Others with refractory ventricular tachycardia will require one of the *nonpharmacologic* modalities mentioned on p. 190.

Differential Diagnosis

Ventricular tachycardia is one of the major tachyarrhythmias. In preceding chapters we saw several other important tachycardias—sinus tachycardia, paroxysmal atrial tachycardia, atrial fibrillation, and atrial flutter. These are all examples of *supraventricular tachycardias*. The differentiation of ventricular tachycardia from these supraventricular tachyarrhythmias is described in Chapter 18.

VENTRICULAR FIBRILLATION

With ventricular fibrillation (Figs. 14-14 and 14-15) the ventricles do not beat in any coordinated fashion but instead fibrillate or quiver asynchronously and ineffectively. There is no cardiac output, and the patient becomes unconscious immediately. Ventricular fibrillation is one of the three major ECG patterns seen with cardiac arrest. The other two are *asystole* and *electromechanical dissociation* (Chapter 17).

The ECG in ventricular fibrillation shows characteristic fibrillatory waves with an irregular pattern that may be either coarse or fine (Fig. 14-14).

Ventricular fibrillation requires immediate defibrillation with an unsynchronized DC shock. Patients who have had runs of ventricular tachycardia or ventricular fibrillation should also be given an immediate dose of an intravenous drug such as lidocaine or procainamide to suppress further ventricular ectopy. Another antiarrhythmic agent, bretylium tosylate, is sometimes effective in treating and preventing ventricular fibrillation.

This tachyarrhythmia can occur in patients with heart disease of any type. It may be preceded by a warning arrhythmia (such as PVCs or ventricular tachycardia) or may occur spontaneously. It is the most common cause of sudden death in patients with an acute MI, although it may occur in normal hearts as well because of drugs (like epinephrine or cocaine), lightning injury, or accidental electrocution.

Some patients, usually those with severe organic heart disease, will have multiple recurrences of sustained ventricular tachycardia or ventricular fibrillation despite aggressive medical therapy. For these individuals a special device, called the *automatic implantable cardioverter defibrillator (AICD)*, has been developed to deliver an electric shock directly to the heart during a life-threatening tachycardia. The generator is implanted under the abdominal wall and attached to an electrode patch sewn to the outer surface of the ventricle. Readers interested in the AICD as well as in other *nonpharmacologic modalities* for treating refractory arrhythmias (surgery, anti-tachycardia pace-

makers, catheter ablation techniques) should consult the Bibliography and other more specialized sources.

ACCELERATED IDIOVENTRICULAR RHYTHM

Figs. 14-16 and 14-17 present a distinctive arrhythmia that has been called "accelerated idioventricular rhythm" (AIVR) or "slow ventricular tachycardia." Recall that with typical ventricular tachycardia the heart rate is generally faster than 100 to 110 beats/min. With AIVR it is usually between 50 and 100 to 110 beats/min, and the ECG shows wide QRS complexes without P waves. (The cutoff between AIVR and ventricular tachycardia based on heart rate is arbitrary, and different au-

ACCELERATED IDIOVENTRICULAR RHYTHM

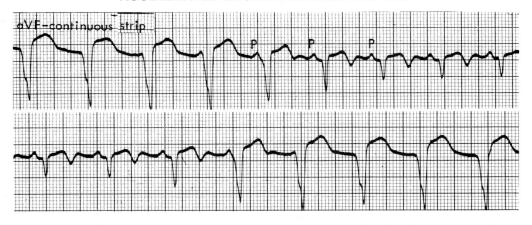

Fig. 14-16. AIVR in a case of inferior wall myocardial infarction. The first four beats show the typical pattern, followed by a return of sinus rhythm, then the reappearance of AIVR.

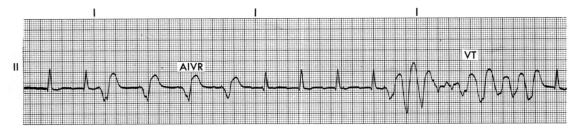

Fig. 14-17. Accelerated idioventricular rhythm (*AIVR*) and ventricular tachycardia (*VT*) occurring together. Notice the similarity between them, but the rate in AIVR is slower.

thors use slightly different rate criteria.)

AIVR is particularly common with acute myocardial infarction. It is generally short lived, lasting for minutes or less, and usually requires no specific therapy. Treatment (for example, with lidocaine) is indicated if it occurs with actual ventricular tachycardia (Fig. 14-17), particularly in the setting of acute MI.

In some cases (Fig. 14-16) AIVR appears to be a benign escape rhythm that competes with the underlying sinus mechanism. When the sinus rate slows, AIVR appears; and when the sinus rate speeds up, the arrhythmia disappears. In other cases (Fig. 14-17) AIVR is initiated by premature beats rather than by escape beats. This latter type of AIVR is more likely to be associated with actual ventricular tachycardia.

TORSADE DE POINTES: A SPECIAL FORM OF VENTRICULAR TACHYCARDIA

A special type of ventricular tachycardia has been called "torsade de pointes," a French term meaning "twisting of the points." Fig. 14-18 shows an example of this distinctive tachycardia. Notice how the vector of the QRS complexes appears to rotate cyclically, pointing downward for several beats and then twisting and pointing upward in the same lead.

Torsade de pointes is important because of its diagnostic and therapeutic implications. As shown in Fig. 14-18, it classically occurs in the setting of delayed ventricular repolarization, evidenced by *prolongation of the QT intervals or the presence*

of prominent U waves. Reported causes include
1. Drug toxicity, particularly that due to quinidine (quinidine syncope, p. 127) and related antiarrhythmic agents (disopyramide and procainamide) as well as psychotropic drugs (phenothiazines and tricyclic antidepressants)
2. Electrolyte imbalance, including hypokalemia, hypomagnesemia, and hypocalcemia, which prolong repolarization
3. Miscellaneous factors such as severe bradyarrhythmias, hereditary QT prolongation syndromes, liquid protein diets, and myocardial ischemia

Recognition of torsade is critical because it is often caused by drugs conventionally recommended in treating ventricular tachycardia (such as quinidine or procainamide). Therapy of torsade therefore should include removing or correcting causative factors (drug toxicity, electrolyte imbalance). In emergency settings a temporary pacemaker may be inserted to accomplish "overdrive" suppression of the arrhythmia by increasing the underlying heart rate and thereby decreasing ventricular repolarization time. Drug therapy with bretylium tosylate, isoproterenol, or lidocaine may be useful in selected cases. Sustained episodes of torsade require attempted cardioversion. However, the arrhythmia will often recur unless causative factors (drug effect, electrolyte imbalance, underlying bradycardia) are corrected. For further discussion of this important topic, readers are referred to the Bibliography.

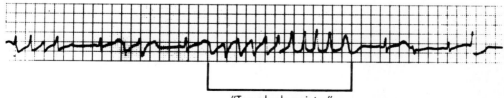

"Torsade de pointes"
ventricular tachycardia

Fig. 14-18. Notice the shifting polarity and amplitude of the QRS complexes during a bout of ventricular tachycardia. This is the hallmark of torsade de pointes. There is also QT prolongation (0.52 sec) in the normal sinus beats.

REVIEW

PVCs have the following characteristics:
1. They are premature and occur before the next normal beat is expected.
2. They have an aberrant shape. The QRS is abnormally wide, usually 0.12 second or more in duration, and the T wave and QRS usually point in opposite directions.

PVCs may occur with varying *frequency*. Two in a row are called a *couplet*. Three in a row are *ventricular tachycardia*. When a PVC occurs regularly after each normal beat, this is called *ventricular bigeminy*. When the rhythm is two normal beats followed by a PVC, this is *ventricular trigeminy*.

A PVC is often followed by a compensatory pause before the next beat.

Uniform PVCs have the same shape in a single lead. *Multiform* PVCs have different shapes in the same lead.

When PVC occurs simultaneously with the apex of the T wave of the preceding beat, this is called an *R on T phenomenon*. It may be the precursor of ventricular tachycardia or ventricular fibrillation, particularly in the setting of acute MI.

PVCs may occur both normally and in patients with organic heart disease.

Treatment of PVCs depends on several considerations. Look for reversible causes (hypoxemia, congestive heart failure, digitalis toxicity or toxicity due to other drugs, hypokalemia, or hypomagnesemia). Frequent PVCs in the presence of acute MI should be promptly suppressed.

Ventricular tachycardia is a run of three or more PVCs. *Sustained* ventricular tachycardia refers to episodes lasting more than 30 seconds, which may lead to syncope or even cardiac arrest.

Ventricular fibrillation occurs when the ventricles stop beating and, instead, fibrillate or twitch in an ineffective fashion. It is one of the three major ECG patterns seen with cardiac arrest; the other two are *asystole* and *electromechanical dissociation* (Chapter 17).

Accelerated indioventricular rhythm (AIVR) is a ventricular arrhythmia that resembles a slow ventricular tachycardia with a rate between 50 and 100 to 110 beats/min. It is commonly seen with myocardial infarction and is usually self-limited.

Torsade de pointes is the name of a form of ventricular tachycardia in which the QRS complexes in the same lead appear to twist periodically and turn in the opposite direction. It is generally seen in the setting of delayed ventricular repolarization (increased QT interval or prominent U waves) due to drugs (quinidine), electrolyte abnormalities (hypokalemia, hypomagnesemia), or other factors.

Questions

1. What is the arrhythmia shown below?

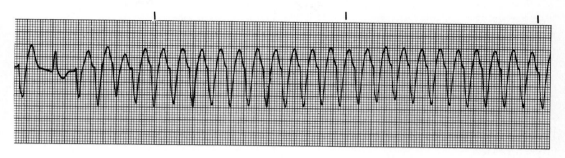

2. Which arrhythmia does this rhythm strip show?

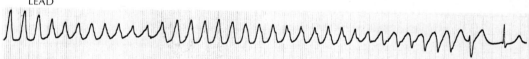

MONITOR
LEAD

3. Name three potentially treatable causes of PVCs.
4. What is the rhythm here?

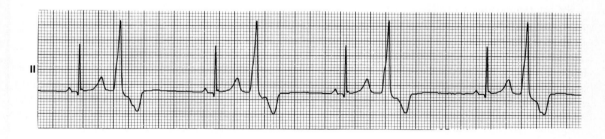

II

Answers

1. Ventricular tachycardia.
2. Torsade de pointes. Notice the changing orientation and amplitude of the QRS complexes. Contrast this with the ECG in Question 1, where all QRS complexes are the same.
3. Hypoxemia, digitalis toxicity, hypokalemia, hypomagnesemia, and so on. (See p. 186.)
4. Sinus rhythm with ventricular bigeminy.

15

AV Heart Block

Heart block is the general term for atrioventricular (AV) conduction disturbances. Normally, the AV junction (node) acts like an apparent bridge between the atria and the ventricles. The PR interval, as mentioned earlier, is primarily a measure of the lag in AV conduction between the initial stimulation of the atria and the initial stimulation of the ventricles. The normal PR interval is between 0.12 and 0.2 second. Heart block occurs when there is impaired transmission through the AV junction, either transiently or permanently. The mildest form is called *first-degree heart block*. Here the PR interval is simply prolonged above 0.2 second. *Second-degree heart block* is an intermediate grade of AV conduction disturbance. The most extreme form is *third-degree* or *complete heart block*. Here the AV junction does not conduct any stimuli between the atria and ventricles. These three degrees of heart block are described in this chapter, along with the related topic *AV dissociation*.

FIRST-DEGREE HEART BLOCK

With first-degree heart block the PR interval is prolonged above 0.2 second and is constant from beat to beat (Fig. 15-1).

First-degree heart block does not produce any symptoms or any significant change in cardiac function. There are numerous causes, and most factors that produce first-degree AV block can also produce second- and third-degree block. For example, digitalis, which has a vagal effect on the AV junction, can produce any degree of heart block. Other drugs such as quinidine, any of the numerous beta blockers, and the calcium blockers (verapamil and diltiazem) can also cause severe depression of AV conduction.

Patients with ischemic heart disease may have heart block of any degree. This may occur with chronic myocardial ischemia over a long time or with an acute myocardial infarction. Varying degrees of heart block are particularly common with inferior wall infarction because the right coronary artery, which generally supplies the inferior wall, also usually supplies the AV junction. In addition, acute inferior MI is often associated with increased vagal tone. Heart block during inferior wall infarction tends to be transient.

Hyperkalemia may cause first-degree heart block. Other signs of hyperkalemia (as mentioned in Chapter 10) include peaking of the T waves and widening of the QRS complexes. First-degree AV block may occur with acute rheumatic fever. Occasionally first-degree AV block may be seen in normal persons.

SECOND-DEGREE AV BLOCK

Second-degree AV block is somewhat more complicated because there are two types—Mobitz type I (also called Wenckebach block) and Mobitz type II. Despite this imposing nomenclature, the two types of second-degree block are actually not too difficult to understand.

FIRST DEGREE AV BLOCK

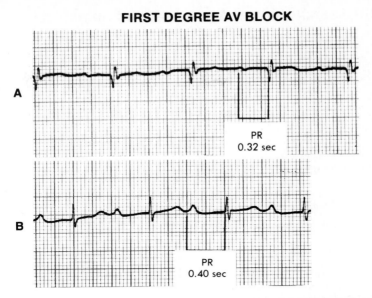

Fig. 15-1. With first-degree AV block the PR interval is uniformly prolonged above 0.2 second with each beat. **A** and **B** are from different patients.

Mobitz Type I (Wenckebach) AV Block

With the Wenckebach pattern, each stimulus from the atria to the ventricles appears to have a more difficult time passing through the AV junction. Finally, a point is reached where the stimulus is not conducted at all. This *blocked beat* is followed by relative recovery of the AV junction, and the whole cycle starts again.

The characteristic ECG picture of Wenckebach block therefore is a progressive lengthening of the PR interval from beat to beat until finally a beat is "dropped." The dropped beat is a P wave that is not followed by a QRS complex, indicating failure of the AV junction to conduct the stimulus from the atria to the ventricles. Fig. 15-2 diagrammatically depicts the Wenckebach phenomenon, and Fig. 15-3 shows an actual example of this pattern. The number of P waves occurring before a beat is dropped may vary. In many cases it will be just two or three. What characterizes the Wenckebach pattern is the general sequence of a progressive lengthening of the PR interval followed by a dropped beat.

As you can see from the examples, the Wenckebach cycle also produces a distinct clustering of QRS complexes separated by a pause that results from the dropped beat. Any time you encounter an ECG with this type of *group beating,* suspect a Wenckebach block and look for the diagnostic pattern of lengthening PR intervals.

Clinically patients with the Wenckebach type of AV block are usually without symptoms unless the ventricular rate is very slow. The pulse rate is irregular.

Common causes of Wenckebach block include drugs (digitalis, beta blockers, calcium channel blockers [diltiazem and verapamil]) and ischemic heart disease. Wenckebach block is not uncommon with acute inferior wall infarction. In such cases it is usually transient and generally does not require any specific treatment except for observation, since these patients may progress into complete heart block. Of note, Wenckebach AV block may also occur in athletes at rest, due to a physiologic increase in vagal tone.

WENCKEBACH (MOBITZ TYPE I) SECOND-DEGREE AV BLOCK

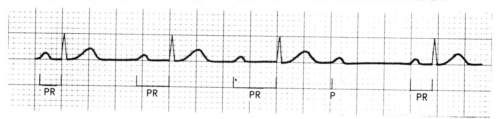

Fig. 15-2. The PR interval lengthens progressively with successive beats until one P wave is not conducted at all. Then the cycle repeats itself.

WENCKEBACH (MOBITZ TYPE I) SECOND-DEGREE AV BLOCK

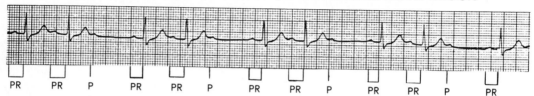

Fig. 15-3. Notice the progressive increase in PR intervals, with the third P wave in each sequence not followed by a QRS. Wenckebach block produces a characteristically syncopated rhythm with grouping of the QRS complexes *(group beating)*.

MOBITZ TYPE II SECOND-DEGREE AV BLOCK

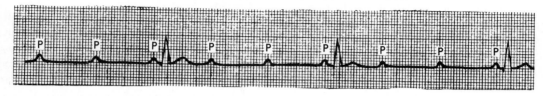

Fig. 15-4. With Mobitz type II block there is a series of nonconducted P waves followed by a P wave that is conducted. In this diagrammatic example 3:1 AV block is present, with three P waves for each QRS complex. The QRS is wide (0.12 sec). (See also Fig. 20-10.)

Mobitz Type II AV Block

Mobitz type II AV block is a rarer and more severe form of second-degree AV block. In most cases the QRS complexes of the conducted beats are wide ($\geq$0.12 sec) due to involvement of the His-Purkinje system and not just the AV node. The characteristic features of Mobitz type II AV block are shown in Fig. 15-4. As you can see, there is a series of nonconducted P waves followed by a P wave that is conducted. For example, with 3:1 block every third P wave is conducted to the ventricles. With 4:1 block every fourth P wave is followed by a QRS complex. Fig. 20-11 shows 2:1 block involving the His-Purkinje system rather than just the AV node.*

Mobitz type II AV block is generally a sign of severe conduction system disease. Since patients with this form of block often progress into complete heart block, cardiologists generally consider this an indication for a pacemaker. Unlike Wenckebach (Mobitz type I) block, Mobitz type II is *not* usually seen with digitalis excess or with inferior wall infarction. However, Mobitz type II may be seen with anterior wall MI, and these patients often progress into complete heart block. Therefore cardiologists generally treat a patient with an anterior wall infarction and Mobitz type II AV block by inserting a pacemaker.

THIRD-DEGREE (COMPLETE) HEART BLOCK

First- and second-degree heart blocks are examples of *incomplete* block because the AV junction

---

*A point of common confusion: It should be noted that 2:1 AV block per se does not always indicate a Mobitz type II block. Not uncommonly 2:1 AV block is due to a Wenckebach (Mobitz I) mechanism in which the block simply occurs after every other P wave. In such cases careful search of a long rhythm strip will often reveal 3:2, 4:3, etc. types of Wenckebach in addition to the 2:1 periods. Furthermore, in most (but not all) cases of AV Wenckebach the QRS complex is of normal duration. By contrast, when 2:1 is due to a Mobitz II mechanism the His-Purkinje system (not just the AV node) is involved and the QRS duration is usually prolonged. Thus 2:1 block with a narrow QRS most likely represents AV Wenckebach. However, 2:1 block with a wide QRS and no other evidence of Wenckebach periodicity is likely Mobitz II, which carries a more serious prognosis for progression to complete heart block.

does conduct stimuli, albeit intermittently, to the ventricles. With complete heart block, there is no transmission of stimuli from the atria to the ventricles. Instead, the atria and the ventricles are paced independently. With complete heart block, atrial and ventricular depolarizations are completely independent. The atria generally continue to be paced by the sinus node. The ventricles, however, are paced by an escape pacemaker located somewhere below the point of block in the AV junction. The ventricular rate with complete heart block may be lower than 30 or as high as 60 beats/min. The atrial rate is generally faster than the ventricular rate.

Examples of complete heart block are shown in Figs. 15-5 and 15-6. The ECG with complete heart block has the following characteristics:

1. P waves are present, with a regular atrial rate faster than the ventricular rate.
2. QRS complexes are present, with a slow (usually fixed) ventricular rate.
3. The P waves bear no relation to the QRS complexes, and the PR intervals are completely variable since the atria and ventricles are electrically disconnected.
4. Complete heart block may occur in a patient whose basic atrial rhythm is flutter or fibrillation. In these patients the ventricular rate is slow and almost completely regular (Fig. 13-8).

With complete heart block the QRS complexes may be either of normal width (Fig. 15-5) or abnormally wide (Fig. 15-6) with the appearance of a bundle branch block pattern. The width of the QRS complexes depends in part on the location of the blockage in the AV junction. If the block is in the first part (the AV node), the ventricles will be stimulated normally by a junctional pacemaker and the QRS complexes will be narrow (Fig. 15-5) unless the patient has an underlying bundle branch block. If the block is lower in the AV junction (bundle of His), the ventricles will be paced by an *idioventricular pacemaker,* producing wide QRS complexes resembling those of a bundle branch block pattern (Fig. 15-6). As a general clinical rule complete heart block with wide QRS complexes tends to be less stable than complete heart block

THIRD-DEGREE (COMPLETE) AV BLOCK

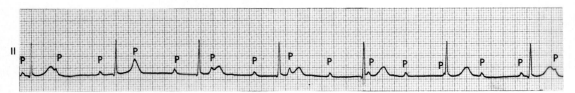

Fig. 15-5. Complete heart block is characterized by independent atrial (P) and ventricular (QRS) activity. The atrial rate is always faster than the ventricular rate. The PR intervals are completely variable. Some P waves fall on the T wave, distorting the shape of the T wave. Other P waves may fall in the QRS complex and be "lost." Notice that the QRS complexes are of normal width, indicating that the ventricles are being paced from the AV junction. Compare this with Fig. 15-6, an example of complete heart block with wide QRS complexes because the ventricles are being paced from below the AV junction (idioventricular pacemaker).

THIRD-DEGREE (COMPLETE) AV BLOCK

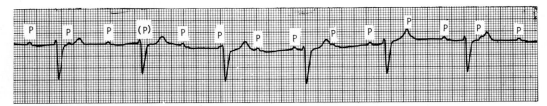

Fig. 15-6. Another example of complete heart block, showing a slow idioventricular rhythm and a faster independent atrial (sinus) rhythm.

with narrow QRS complexes, since the ventricular rate is usually slower.

Complete heart block can occur for a number of reasons. It is most commonly seen in older patients who have chronic degenerative changes in their conduction systems *not* related to an acute myocardial infarction. Such chronic degenerative conduction disease is the most common cause of complete heart block. Digitalis intoxication, which can cause first- and second-degree heart block, may also lead to complete heart block (Chapter 16). Varying degrees of AV block, including some cases of complete block, have been reported with Lyme disease (arthritis).

Complete heart block may be seen acutely as a complication of myocardial infarction. The course

and therapy of complete heart block with MI depend to a large extent on whether the infarct is anterior or inferior. Transient AV conduction disturbances are commonly seen with acute inferior wall MI because of the common blood supply to the AV junction and inferior wall (via the right coronary artery). Occlusion of the right coronary artery with inferior MI also often leads to temporary ischemia of the AV junction, sometimes resulting in complete heart block. (In addition, acute inferior MI may cause an increase in vagal tone.) Complete heart block occurring with inferior wall MI is often a transient and reversible complication that may respond to atropine and therefore not require a temporary pacemaker.

With acute anterior myocardial infarction and

complete heart block, the situation is more serious. Patients with anterior wall and complete heart block generally have extensive myocardial damage. The idioventricular escape rhythm that develops is usually slow and unstable. Therefore, if complete heart block occurs with an acute anterior MI, the cardiologist will generally insert a temporary pacemaker (and subsequently a permanent one).

Regardless of its cause, complete heart block is a serious and potentially life-threatening arrhythmia. If the ventricular rate becomes too slow, the cardiac output will drop and the patient may faint. Fainting spells associated with complete heart block (or other types of bradycardia) are referred to as *Stokes-Adams attacks*. In some patients complete heart block is a chronic and persistent finding. In others the block may occur transiently and be recognized only with continuous ambulatory (Holter) monitoring for a period of 24 hours or longer.

Complete heart block resulting from digitalis toxicity or acute inferior MI is often transient and can sometimes be treated medically without insertion of a pacemaker. However, chronic complete heart block (or intermittent complete heart block not due to some reversible cause) calls for an implanted (permanent) pacemaker (Chapter 20).

BIFASCICULAR BLOCKS AND COMPLETE HEART BLOCK

Cardiologists have been interested in developing criteria to predict which patients with acute myocardial infarction (particularly anterior wall infarcts) will go on to complete heart block. Current information suggests that certain high-risk patients can be identified. Specifically, it has been found that patients with an acute anterior wall MI and complete heart block often have other conduction disturbances before the onset of the heart block: (1) new left bundle branch block, (2) new right bundle branch block with left axis deviation, or (3) new right bundle branch block with right axis deviation. These are all examples of *bifascicular blocks*.

Recall, from Chapter 7, that the ventricular conduction system is trifascicular, consisting of the right bundle branch and the left bundle branch, the latter further dividing into left anterior and left posterior fascicles. Blockage of just the left anterior fascicle produces left anterior hemiblock with left axis deviation. Blockage of just the left posterior fascicle produces left posterior hemiblock with right axis deviation. Bifascicular block indicates blockage of any two of the three fascicles. For example, right bundle branch block with left anterior hemiblock produces a right bundle branch block pattern with marked left axis deviation (Figs. 8-20 and 15-7); right bundle branch block with left posterior hemiblock produces a right bundle branch block pattern with right axis deviation (provided other causes of right axis deviation are excluded). Similarly, a complete left bundle branch block may indicate blockage of both the anterior and the posterior fascicles.

Bifascicular blocks are significant because they make ventricular conduction dependent on the single remaining fascicle. Additional damage to this third remaining fascicle may completely block AV conduction, producing complete heart block (trifascicular block). Therefore the acute development of bifascicular block during an acute anterior wall MI is a warning signal of possible impending complete heart block. If bifascicular block occurs in the setting of acute anterior infarction (Fig. 8-20), cardiologists may insert a temporary pacemaker as a prophylactic measure.

An important distinction must be made between *acute* bifascicular blocks occurring with anterior wall (Fig. 8-20) and *chronic* bifascicular blocks (Fig. 5-7). Many people without any symptoms at all may have ECGs resembling Fig. 15-7. Patients with chronic bifascicular block do not generally require a pacemaker, unless they develop high-degree AV block. The risk of complete heart block in patients with chronic bifascicular block seems to be quite low. By contrast, patients with acute anterior infarction in whom bifascicular block suddenly occurs have a poor prognosis and are at much higher risk of complete heart block.

BIFASCICULAR BLOCK (RIGHT BUNDLE BRANCH BLOCK WITH LEFT ANTERIOR HEMIBLOCK)

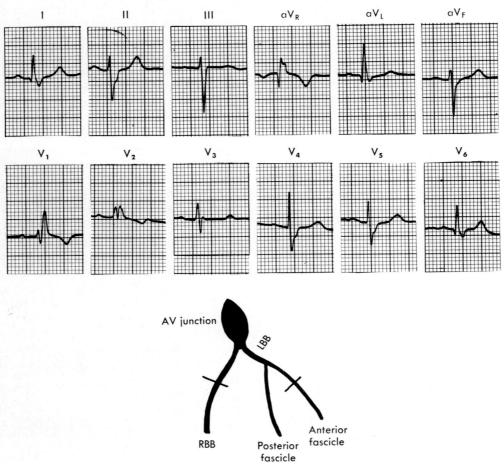

Fig. 15-7. Notice that the chest leads show the typical RBBB pattern (rSR' in lead V_1 and qRS in V_6). The extremity leads show marked left axis deviation (mean QRS axis about $-60°$), consistent with left anterior hemiblock. Thus a bifascicular block, involving the bundle and the anterior fascicle of the left bundle, is present (as shown in the diagram).

AV DISSOCIATION (AVD)

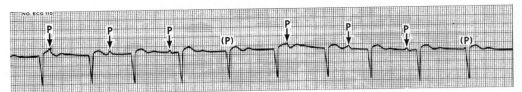

Fig. 15-8. AV dissociation is characterized by independent atrial and ventricular rhythms, with the ventricular rate usually the same as (or slightly faster than) the atrial rate. Notice that the first and fifth P waves are partially hidden in the T waves and that the fourth and eighth P waves are lost in the QRS complexes. (See Question 141, p. 294).

AV DISSOCIATION

AV dissociation is a distinctive arrhythmia, mentioned here because it is often confused with complete heart block.

With AV dissociation the sinus node and AV junction get "out of synch"; thus the sinus node loses its normal control of the ventricular rate. As a result the atria and ventricles are paced independently—the atria from the sinus node, the ventricles from the AV junction. This is similar to what occurs with complete heart block. *However, with AV dissociation the ventricular rate is slightly faster than the atrial rate.* In some instances the atrial and ventricular rates are almost the same (*isorhythmic* AV dissociation).

AV dissociation usually occurs when the sinus node has been depressed by increased vagal tone, (for example, with acute MI, digitalis toxicity, or other pathologic states). Occasionally AV dissociation is seen in normal people.

Fig. 15-8 presents an example of AV dissociation. Notice the P waves with a variable PR interval, because the ventricular (QRS) rate is slightly faster than the atrial rate. At times the P waves may merge with the QRS and become imperceptible for several beats. If the sinus rate speeds up sufficiently (or the AV junctional rate slows), the stimulus may be able to penetrate the AV junction, reestablishing sinus rhythm.

There are two major differences between AV dissociation and complete heart block:

1. The atrial (P wave) rate with AV dissociation is nearly the same as or somewhat slower than the ventricular (QRS) rate. With complete heart block the ventricular rate is usually much slower than the atrial rate.

2. With AV dissociation, although the atria and ventricles beat independently, a stimulus from the atria can penetrate the AV junction if it comes at the right time. With complete heart block, however, the atria and ventricles beat independently because there is a block somewhere in the AV junction, and stimuli *cannot* pass from the atria to the ventricles. In other words, with AV dissociation the sinus node and AV junction are only desynchronized while with complete heart block they are electrically disconnected.

Thus, compared to complete heart block,* AV dissociation is a minor usually transient arrhythmia. Generally no special treatment is required. If it is caused by a drug, the drug may be stopped or its dosage lowered.

---

*There is understandable confusion among students and clinicians regarding the term "*AV dissociation.*" This confusion arises because the term is actually used in two related, though not identical, ways in the ECG literature. As used in this chapter, *AV dissociation* refers to a distinctive arrhythmia that is different from complete heart block. Some authors use "AV dissociation" in a more general sense to refer to any arrhythmia in which the atria and ventricles are paced from separate sites. This second definition will obviously also include complete heart block as well as some cases of ventricular tachycardia in which the atria remain in sinus rhythm (pp. 228 and 238).

REVIEW

There are three types of AV heart block:
1. *First-degree AV block*—the PR interval uniformly prolonged beyond 0.2 second
2. *Second-degree AV block*—two subtypes:
    a. *Wenckebach (Mobitz type I) AV block*—increasing prolongation of the PR interval until a P wave is blocked and not followed by a QRS; this produces a distinctive clustering of QRS complexes separated by a pause resulting from the dropped beat (known as *group beating*)
    b. *Mobitz type II AV block*—a series of P waves without QRS complexes, followed by a P wave and a QRS (for example, with 3:1 block, every third P wave is conducted and followed by a QRS complex); the conducted P waves have the same PR interval, and QRS complexes are usually wide
3. *Third-degree (complete) AV block*—showing
    a. The atria and ventricles beating independently because stimuli cannot pass through the AV junction
    b. The atrial rate faster than the ventricular rate
    c. The PR interval constantly changing

Complete heart block with acute anterior wall MI is sometimes preceded by the sudden appearance of *bifascicular block* (right bundle branch block with left anterior or posterior hemiblock or complete left bundle branch block). However, patients with *chronic* bifascicular block who have no symptoms usually do not require any special therapy.

The significance of complete heart block with acute MI depends on the location of the infarct. Complete heart block occurring with acute inferior wall MI is not uncommon, is usually transient, and can sometimes be managed without a pacemaker. By contrast, complete heart block with acute anterior wall MI is usually associated with a very poor prognosis and requires a pacemaker.

Complete heart block must be distinguished from *AV dissociation*. With AV dissociation, the atria and ventricles beat independently; however, the ventricular rate is about the same as or faster than the atrial rate. AV dissociation is a minor, usually transient, arrhythmia.

Questions

True or false (1 to 5):
1. With first-degree AV block, the heart rate will be very slow.
2. Bifascicular block always leads to complete heart block.
3. The PR interval is constant in complete heart block.
4. Digitalis toxicity may cause complete heart block.
5. Complete heart block may occur with atrial fibrillation.

6. The rhythm strip below shows sinus rhythm with which of the following?
   a. Wenckebach type second-degree AV block
   b. Complete heart block
   c. 3:1 AV block
   d. AV dissociation
   e. Blocked premature atrial contractions

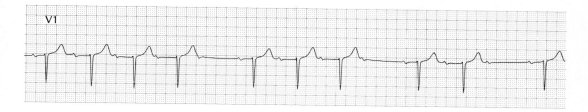

7. In the rhythm strip below
   a. What is the approximate atrial (P wave) rate?
   b. What is the approximate ventricular (QRS) rate?
   c. Is the PR interval constant?
   d. What is the ECG abnormality shown?

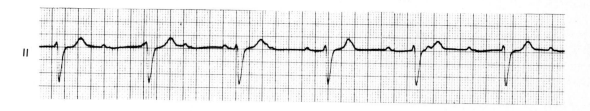

Answers

1. False. The heart rate may be slow, fast, or normal.
2. False.
3. False.
4. True. Digitalis toxicity may cause any degree of AV block.
5. True. (See Fig. 3-9.)
6. a. Wenckebach block. Notice the succession of P waves, with increasing PR intervals, followed by a dropped (nonconducted) P wave. This pattern leads to "group beating." Blocked premature atrial contractions can also cause group beating, but then the nonconducted P wave comes early, before the next sinus P wave is due. The P waves in this example come on time.
7. a. 100 beats/min.
   b. 42 beats/min.
   c. No.
   d. Sinus rhythm with complete heart block. Notice that some of the P waves are hidden in QRS or T waves.

16

Digitalis Toxicity

This chapter focuses on the arrhythmias and conduction disturbances caused by digitalis intoxication. There are several reasons for discussing this topic in an introductory textbook. The most important is that digitalis is a frequently prescribed drug and digitalis toxicity is a common clinical problem. Furthermore, digitalis toxicity can cause fatal arrhythmias. Early recognition of digitalis toxicity therefore should be a preoccupation of everyone in clinical medicine. Finally, because digitalis toxicity can produce virtually any arrhythmia and all degrees of heart block, this topic provides a convenient review of material presented in previous chapters.

CLINICAL BACKGROUND

Digitalis refers to a class of cardiac drugs with specific effects on the mechanical and electrical function of the heart. The most commonly used digitalis preparation is digoxin.

Digitalis is used in clinical practice for two major reasons. First, in selected patients with congestive heart failure it increases the strength of myocardial contractions. This is its *mechanical* action. Second, it affects the *electrical* function of the heart, making it useful for treating certain arrhythmias. The antiarrhythmic action of digitalis results primarily because it slows conduction through the AV junction due to increased vagal tone. Consequently it is extremely useful in treating such supraventricular tachycardias as PAT, atrial fibrillation, and atrial flutter, in all of which there is excessive transmis-

sion of stimuli from the atria to the ventricles through the AV junction.

Unfortunately, although digitalis has wide use in the treatment of heart failure and certain arrhythmias, it also has a relatively low margin of safety. The difference between therapeutic and toxic concentrations is very narrow.

SIGNS OF DIGITALIS TOXICITY

Digitalis toxicity can produce general systemic symptoms as well as specific cardiac arrhythmias and conduction disturbances. The most common extracardiac symptoms are anorexia, nausea, and vomiting. Visual effects (altered color perception) and mental changes have also been reported. In this section we will concentrate on the arrhythmias and conduction disturbances produced by digitalis excess.

As a general clinical rule *virtually any arrhythmia and all degrees of heart block can be produced by digitalis intoxication*. Of all the arrhythmias we have discussed, atrial fibrillation and atrial flutter with a rapid ventricular response are *least* likely to be caused by digitalis toxicity. However, there remain a number of arrhythmias that are commonly seen with digitalis toxicity.

Ventricular Arrhythmias

Premature ventricular contractions (PVCs) are often the first sign of digitalis toxicity. Isolated PVCs may occur at first. Ventricular bigeminy (Fig. 16-1), with each normal beat followed by a PVC,

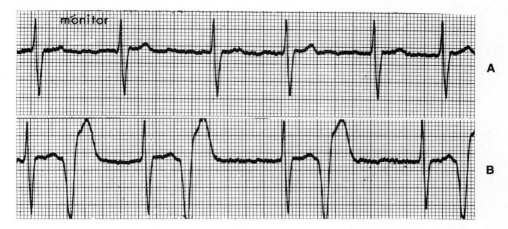

Fig. 16-1. Ventricular bigeminy caused by digitalis toxicity. Ventricular ectopy is one of the most common signs of digitalis toxicity. The underlying rhythm in **A** is atrial fibrillation. In **B** each normal QRS is followed by a PVC.

BIDIRECTIONAL TACHYCARDIA

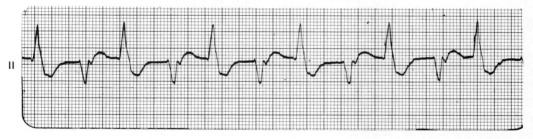

Fig. 16-2. This digitalis-toxic arrhythmia is a special type of ventricular tachycardia with QRS complexes that alternate in direction from beat to beat. No P waves are present.

is common. Ventricular tachycardia and fatal ventricular fibrillation may occur if the digitalis toxicity is not recognized and treated. (See Chapter 17.)

Bidirectional Ventricular Tachycardia

Bidirectional ventricular tachycardia (Fig. 16-2) resembles ventricular tachycardia, except that each successive beat in any lead alternates in direction. This distinctive tachyarrhythmia should always raise the question of digitalis intoxication.

AV Junctional (Nodal) Rhythms

AV junctional rhythms are frequently a sign of digitalis toxicity. Most AV junctional rhythms resulting from excessive digitalis have a rate of less than 120 beats/min.

Sinus Bradycardia and Sinoatrial (SA) Block

Sinus bradycardia may be one of the earliest signs of digitalis excess. SA block with sinus arrest may also occur.

PAROXYSMAL ATRIAL TACHYCARDIA WITH BLOCK

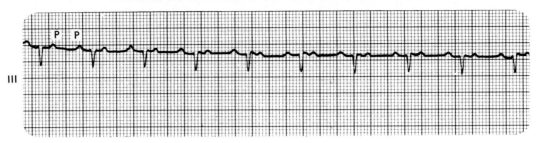

Fig. 16-3. This rhythm strip shows PAT (atrial rate about 200 beats/min) with 2:1 block, producing a ventricular rate of about 100 beats/min.

Paroxysmal Atrial Tachycardia with AV Block

PAT with block is another tachyarrhythmia that has not been discussed in earlier chapters. (An example appears in Fig. 16-3.) PAT with block shows the following: an atrial tachycardia with P waves occurring at a rate usually between 150 and 250 beats/minute and, because of the AV block, a slower ventricular rate. Not uncommonly 2:1 AV block is present, so the ventricular rate will be half the atrial rate. Digitalis toxicity is an important, but not the only, cause of this arrhythmia. Superficially PAT with block may resemble atrial flutter; however, in PAT with block the baseline between P waves is isoelectric. Furthermore, when atrial flutter is present the atrial rate is faster (usually 250 to 350 beats/min).

AV Heart Block and AV Dissociation

Because digitalis slows conduction through the AV junction, it is not surprising that toxic doses can result in any degree of AV heart block.

First-degree block. With first-degree AV block there is uniform prolongation of the PR interval greater than 0.2 second. Some degree of PR lengthening may be expected with digitalis therapy. More marked widening of the PR interval suggests early digitalis toxicity.

Second-degree block. With higher doses of digitalis, first-degree AV block may progress to second-degree block of the Mobitz type I (Wenckebach) variety.

Complete heart block. Third-degree, or complete, heart block may also occur with digitalis toxicity.

In addition, digitalis toxicity may cause AV dissociation. (See Chapter 15.)

Atrial Fibrillation with Slow Ventricular Rate

Although atrial fibrillation and atrial flutter with a rapid ventricular response are the two arrhythmias least likely to be caused by digitalis toxicity, digitalis toxicity can still occur in patients with atrial fibrillation or flutter. In such cases the toxicity is often shown by marked slowing of the ventricular rate (less than 50 beats/min) (Fig. 16-4) and/or the appearance of PVCs. (In some cases the earliest sign of digitalis toxicity in a patient with atrial fibrillation may be a subtle *regularization* of the ventricular rate.)

• • •

The spectrum of digitalis toxic arrhythmias and conduction disturbances is obviously broad. It is simpler to list the patterns *not* caused by digitalis toxicity. Although digitalis may be responsible for any degree of AV heart block, it does not produce intraventricular conduction disturbances (bundle branch block patterns).

As a general rule digitalis toxicity should be suspected in any patient with a bradyarrhythmia (sinus bradycardia, SA block, second- or third-degree heart block, atrial fibrillation with a slow ventricular rate, slow AV junctional rhythms). Also

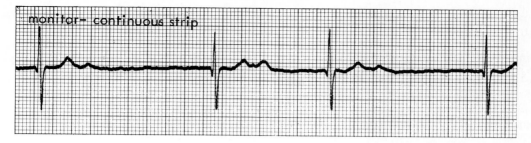

Fig. 16-4. Atrial fibrillation with an excessively slow ventricular rate because of digitalis toxicity. Atrial fibrillation with a rapid ventricular rate is rarely caused by digitalis toxicity. However, in patients with underlying atrial fibrillation, digitalis toxicity is often manifested by excessive slowing or regularization of the QRS rate.

look for digitalis toxicity in any patient with ventricular ectopy (PVCs, ventricular bigeminy, ventricular tachycardia, ventricular fibrillation). Bidirectional ventricular tachycardia and PAT with block are two special arrhythmias often associated with digitalis toxicity. Of all these arrhythmias just mentioned, ventricular ectopy and AV junctional rhythms are probably the most common ECG signs of digitalis toxicity.

Because of its frequency and potential lethality, digitalis toxicity should be suspected in any patient taking digitalis who has an unexplained arrhythmia until you can prove otherwise. The list below summarizes the most common arrhythmias and conduction disturbances seen with digitalis toxicity.

1. Ventricular ectopy: isolated PVCs, ventricular bigeminy, ventricular tachycardia, bidirectional ventricular tachycardia, ventricular fibrillation
2. AV junctional (nodal) rhythms
3. Sinus bradycardia and SA block
4. AV heart block (first, second, third degree) and AV dissociation
5. Atrial fibrillation with a slow or regularized ventricular response
6. PAT with block

FACTORS PREDISPOSING TO DIGITALIS TOXICITY

There are a number of factors that significantly increase the hazard of digitalis intoxication.

Hypokalemia. A low serum potassium concentration makes certain digitalis-induced arrhythmias (particularly ventricular ectopy and PAT with block) more likely. Hypokalemia is not uncommon in digitalized patients because these patients frequently receive diuretics for treatment of heart failure and edema. The serum potassium concentration must be checked periodically in any patient taking digitalis and in every patient suspected of having digitalis toxicity.

Hypomagnesemia and hypercalcemia. Hypomagnesemia is seen in a variety of settings—including alcoholism, intestinal malabsorption, and diuretic therapy. Hypercalcemia is seen with hyperparathyroidism and certain tumors, among other conditions.

Hypoxemia and chronic lung disease. Hypoxemia and chronic lung disease also increase the risk of digitalis toxicity.

Myocardial infarction. Patients with acute myocardial infarction appear to be more sensitive to digitalis, and lower doses are recommended in the first few days for these patients.

Old age. Elderly patients are, in general, more sensitive to digitalis.

Renal insufficiency. Digoxin, the most widely used preparation of digitalis, is excreted primarily in the urine. Therefore any degree of renal insufficiency, as measured by increased blood urea nitrogen (BUN) and creatinine concentration, requires a lower maintenance dose of digoxin.

Hypothyroidism. Patients with hypothyroidism

(myxedema) appear to be more sensitive to the effects of digitalis.

TREATMENT OF DIGITALIS TOXICITY

The first step in treatment is prevention. Before starting any patient on digitalis, you should have a baseline ECG, serum electrolytes, and BUN and creatinine measurements. (Serum magnesium blood levels are usually not required unless clinically indicated by diuretic therapy, etc.) In addition, take into consideration the patient's age, pulmonary status, and whether he is having an acute myocardial infarction. Early signs of digitalis toxicity, such as PVCs, sinus bradycardia, or increasing AV block, should be carefully checked. Furthermore, concomitant quinidine administration increases the digoxin level in patients taking both drugs. A similar effect occurs with verapamil.

Definitive treatment of digitalis toxicity depends on the particular arrhythmia seen. In cases of minor arrhythmias, such as occasional PVCs, sinus bradycardia, first-degree or Wenckebach AV block, or AV junctional rhythms, stopping the digitalis and observing the patient are usually adequate. More serious arrhythmias, such as ventricular tachycardia, may require suppression with an intravenous drug (for example, lidocaine or procainamide). Potassium chloride should be given to raise the serum potassium level well within normal limits (unless complete heart block is present). Patients with complete heart block from digitalis toxicity may require a temporary pacemaker to tide them over while the effect of the digitalis dissipates, particularly if they have symptoms of syncope, hypotension, or congestive heart failure. In other cases, complete heart block can be managed conservatively while the digitalis wears off. PAT with block can often be treated with potassium chloride.

Occasionally a patient will present with a massive overdose of digitalis, taken either inadvertently or in a suicide attempt. In such cases the serum digoxin level will be markedly elevated and refractory brady- or tacharrhythmias may develop. In addition, massive digitalis toxicity may cause life-threatening hyperkalemia since the drug blocks the cellular mechanism that pumps potassium into the cells. Patients with massive overdose of digi-

talis can be treated with a special digitalis-binding antibody (Digibind) given intravenously. A detailed account of the treatment of digitalis toxicity is given in selected references in the Bibliography.

Finally, it must be emphasized that electrical cardioversion of arrhythmias in patients who have digitalis toxicity is extremely hazardous and may precipitate fatal ventricular tachycardia and fibrillation. Therefore you should avoid trying to cardiovert electrically any patient who has PAT with block, atrial fibrillation, or atrial flutter and is suspected of having digitalis toxicity.

SERUM DIGOXIN LEVELS

The concentration of digoxin in the serum can be measured by means of radioimmunoassay. Therapeutic concentrations range between 0.5 and 2 ng/ml in most laboratories. Concentrations exceeding 2 ng/ml are associated with a high incidence of digitalis toxicity. In ordering a test of digoxin level in a patient, it is important to recognize that therapeutic levels do not rule out the possibility of digitalis toxicity. Some patients, as mentioned, are more sensitive to digitalis. In other patients factors such as hypokalemia may produce digitalis toxicity despite a "therapeutic" serum level. Conversely, still other patients, particularly those in atrial fibrillation with a rapid ventricular response, will require higher levels of digitalis to control their ventricular rate. A high digitalis level therefore does not necessarily indicate digitalis toxicity. However, patients with high digitalis levels should be examined for evidence of digitalis excess, including extracardiac symptoms (for example, gastrointestinal distress) and all the cardiac effects that have been discussed.

DIGITALIS TOXICITY AND DIGITALIS EFFECT

Do not confuse digitalis toxicity (which refers to the arrhythmias and conduction disturbances produced by this drug) with digitalis effect. *Digitalis effect* (Fig. 10-1) refers to the distinct scooping of the ST-T complex seen in some patients taking digitalis. The presence of digitalis effect does not imply digitalis toxicity.

REVIEW

Digitalis toxicity can produce almost any arrhythmia and all degrees of AV heart block. The following arrhythmias are commonly seen:

1. Ventricular ectopy (PVCs)—isolated at first, often followed by ventricular bigeminy (a PVC following each normal beat); fatal ventricular tachycardia and ventricular fibrillation can occur if digitalis toxicity is not recognized and treated
2. Bidirectional ventricular tachycardia—resembling conventional ventricular tachycardia, except that each successive beat in any lead points in the opposite direction
3. AV junctional (nodal) rhythms
4. Sinus bradycardia and SA block—actual sinus arrest may also occur
5. PAT with block (paroxysmal atrial tachycardia with AV block)
6. AV heart block—first-degree initially, sometimes followed by second-degree Wenckebach-type block; complete heart block or AV dissociation may also be seen
7. Atrial fibrillation or flutter with a slow ventricular response—occurring when patients with atrial fibrillation or flutter are given excess digitalis; the ventricular rate may slow to 50 beats/min or less and will often become very regular

Atrial fibrillation or atrial flutter with a rapid ventricular response rarely occurs as a result of digitalis toxicity. Furthermore, digitalis toxicity does not produce bundle branch blocks.

Factors such as renal failure, hypokalemia, hypercalcemia, hypomagnesemia, hypoxemia, old age, and acute myocardial infarction may predispose to digitalis toxicity. Concomitant administration of quinidine or verapamil will also increase serum digoxin levels.

Digitalis toxicity should not be confused with digitalis effect. *Digitalis effect* refers to the shortening of the QT interval and scooping of the ST-T complex produced by *therapeutic* doses of digitalis.

Questions

1. Name three factors that can potentiate digitalis toxicity.

True or false (2 to 5):

2. PVCs are a frequent manifestation of digitalis toxicity.
3. Atrial fibrillation with a rapid ventricular response is a common manifestation of digitalis toxicity.
4. Left bundle branch block may result from digitalis toxicity.
5. Complete heart block may be caused by digitalis toxicity.
6. The rhythm strip shown below is from a patient with digitalis toxicity. Identify the arrhythmia.

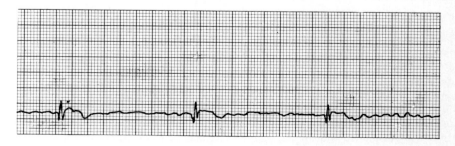

Answers

1. Hypokalemia, hypomagnesemia, hypoxemia, acute myocardial infarction, renal failure. (See p. 207 for other answers.)
2. True.
3. False.
4. False.
5. True.
6. Atrial fibrillation with an excessively slow ventricular rate (probably resulting from complete heart block).

17

Cardiac Arrest

In the preceding chapters the major disorders of heart rhythm and atrioventricular conduction have been systematically discussed. In this chapter, instead of considering entirely new ECG patterns, we will review some earlier topics, placing them in a special clinical perspective. The subject of this chapter is the recognition of life-threatening arrhythmias causing cardiac arrest. *Cardiac arrest occurs when the heart stops contracting effectively and ceases to pump blood.*

CLINICAL ASPECTS OF CARDIAC ARREST

The patient in cardiac arrest loses consciousness within seconds and may even have a seizure as a result of inadequate blood flow to the brain. Irreversible brain damage will usually occur within 4 minutes and sometimes sooner. Furthermore, shortly after the heart stops pumping, spontaneous breathing will also cease *(cardiopulmonary arrest)*. Sometimes, when respirations stop first (primary respiratory arrest), cardiac activity will stop very shortly thereafter.

The diagnosis of cardiac arrest should be made clinically even before the patient is connected to an electrocardiograph. Cardiac arrest should be recognized immediately in any unconscious person who does not have palpable pulses. The patient is quickly examined by trying to feel for pulses in the carotid arteries. The patient in cardiac arrest will become cyanotic (bluish gray) from lack of oxygenated blood. No heart tones will be audible

with a stethoscope on the chest, and the blood pressure will, of course, be unobtainable. The arms and legs become cool; and if the brain becomes severely hypoxic, the pupils will be fixed and dilated. Seizure activity may occur. *The absence of pulses in an unconscious person, however, is the major diagnostic sign of cardiac arrest.*

Once cardiac arrest is recognized, treatment must be immediately started. The basic method of *cardiopulmonary resuscitation* (CPR) has been described by the National Academy of Sciences. In capsule form the initial treatment of any cardiac arrest consists of the following four steps:

A—Establish an *A*irway.

B—*B*reathe for the patient, either by mouth-to-mouth or mouth-to-mask methods or by manually compressing a bag-valve device, forcing air into the patient's nose or mouth.

C—Maintain *C*irculation by external cardiac compression (rhythmic compression of the lower sternum with the heels of the palms).

D—Begin *D*efinitive treatment with whatever intravenous, endotracheal, or intracardiac drugs are needed, with electrical defibrillation, with a temporary pacemaker when indicated, and so on.

While the above steps are being done by two or more rescuers, another rescuer can raise the patient's lower extremities to a vertical position and keep them elevated for 15 seconds. This brings blood back to the circulation. The details of CPR, including drug dosages, the use of defibrillators, and so on, lie outside the scope of this book but are discussed in selected references in the Bibliography. In this chapter we will concentrate primarily on the particular ECG patterns seen during cardiac arrest and on the clinical implications of these patterns. It is important to reemphasize that initial treatment of the patient with ventilation and external cardiac compression should *never* be delayed while the patient is being connected to the electrocardiograph.

THE THREE BASIC ECG PATTERNS IN CARDIAC ARREST

There are only three basic ECG patterns seen with cardiac arrest, and they have been mentioned in earlier chapters. Cardiac arrest may be associated with

1. Ventricular tachyarrhythmia (ventricular fibrillation or a sustained type of ventricular tachycardia)
2. Ventricular standstill (brady-asystolic patterns)
3. Electromechanical dissociation

We will review each of these patterns again briefly, stressing the clinical implications of each in cardiac arrest (Figs. 17-1 to 17-7).

Ventricular Tachyarrhythmia

With ventricular fibrillation (VF) the ventricles do not contract but instead twitch in a completely ineffective way. There is no cardiac output, and the patient loses consciousness within seconds. The characteristic ECG pattern, with its unmistakable oscillatory waves, is illustrated in Fig. 17-1.

Of the three basic ECG patterns seen with cardiac arrest, ventricular fibrillation is the most common one initially encountered. It may appear spontaneously, although (as noted in Chapter 14) it often is preceded by another ventricular arrhythmia (usually ventricular tachycardia or premature ventricular contractions). Fig. 17-2 shows a ventricular tachycardia degenerating into ventricular fibrillation during cardiac arrest.

Treatment of ventricular fibrillation was mentioned in Chapter 12. The patient should be immediately defibrillated using a DC *defibrillator*

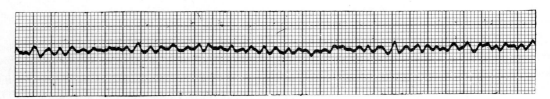

Fig. 17-1. Ventricular fibrillation causing cardiac arrest.

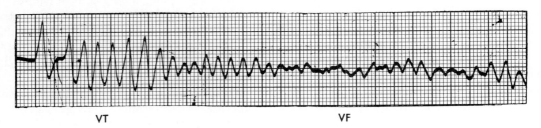

VT   VF

Fig. 17-2. Ventricular tachycardia *(VT)* and ventricular fibrillation *(VF)* recorded during cardiac arrest. The rapid sine-wave type of ventricular tachycardia seen here is sometimes referred to as ventricular flutter.

(*cardioverter*) to administer a direct-current electric shock to the heart by means of paddles placed on the chest wall (p. 164). Fig. 17-7, *D*, shows an example of a successful defibrillation.

The drug bretylium tosylate (Bretylol) may be helpful in treating or preventing ventricular fibrillation. Drugs like lidocaine or procainamide are not usually effective in direct treatment, although they may be useful in preventing further episodes once normal sinus rhythm is restored.

Success in defibrillating any patient depends on a number of factors. The single most important is haste. The less delay in defibrillation, the greater will be the chance of success.

In fact, if a defibrillator is immediately available, a defibrillatory shock should be given to any patient in cardiac arrest, even before connection is made to the electrocardiograph. * The reason for this priority is that the most common cause of cardiac arrest is ventricular fibrillation, as mentioned before. (Even if the patient has ventricular standstill, the second most likely arrhythmia in cardiac arrest, a DC shock will not be harmful.) In some cases epinephrine, given intravenously, via endotracheal tube, or by direct intracardiac injection, may make it easier to defibrillate a patient. Sometimes it may take repeated shocks before the patient is successfully defibrillated. In other cases all attempts will fail. Finally, it is important to stress that external cardiac compression must be continued between attempts at defibrillation.

Cardiac arrest may also occur during a sustained episode of other ventricular tachyarrhythmias, including conventional ventricular tachycardia, torsade de pointes, and ventricular flutter. These arrhythmias were described in Chapter 14.

Ventricular Standstill (Brady-Asystolic Patterns)

Ventricular standstill and escape rhythms were described in Chapter 11. The normal pacemaker of the heart is the sinus node, located in the right atrium. Failure of the sinus node to function (sinus arrest) will lead to ventricular standstill (asystole) if no other subsidiary pacemaker (for example, in the atria, AV junction, or ventricles) takes over. In such cases the ECG will record a *straight-line pattern* (as seen in Fig. 17-3), indicating asystole.*

Treatment of ventricular standstill also requires continued external cardiac compression. Sometimes spontaneous cardiac electrical activity will resume. Drugs such as epinephrine may help stimulate cardiac activity. Finally, if all else fails, patients with refractory ventricular standstill will require a *temporary pacemaker,* inserted as an emergency at the bedside. As described in Chapter 20, a temporary pacemaker is simply a special catheter wire electrode usually inserted through a vein (*transvenous* pacemaker) into the right ventricle and connected to a battery outside the body. In a dire emergency the pacemaker wire is sometimes inserted directly into the heart through the chest wall (*transthoracic* temporary pacemaker). In recent years a new type of temporary pacemaker

---

*At this point it should be mentioned that sometimes a strong thump on the sternum with your fist ("thump version") may itself restore normal rhythm during cardiac arrest, particularly if the patient is having a sustained run of VT or VF (Fig. 14-13) and a defibrillator is not immediately available.

*Whenever you encounter a straight-line pattern, always check to see that all the electrodes are connected to the patient. They often become disconnected during a cardiac arrest, leading to the mistaken diagnosis of asystole. Very low-amplitude ventricular fibrillation may also mimic a straight-line pattern.

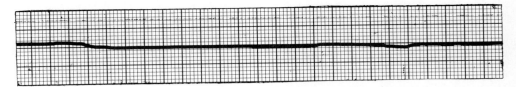

Fig. 17-3. Complete ventricular standstill (asystole) producing a straight-line pattern during cardiac arrest.

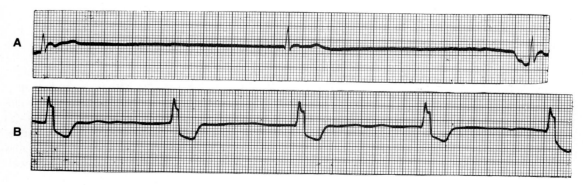

Fig. 17-4. Escape rhythms with underlying ventricular standstill: **A,** junctional escape rhythm with narrow QRS complexes; **B,** idioventricular escape rhythm with wide QRS complexes. Treatment should include the use of intravenous atropine and, if needed, isoproterenol or other sympathomimetic drugs in an attempt to speed up these bradycardias, which cannot support the circulation.

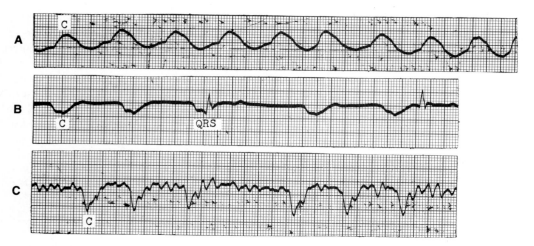

Fig. 17-5. External cardiac compression artifact. External cardiac compression during a resuscitation produces artifactual ECG complexes (marked *C*), which may be mistaken for actual QRS complexes: **A,** ventricular standstill with external cardiac compression; **B,** straight-line pattern interrupted by external cardiac compression artifacts and two escape beats *(QRS)*; **C,** ventricular fibrillation with cardiac compression.

has become available that does not require intravenous insertion. This *external* pacemaker utilizes special electrodes, which can be pasted on the chest wall.

Not uncommonly in ventricular standstill, you will also see *occasional* ORS complexes appearing at infrequent intervals against the background of the basic straight-line rhythm. These are *escape beats* (Chapter 11) and represent the attempt of intrinsic cardiac pacemakers to restart the heart's beat. Examples of escape rhythms with underlying ventricular standstill are shown in Fig. 17-4. In some cases the escape beats are narrow (Fig. 17-4, *A*), indicating their origin from either the atria or the AV junction. In others they come from a lower focus in the ventricles, producing a slow *idioventricular* rhythm with wide QRS complexes (Fig. 17-4, *B*). The term *"brady-asystolic pattern"* is sometimes used to describe this type of cardiac arrest ECG.

When a slow escape rhythm appears during cardiac arrest, drugs such as atropine (a vagal blocker) and isoproterenol or epinephrine (sympathetic stimulants) may be given intravenously to speed up the heart rate.

These escape beats should not be confused with *artifacts* produced by cardiac compression. Artifacts are large wide deflections that occur with each cardiac compression (Fig. 17-5). Their size varies with the strength of the compression, and their direction varies with the lead in which they appear (negative in leads I, II, III, and aV_F, positive in aV_R and aV_L). They should not be mistaken for spontaneous electrical activity of the heart.

Electromechanical Dissociation

The large majority of patients with cardiac arrest will have an ECG showing either a sustained ventricular tachyarrhythmia or ventricular standstill (sometimes with escape beats). Occasionally, however, the ECG of a patient in cardiac arrest will continue to show identifiable QRS complexes at a normal rate. The actual heart rhythm in such cases may be a sinus rhythm, AV junctional (nodal) rhythm, or heart block. However, despite the presence of regularly recurring QRS complexes and even P waves on the ECG, the patient is uncon-

scious and does not have a palpable pulse or blood pressure. In other words, the patient has cardiac electrical activity but no mechanical heart contractions to effectively pump blood. The term *"electromechanical dissociation"* (EMD) is used in such cases.

Electromechanical dissociation can arise in a number of settings.

When assessing a patient with EMD, it is essential to consider the potentially *reversible* causes first. One of the most important of these is pericardial effusion (in which the pericardial sac fills up with an excessive amount of blood or other fluid). This serves to "choke off" the heart, preventing it from adequately filling and emptying. The term *"pericardial tamponade"* ("tamp" meaning "to plug up") is used to describe situations when pericardial effusion produces decreased cardiac output and ultimately cardiac arrest. Pericardial tamponade can be treated by removal of some of the fluid from the pericardial sac with a special needle inserted through the chest wall (pericardiocentesis). Because the disease process is primarily extracardiac (involving the pericardium), the ECG generally shows relatively normal electrical activity, despite the impaired mechanical function of the heart. (While on the subject of pericardial effusion, recall from Chapter 10 the major ECG pattern seen with pericardial effusion: low voltage complexes.) Tension pneumothorax and massive pulmonary embolism are two other causes of EMD, both also potentially reversible.

Probably the most common setting in which electromechanical dissociation occurs is when the myocardium has sustained severe generalized injury that may not be reversible (for example, myocardial infarction). In such cases, even though the heart's conduction system may be intact enough to generate a relatively normal rhythm, there is not sufficient functional ventricular muscle to respond to this electrical signal with an adequate contraction. Sometimes the myocardial depression will be temporary and reversible ("stunned myocardium") and the patient may respond to resuscitative efforts.

Fig. 17-6 shows an example of EMD in which there was sinus rhythm and yet no pulse or blood

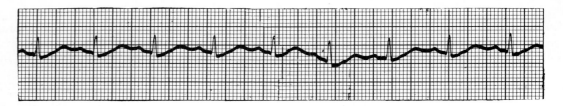

Fig. 17-6. Sinus rhythm with electromechanical dissociation (EMD). Although the ECG showed sinus rhythm, the patient had no pulse or blood pressure. In this case the EMD was a result of depression of myocardial function after a cardiac arrest. (Pericardial tamponade may also cause EMD.)

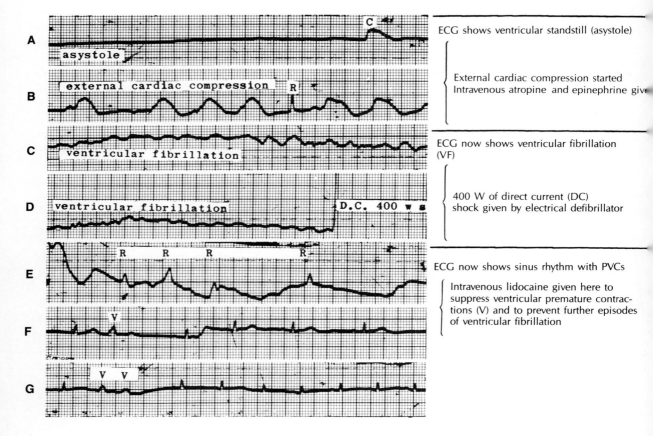

ECG shows ventricular standstill (asystole)

External cardiac compression started
Intravenous atropine and epinephrine give

ECG now shows ventricular fibrillation (VF)

400 W of direct current (DC) shock given by electrical defibrillator

ECG now shows sinus rhythm with PVCs

Intravenous lidocaine given here to suppress ventricular premature contractions (V) and to prevent further episodes of ventricular fibrillation

Fig. 17-7. ECG history of cardiac arrest and successful resuscitation. The left panel shows the ECG sequence during an actual cardiac arrest. The right panel shows sequential therapy appropriate for the different ECG patterns. Initially, **A** and **B,** there is ventricular standstill (asystole) with a straight-line pattern, treated by external cardiac compression. This is followed, **C** and **D,** by ventricular fibrillation. Sinus rhythm, **E** to **G,** appears after defibrillation with 400 watt-seconds of direct-current electric shock. *C* is an external cardiac compression artifact; *R* is an R wave from the spontaneous QRS complex; *V* is a premature ventricular contraction.

pressure following severe depression of myocardial contractility.

• • •

The three basic ECG patterns seen with cardiac arrest—ventricular tachyarrhythmia, ventricular standstill, and electromechanical dissociation—have all been described separately. However, during the course of resuscitating any patient, it is not unusual to see two or even all three of these ECG patterns at different times during the arrest.

Fig. 17-7 shows an actual ECG history of a cardiac arrest.

CAUSES OF CARDIAC ARREST

Cardiac arrest resulting from any of the three mechanisms—ventricular tachyarrhythmia, ventricular standstill, or electromechanical dissociation—may occur in numerous settings. It can be due to any type of organic heart disease. For example, a patient with an acute MI may have cardiac arrest for several reasons. Myocardial ischemia and increased ventricular irritability may precipitate ventricular fibrillation. Damage to the conduction system may result in ventricular standstill. Finally, electromechanical dissociation may occur with extensive myocardial injury. Occasionally, actual rupture of the ventricular wall will occur, leading to fatal pericardial tamponade.

Cardiac arrest also occurs in people with *chronic* heart disease, most often due to ischemia or infarction, valvular abnormalities, or a cardiomyopathy.

Lightning strike or electric shock may produce cardiac arrest in normal hearts. Cardiac arrest may also occur during surgical procedures. Drugs such as epinephrine can produce ventricular fibrillation. Quinidine and related drugs may lead to torsade de pointes (described in Chapter 14). Excessive digitalis can also lead to fatal ventricular arrhythmias. Recognition of arrhythmias caused by digitalis intoxication was discussed in the preceding chapter. Other cardiac drugs may precipitate sustained ventricular tachyarrhythmias through the so-called *proarrhythmic effect* (Chapter 14). The recreational use of *cocaine* has been known to precipitate a fatal arrhythmia.

Marked elevation of the serum potassium concentration (Chapter 10) will ultimately lead to cardiac arrest with ventricular standstill. A very low serum potassium may cause fatal ventricular arrhythmias in a patient taking digitalis. Hypokalemia (as well as hypomagnesemia and hypocalcemia) can also lead to torsade de pointes.

Brady-asystolic cardiac arrest may occur with the sick sinus syndrome (Chapters 11 and 18) or with high-degree AV block (Chapter 15).

Following successful resuscitation of the patient in cardiac arrest, an intensive search for the cause must be started. Serial 12-lead ECGs, along with serum cardiac enzymes, will help diagnose MI. A complete blood count and serum electrolytes should be obtained, as well as an arterial blood gas sample. A portable chest x-ray unit can be brought to bedside. In addition, a pertinent medical history should be obtained from every available source, with particular attention to drug usage (digitalis, quinidine, etc.) and previous cardiac problems.

REVIEW

Cardiac arrest occurs when the heart stops pumping blood. The diagnosis should be made clinically even before the patient is connected to an electrocardiograph. The major clinical sign of cardiac arrest is the absence of pulses in an unconscious patient.

Cardiac arrest may be associated with one or more of the following ECG patterns:

1. *Ventricular tachyarrhythmia*—runs of ventricular fibrillation, sustained typical ventricular tachycardia, torsade de pointes, or ventricular flutter

2. *Ventricular standstill (asystole)* or *brady-asystolic pattern*—a straight-line pattern with inter-ruptions by occasional junctional or ventricular escape beats.
3. *Electromechanical dissociation* (EMD)—regularly recurring QRS complexes, sometimes even P waves, not associated with a palpable pulse or blood pressure; usually caused by diffuse myocardial injury, although may be due to pericardial tamponade, tension pneumothorax, or massive pulmonary embolism

During the course of resuscitating a patient, you may see any or all of the above patterns.

In addition, the ECG with cardiac arrest will show distinctive *artifacts* caused by external cardiac compression (wide complexes that should not be mistaken for the intrinsic electrical activity of the heart).

For a review of the general treatment principles in cardiac arrest, reread pp. 212 to 217.

Questions

1. Would a pacemaker be of any value in treating a patient with cardiac arrest and electromechanical dissociation (EMD)?
2. The rhythm strip below was obtained from a patient during the course of a cardiac arrest and attempted resuscitation.
   a. What is the basic rhythm?
   b. What are the complexes marked **X** caused by?

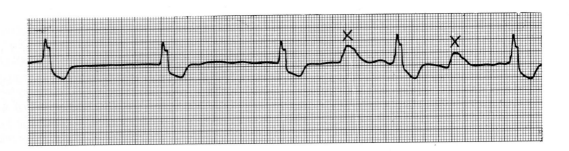

3. Name four drugs that can produce cardiac arrest associated with a sustained ventricular tachyar-rhythmia (ventricular fibrillation, typical ventricular tachycardia, torsade de pointes, or ventricular flutter).

Answers

1. No. By definition, patients with EMD have relatively normal electrical activity. The problem is that this electrical activity is not associated with adequate mechanical (pumping) action, usually because of diffuse myocardial injury, pericardial tamponade, or severe loss of intravascular volume. A pacemaker would not be of help in this situation because the patient already has adequate electrical stimulation.
2. a. Idioventricular escape rhythm.
   b. External cardiac compression artifacts.
3. Digitalis (digoxin), epinephrine, cocaine, quinidine (also procainamide, disopyramide, and other antiarrhythmic agents).

18

Bradycardias and Tachycardias

REVIEW AND DIFFERENTIAL DIAGNOSIS

The preceding chapters have described the major arrhythmias and AV conduction disturbances. There are several ways of classifying these abnormalities. In this section we will simply divide them into two groups, bradycardias and tachycardias, and discuss the differential diagnosis of each group.

BRADYCARDIAS (BRADYARRHYTHMIAS)

We have discussed several arrhythmias and conduction disturbances associated with a slow heart rate. The term *"bradycardia"* or *"bradyarrhythmia"* is used here to refer to arrhythmias and conduction abnormalities producing a heart rate of less than 60 beats/min. Fortunately, the differential diagnosis of a patient with a slow pulse is relatively simple since there are only a handful of possible causes. Specifically, we can cite five general types of bradyarrhythmias.

Sinus bradycardia, including SA block
AV junctional (nodal) escape rhythm
AV heart block (second or third degree) or AV dissociation
Atrial fibrillation (or flutter) with slow ventricular response
Idioventricular escape rhythm

Sinus bradycardia. Sinus bradycardia (Fig. 18-1) is sinus rhythm with a rate less than 60 beats/min. Each QRS is preceded by a P wave, and the P wave is negative in lead aV_R and positive lead II, indicating that the sinus node is the pacemaker. Some patients may have a sinus bradycardia as slow as 40 beats/min or less.

Sinus bradycardia may be related to a decreased firing rate of the sinus node or to actual SA block. The most extreme example is sinus node arrest (Chapter 11).

AV junctional (nodal) escape rhythm. With a slow junctional escape rhythm (Fig. 18-2) either the P waves are *retrograde* (inverted in lead II, upright in lead aV_R) or else no P waves are apparent if the atria and ventricles are stimulated simultaneously.

AV heart block (second or third degree) or AV dissociation (Fig. 18-3). A slow ventricular rate of 60 beats/min or less (even as low as 20 beats/min) is the rule with complete heart block, owing to the slow intrinsic rate of the junctional or idioventricular pacemaker. Patients with second-degree AV block (either Wenckebach or Mobitz type II) also often have a bradycardia because of the dropped beats (Figs. 15-3 and 15-4). AV dissociation, which may be confused with complete heart block (pp. 201 and 238), is also often associated with a heart rate of less than 60 beats/min.

SINUS BRADYCARDIA

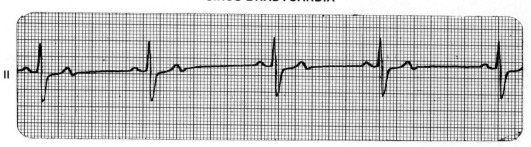

Fig. 18-1. Sinus bradycardia with a slight sinus arrhythmia.

AV JUNCTIONAL RHYTHM

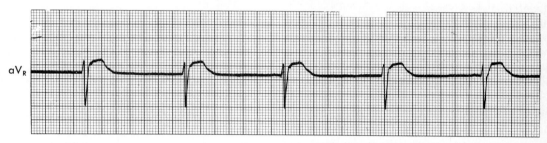

Fig. 18-2. The heart rate is about 43 beats/min. The baseline between complexes is perfectly flat (no P waves evident).

COMPLETE HEART BLOCK

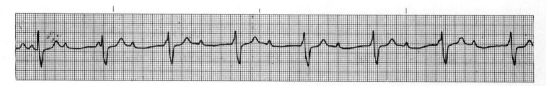

Fig. 18-3. The atrial (P wave) rate is about 80 beats/min. The ventricular (QRS) rate is about 43 beats/min. The atria and ventricles are beating independently, so the PR intervals are variable. The QRS complex is wide because the ventricles are paced by an idioventricular pacemaker.

ATRIAL FIBRILLATION WITH A SLOW VENTRICULAR RATE

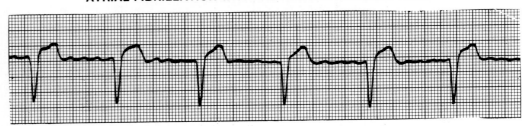

Fig. 18-4. Regularization and excessive slowing of the ventricular rate with atrial fibrillation are sometimes a sign of digitalis toxicity. (See Chapter 16.)

Atrial fibrillation or flutter with a slow ventricular rate (Fig. 18-4). Paroxysmal atrial fibrillation is generally associated with a rapid ventricular rate, which may become excessively slow (less than 50 to 60 beats/min) because of drug effects or toxicity (beta blocker, calcium channel blocker, digitalis) or if the patient has underlying disease of the AV junction. In such cases the ECG shows the characteristic atrial fibrillatory waves with a slow ventricular (QRS) rate. The f waves may be very fine and easily overlooked.

Idioventricular escape rhythm. In some cases, where the SA nodal and AV junctional escape pacemakers fail to function, a very slow pacemaker in the ventricular conduction (His-Purkinje) system may take over. This rhythm is referred to as an idioventricular escape rhythm. The rate is usually very slow (<45 beats/min) and the QRS complexes are wide without any preceding P wave (see Fig. 17-4, *B*).

Clinical Significance

With the exception of sinus bradycardia, which is a common normal variant, the other bradycardias are often abnormal.* The possible causes of AV junctional rhythms, heart block, and atrial fibrillation were all described in earlier chapters. *It is worth reemphasizing that in any patient with a bradycardia the possibility of digitalis intoxication*

must always be considered. Sinus bradycardia, AV junctional rhythm, second- and third-degree AV block, and atrial fibrillation or flutter with an excessively slow ventricular response are all frequent signs of digitalis toxicity.

Patients with any of the bradycardias listed may have no symptoms or may complain of light-headedness or fainting resulting from decreased cardiac output. Treatment depends on the particular arrhythmia and the clinical setting.

To summarize: Most patients with an ECG heart rate of less than 60 beats/min will have one of the five following arrhythmias: sinus bradycardia (including SA block), AV junctional rhythm, AV heart block (or AV dissociation), atrial fibrillation or flutter with a very slow ventricular rate, or idioventricular escape rhythm.*

TACHYCARDIAS (TACHYARRHYTHMIAS)

At the opposite end of the spectrum are those patients with rapid heart rates. The term *"tachycardia"* or *"tachyarrhythmia"* refers to rhythm disturbances producing a heart rate faster than 100 beats/min. The differential diagnosis of tachycardias is more complicated than the straightforward list for bradycardias. Still, the possible list of tachyarrhythmias is not long, and the correct diagnosis can generally be deduced in a rational fashion.

---

*Occasionally normal subjects (in particular, athletes with increased vagal tone at rest) may show junctional rhythms or even AV Wenckebach.

*Bradycardia can also be due to a wandering atrial pacemaker (Fig. 18-14).

In approaching tachyarrhythmias we must first make a basic distinction between *supraventricular tachycardia* (SVT) and *ventricular tachycardia* (VT). These terms have already been defined (Chapters 11, 12, and 14). There are five major SVTs; sinus tachycardia, paroxysmal atrial tachycardia (PAT) (including AV junctional tachycardia), atrial fibrillation, atrial flutter, and multifocal atrial tachycardia.* With each of these tachyarrhythmias the pacemaker is located in either the atria or the AV junction, above the ventricles (hence *supra*ventricular). This is in contrast to ventricular tachycardia; with VT the stimulus starts in the ventricles themselves. VT is simply a run of three or more consecutive premature ventricular contractions (Fig. 14-5). The QRS complexes are always wide because the ventricles are not being stimulated simultaneously. The rate of VT is usually between 100 and 200 beats/min. With SVT, by contrast, the ventricles are stimulated normally (simultaneously) so the QRS will be narrow (unless a bundle branch block is also present).

The first step in analyzing a tachyarrhythmia is to look at the width of the QRS complex in all 12 leads if possible. If the QRS is narrow (0.1 sec or less), you are dealing with SVT and not VT. If it is wide, then consider the rhythm to be VT unless it can be proved otherwise.

---

*Be aware of a possible confusion in terminology when cardiologists also use the term *paroxysmal supraventricular tachycardia* (PSVT) to refer more specifically to various types of PAT or AV junctional tachycardia. (See p. 162.)

Differential Diagnosis of SVTs

Let us begin with the differential diagnosis of SVTs. The heart rate is greater than 100 beats/min, and the QRS complexes are narrow. The four most common supraventricular arrhythmias have already been mentioned. They are (1) sinus tachycardia, (2) PAT (including AV junctional tachycardia), (3) atrial fibrillation, and (4) atrial flutter. A fifth possibility, to be discussed, is multifocal atrial tachycardia.

The characteristics of these four arrhythmias have already been described in previous chapters. *Sinus tachycardia* in adults generally produces a heart rate between 100 and 180 beats/min. Finding an SVT with a rate of 180 beats/min or more means that you are almost certainly dealing with one of the other three arrhythmias listed. *PAT* (or AV junctional tachycardia) and *atrial fibrillation* can be distinguished on the basis of regularity. PAT is usually an almost perfectly regular tachycardia with a ventricular rate between 140 and 250 beats/min. Of all the arrhythmias, it is one of the most regular. Atrial fibrillation, on the other hand, is distinguished by its irregularity. Remember that with rapid atrial fibrillation (Fig. 18-5) the fibrillatory waves may not be clearly visible but the diagnosis of atrial fibrillation can be made in almost every case by noting the absence of P waves and the haphazardly irregular QRS complexes. *Atrial flutter* (Fig. 18-6) is characterized by sawtooth flutter waves between QRS complexes. However, when atrial flutter is present with 2:1 block (that is, when the atrial rate is 300 beats/min and the ventricular

ATRIAL FIBRILLATION WITH A RAPID VENTRICULAR RATE

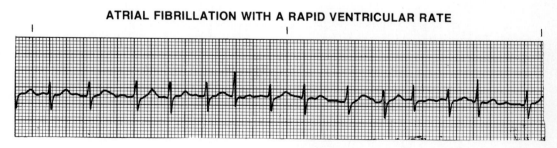

Fig. 18-5. The ventricular rate is about 130 beats/min (13 QRS cycles/6 sec). Notice the characteristic haphazardly irregular rhythm.

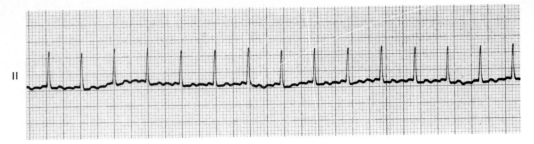

Fig. 18-6. This strip shows atrial flutter with 2:1 conduction.

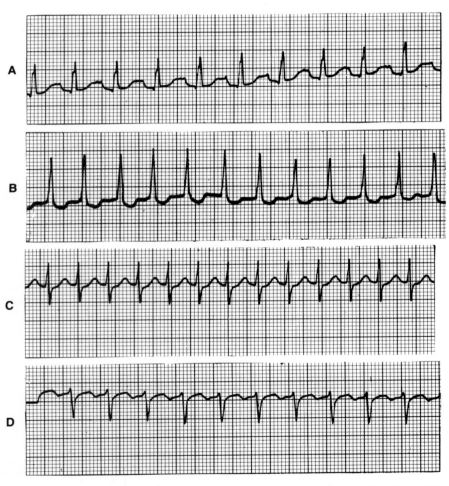

Fig. 18-7. Four look-like supraventricular tachyarrhythmias: **A,** sinus tachycardia; **B,** atrial fibrillation; **C,** paroxysmal atrial (junctional) tachycardia (PAT); **D,** atrial flutter with 2:1 block. When the ventricular rate is about 150 beats/min, these four arrhythmias may be difficult if not impossible to tell apart. In this example of sinus tachycardia the P waves can barely be seen. Notice the irregularity of the atrial fibrillation. In PAT the rate is very regular without evident P waves. In atrial flutter the F waves cannot be seen clearly.

response is 150 beats/min), the flutter waves are often hidden. Atrial flutter at 150 beats/min therefore can be confused with sinus tachycardia, PAT, or atrial fibrillation (Fig. 18-7). Atrial fibrillation can be excluded because atrial flutter with 2:1 conduction is generally very regular.

Nevertheless, the differential diagnosis of sinus tachycardia, PAT with a ventricular rate of 150 beats/min, atrial fibrillation, and atrial flutter can be a problem (Fig. 18-7). Recall that at a rate of 150 beats/min the P waves with sinus tachycardia and PAT may be hidden. One way of separating these possibilities is to use carotid sinus massage (CSM).* Pressure on the carotid sinus produces a reflex increase in vagal tone. The effects of CSM on sinus tachycardia, PAT, and atrial flutter are described next.

Sinus tachycardia. Sinus tachycardia generally slows slightly with CSM. However, there is no abrupt change in heart rate. Slowing of sinus tachycardia may make the P waves more evident. Sinus tachycardia generally begins and ends gradually, not abruptly.

PAT. PAT and AV junctional tachycardia usually have an *all or none* response to CSM. In successful cases PAT will break suddenly and sinus rhythm will resume following CSM (Fig. 12-5). In other cases CSM has no effect and the tachycardia continues at the same rate.

---

*However, carotid sinus massage is not without risks, particularly in elderly patients. For details regarding this maneuver, readers are referred to the Bibliography.

Atrial flutter. CSM will often increase the degree of block in atrial flutter, converting flutter with a 2:1 response to 3:1 or 4:1 flutter with a ventricular rate of 100 or 75 beats/min. Slowing of the ventricular rate will unmask the characteristic flutter waves (Fig. 13-2).

• • •

The final SVT, which we have not yet discussed, is *multifocal atrial tachycardia* (MAT). An example of MAT is shown in Fig. 18-8. This tachyarrhythmia is characterized by multiple ectopic foci stimulating the atria. To diagnose MAT, it is necessary to find three or more P waves with different shapes. The PR intervals often will vary. This arrhythmia is most commonly seen in patients with chronic lung disease. Because the ventricular rate is irregular and rapid, MAT is most likely to be mistaken for atrial fibrillation.

Differential Diagnosis of VT

Tachycardias are divided into SVTs and VT. This section describes the differential diagnosis of VT. A tachycardia with widened QRS complexes indicates two possible diagnoses. The first and more important is VT, a potentially life-threatening arrhythmia. As noted, VT is a consecutive run of three or more PVCs at a rate generally between 100 and 200 or more beats/min. It is usually very regular. The second possible cause of a tachycardia with widened QRS complexes is so-called "SVT with aberration." The term *"aberration"* simply means that some abnormality in ventricular acti-

MULTIFOCAL ATRIAL TACHYCARDIA

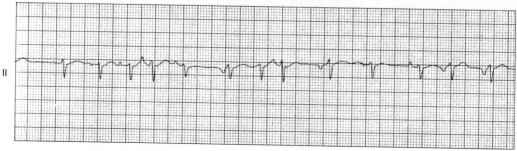

Fig. 18-8. The P waves show variable shapes or variable PR intervals, or both.

vation is present and causing widened QRS complexes.

Differential Diagnosis of SVT with Aberrancy from VT

There are only two major mechanisms for aberrancy with an SVT: (1) a bundle branch block and (2) the Wolff-Parkinson White (WPW) preexcitation syndrome.

SVT with a bundle branch block. If a patient has any of the five major SVTs just listed in association with a bundle branch block, the ECG will show a wide-complex tachycardia that may be mistaken for VT. For example, a patient with sinus tachycardia, atrial fibrillation, atrial flutter, PAT, or MAT who also has a right or left bundle branch block will show a wide-complex tachycardia.

Fig. 18-9, *A*, gives an example of atrial fibrillation with a rapid ventricular response occurring with LBBB. Fig. 18-9, *B*, gives an example of VT. There is an obvious resemblance, making it difficult to tell these patterns apart. The major distinguishing feature is the irregularity of the atrial fibrillation as opposed to the regularity of the VT.

However, in some cases VT may be irregular.

It is important to recognize that in some cases of SVT with aberration, the bundle branch block is seen only during the episodes of tachycardia. Such rate-related bundle branch blocks are said to be "tachycardia dependent."

SVT with the WPW syndrome. The second mechanism responsible for a wide-complex tachycardia is SVT with the WPW syndrome (described in Chapter 10). As noted, patients with WPW preexcitation have an accessory pathway (bundle of Kent) connecting either atrium with either ventricle, thus bypassing the AV junction. Such patients are especially prone to PAT with a narrow (normal) QRS complex for the reason described on p. 142. Sometimes, however, particularly if atrial fibrillation (or atrial flutter) develops, a wide-complex tachycardia may result from conduction down the bypass tract at very high rates. This kind of wide-complex tachycardia will also, obviously, mimic VT. An example of WPW with atrial fibrillation is shown in Fig. 18-10.

The possible diagnosis of WPW with atrial fibrillation should be strongly suspected if you en-

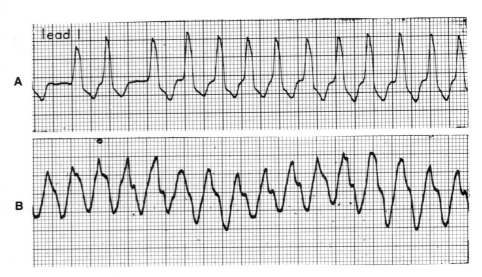

Fig. 18-9. Supraventricular tachycardia with bundle branch block compared to ventricular tachycardia. **A,** Atrial fibrillation with LBBB pattern. **B,** Ventricular tachycardia. It may be difficult and sometimes impossible to tell from the ECG if a patient has actual ventricular tachycardia or a supraventricular tachycardia with bundle branch block.

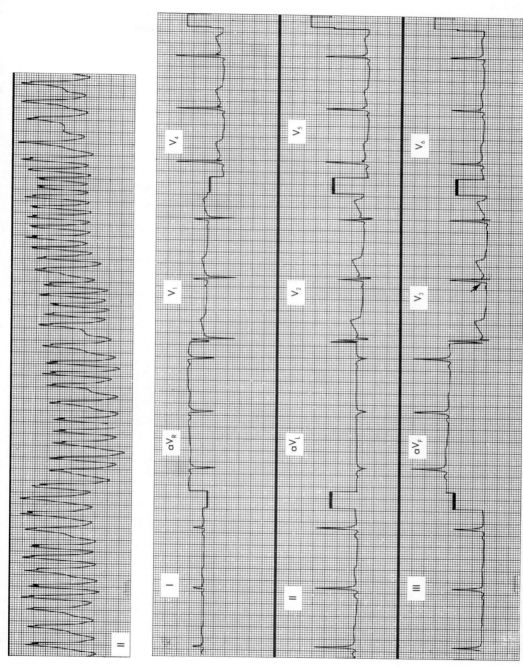

Fig. 18-10. A, Atrial fibrillation with the Wolff-Parkinson-White (WPW) syndrome may lead to a wide-complex tachycardia with very rapid rate. Notice that some of the RR intervals are less than 0.20 second. Irregularity is due to the underlying atrial fibrillation. **B,** After conversion to sinus rhythm the classic WPW triad is visible: relatively short PR interval, wide QRS, and delta wave (*arrow* in V_3).

counter a wide-complex tachycardia that is irregular and has a very high rate (very short RR intervals). In particular, RR intervals of 0.20 second or less are rarely seen with conventional atrial fibrillation and are also rare with ventricular tachycardia. They relate to the ability of the bypass tract (in contrast to the AV junction) to conduct impulses in extremely rapid succession (Fig. 18-10, *A*).

The recognition of WPW with atrial fibrillation is of considerable clinical importance because digitalis may, paradoxically, enhance conduction down the bypass tract. As a result the ventricular response may increase, leading to possible myocardial ischemia and in some cases to ventricular fibrillation. A similar effect has been reported with verapamil.

• • •

An important clue that may be helpful in differentiating SVT with aberrancy from VT is the *presence of AV dissociation.*

Recall from Chapter 15 that with AV dissocia-

tion the atria and ventricles are paced from separate sites, with a faster ventricular rate. Some, but not all, patients with VT will also have AV dissociation; in other words, the ventricles will be paced from an *ectopic* site at a rapid rate while the atria continue to be paced independently by the sinus node. In such cases you may be able to see P waves occurring at a slower rate than the rapid wide QRS complexes shown in Fig. 18-11. Some of the P waves may be "buried" in the QRS complexes and be difficult to discern. Unfortunately, only a minority of cases of VT clearly show AV dissociation. Therefore the absence of AV dissociation does not exclude VT. However, the presence of AV dissociation in a patient with wide complexes at a rapid rate is diagnostic of VT. Furthermore, in some cases of VT with AV dissociation the sinus node may transiently "capture" the ventricles, producing a beat with normal QRS duration ("capture beat") or a "fusion beat," in which case the sinus beat and ventricular beat will coincide to produce

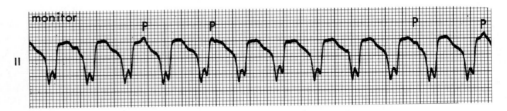

Fig. 18-11. Ventricular tachycardia with AV dissociation. Note the independent atrial rate (75/min) and ventricular rate (140/min). (From Goldberger E: Treatment of cardiac emergencies, ed 4, St Louis, 1985, The CV Mosby Co.)

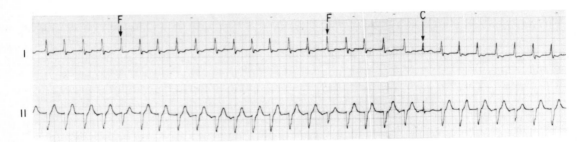

Fig. 18-12. Ventricular tachycardia with AV dissociation producing fusion *(F)* and capture *(C)* beats. Leads I and II were recorded simultaneously. (Courtesy Dr. Robert Engler.)

a hybrid complex. Fig. 18-12 illustrates capture and fusion beats in a case of VT.

What other ECG clues are helpful in distinguishing SVT with aberration from VT? Over the years cardiologists have tried to develop precise criteria to assist in this important differential diagnosis. Unfortunately, no single criterion has proved absolutely reliable. In addition to AV dissociation, the following criteria are strongly suggestive of VT when you are confronted with a wide-complex tachycardia (Akhtar et al., 1988):

1. A QRS duration of more than 0.14 second with an RBBB morphology or more than 0.16 second with an LBBB morphology (However, in some cases of VT the QRS is less than 0.14 sec; also, in some cases of WPW, it may be more than 0.16 sec.)
2. A positive QRS concordance in the chest leads (wide R waves in V_1 to V_6) (However, not all VT episodes will show this.)
3. Extreme axis deviation, that is, between $-90°$ and $+180°$ (Fig 5-14) (However, not all VT causes this kind of axis deviation.)
4. An LBBB pattern with right axis deviation

It will be impossible at times to distinguish between VT and SVT with aberration from the 12-lead ECG. In such cases clinical judgment must be used. For example, if the patient is hypotensive the tachycardia is generally treated as VT (Table 2). On the other hand, remember that not all patients with VT will be hypotensive. Indeed, occasional patients may have minimal symptoms when they are in sustained VT.

Caution: *Intravenous verapamil should **not** be used in undiagnosed wide-complex tachycardias. It may cause hemodynamic collapse in patients with VT or atrial fibrillation with WPW.*

Clinical Significance

As mentioned earlier, the first question to ask in looking at any tachyarrhythmia is if the rhythm is VT or not. If sustained VT is present, then emergency treatment is required (as described in Chapter 14).

With SVT the therapy depends on the clinical setting. In the case of sinus tachycardia (Chapter 11) treatment is directed at the underlying cause (for example, fever, sepsis, congestive heart failure, or hyperthyroidism). Similarly treatment of MAT should be directed at the underlying problem (usually chronic pulmonary disease). Electrical cardioversion should *not* be used with MAT, since it is not likely to be helpful and may induce serious ventricular arrhythmias. The calcium channel blocker verapamil can be used to slow the ventricular response in MAT.

When treating the other three major SVTs (PAT, atrial fibrillation, and atrial flutter), a decision must first be made whether initially to treat with electrical cardioversion or with drug therapy. There are no absolute rules for making such decisions, In assessing any patient with an SVT, you should ask the following three key questions relating to the effects of the tachycardia on the heart and circulation:

1. Is the patient's blood pressure abnormally low? In particular, is he in shock?
2. Is the patient having an acute myocardial infarction or severe ischemia?
3. Is the patient in severe congestive heart failure (pulmonary edema)?

Table 2. Differential Diagnosis of Tachycardias

Narrow QRS Complexes	Wide QRS Complexes
A. Supraventricular tachycardia	A. Ventricular tachycardia
1. Sinus tachycardia	B. Supraventricular tachycardia with aberration
2. Paroxysmal atrial tachycardia or AV junctional tachycardia*	1. Bundle branch block
3. Atrial fibrillation	2. Wolff-Parkinson-White (WPW) syndrome
4. Atrial flutter	
5. Multifocal atrial tachycardia	

*Including reentrant AV nodal tachycardia and narrow-complex tachycardias involving a bypass tract (Wolff-Parkinson-White syndrome). These arrhythmias are sometimes labeled as different types of paroxysmal supraventricular tachycardia (PSVT, see pp. 162 and 168, footnote).

Patients in any one of these categories with atrial fibrillation or atrial flutter with a rapid ventricular response or PAT require emergency therapy. If they do not respond promptly to initial drug administration, then electrical cardioversion should be considered.

Another major question to ask about any patient having a tachyarrhythmia (or any arrhythmia for that matter) is whether the patient is taking digitalis or other drugs. Some arrhythmias, such as PAT with block, may be digitalis toxic rhythms, disturbances for which electrical cardioversion is contraindicated (Chapter 16). Finally, in the case of atrial fibrillation you should check to see if the arrhythmia is chronic or acute, remembering that, although chronic atrial fibrillation can sometimes be converted to normal sinus rhythm, the rhythm often reverts to atrial fibrillation.

SICK SINUS SYNDROME AND THE BRADY-TACHY SYNDROME

We continue this discussion of arrhythmias with an interesting group of patients who have bradyarrhythmias and sometimes alternating attacks of brady- and tachyarrhythmias.

The term *"sick sinus syndrome"* has been coined to describe patients with sinus node dysfunction that causes marked sinus bradycardia, sinus arrest, or junctional escape rhythms, which may lead to symptoms of light-headedness and even syncope.

In some patients with the sick sinus syndrome these bradycardic episodes alternate with periods of tachycardia (for example, PAT, atrial fibrillation, or even VT). Sometimes the bradycardia will occur immediately after spontaneous termination of the tachycardia. The term *"brady-tachy syndrome"* has been used to describe this subset of patients with sick sinus syndrome who have tachyarrhythmias as well as bradyarrhythmias (Fig. 18-13).

Diagnosis of the sick syndrome and, in particular, the brady-tachy variant often requires monitoring the patient's heartbeat over several hours or even days. A single ECG strip may be normal or may reveal only the bradycardic or tachycardic episode. Only long-term monitoring may reveal both sides of these patients' problem: the bradyarrhythmias and tachyarrhythmias. The use of continuous ECG (Holter) monitoring in evaluating elderly patients with light-headedness and syncope has shown a surprisingly high frequency of sick sinus syndrome. Treatment generally requires a permanent pacemaker to prevent sinus arrest and drugs, such as digitalis, quinidine, verapamil, or a beta blocker, to control the tachycardias after the pacemaker has been inserted.

WANDERING ATRIAL PACEMAKER

We conclude this chapter with a less common arrhythmia, wandering atrial pacemaker, that has

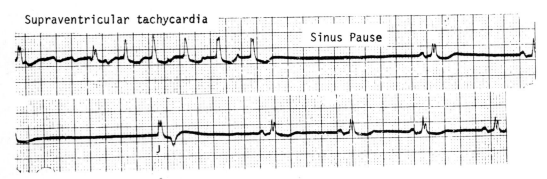

Fig. 18-13. Brady-tachy (sick sinus) syndrome. This rhythm strip shows supraventricular tachycardia (probably atrial flutter) followed by a sinus pause, an AV junctional escape beat *(J)*, and then sinus rhythm.

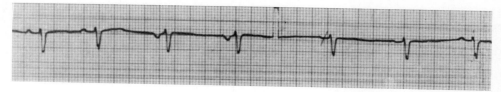

Fig. 18-14. Wandering atrial pacemaker. Notice the variability of P wave configuration in this lead II rhythm strip caused by shifting of the pacemaker site. (From Phibbs B: The cardiac arrhythmias, ed 3, St Louis, 1978, The CV Mosby Co.)

not been mentioned to this point because it is somewhat difficult to classify. As shown in Fig. 18-14, wandering atrial pacemaker is characterized by multiple P waves of varying configuration with a relatively normal or slow heart rate. This pattern reflects shifting of the pacemaker between the sinus node, other atrial sites, and sometimes the AV junction. Wandering atrial pacemaker may be seen in a variety of settings. Occasionally it develops in normal subjects, and it may be seen with digitalis excess as well as with a variety of different types of organic heart disease.

Wandering atrial pacemaker is distinct from MAT (p. 225), another arrhythmia with multiple different P waves. In wandering atrial pacemaker the rate is normal or slow. In MAT it is rapid.

REVIEW

Arrhythmias can be grouped into *bradycardias* (with a heart rate *slower* than 60 beats/min) and *tachycardias* (with a heart rate *faster* than 100 beats/min).

Bradycardias include five major arrhythmias: (1) sinus bradycardia, (2) AV junctional (nodal) rhythm, (3) second- or third-degree heart block or AV dissociation, (4) atrial fibrillation (or flutter) with a slow ventricular rate, and (5) idioventricular escape rhythm. Digitalis or other drug toxicity may be responsible for any of these arrhythmias.

Tachycardias can be subdivided into (1) those with a *narrow* QRS complex and (2) those with a *wide* QRS. The narrow-QRS tachycardias are always *supraventricular* (SVT)—the five most common being (1) sinus tachycardia, (2) paroxysmal atrial tachycardia (or AV junctional tachycardia), (3) atrial fibrillation, (4) atrial flutter, and (5) multifocal atrial tachycardia (MAT). Carotid sinus massage is sometimes helpful in differentiating these arrhythmias at the bedside. Tachycardias with a wide QRS complex may be either *ventricular* or any of the SVTs in association with a *bundle branch block* or *Wolff-Parkinson-White* pattern.

The term *"sick sinus syndrome"* describes patients with sinus node dysfunction who may have a marked sinus bradycardia, sometimes with sinus arrest or slow junctional rhythms, that causes light-headedness or syncope. Some patients with the sick sinus syndrome will have periods of tachycardia alternating with the bradycardia *(brady-tachy syndrome)*.

Wandering atrial pacemaker is an arrhythmia characterized by multiple P waves of varying configuration, usually with a relatively normal or slow heart rate.

Questions

1. Answer the following questions concerning the lead II rhythm strip below:
   a. Does it show an SVT or a VT?
   b. Are there P waves present?
   c. What is this arrhythmia?

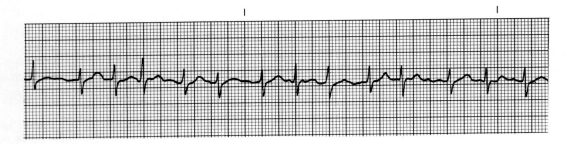

2. What is the most likely diagnosis for the arrhythmia shown below (monitor lead)?

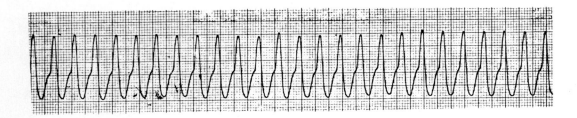

3. A 40-year-old man complaining of occasional palpitations with a fast heartbeat is found to have runs of SVT with a rate of 200 beats/min on his Holter monitor tracing. The rhythm is very regular. What is the most likely diagnosis?
4. What is the cause of the bradycardia in the rhythm strip shown below?

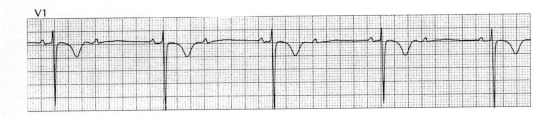

5. Name three readily reversible causes of bradycardia.

Answers

1. a. SVT because of the narrow QRS complexes.
   b. No. The baseline shows an irregular fibrillatory pattern.
   c. Atrial fibrillation.
2. VT.
3. PAT. The rate is too fast for sinus tachycardia and too regular for atrial fibrillation.
4. Sinus rhythm with 2:1 AV block, with a sinus rate of about 74/min and a ventricular rate of about 37/min.
5. Digitalis toxicity, hyperkalemia, excess beta blocker, excess calcium blocker, hypothyroidism.

19

Limitations and Uses of the ECG

Throughout this book the clinical uses of the ECG have been stressed. The purpose of this review chapter is threefold: to underscore some important limitations of the ECG, to reemphasize its utility, and to review some common pitfalls in its interpretation.

IMPORTANT LIMITATIONS OF THE ECG

Like most clinical tests, the ECG yields both *false-positive* and *false-negative* results. A false-positive result is an apparently abnormal ECG in a normal subject. For example, prominent precordial voltage may occur in the absence of LVH (p. 72). Furthermore, Q waves may occur as a normal variant and therefore do not always indicate heart disease (p. 103). False-negative results, on the other hand, occur when the ECG fails to show evidence of some cardiac abnormality. For example, some patients with acute MI may not show diagnostic ST-T changes, or patients with chronic coronary artery disease may not show ST depressions during stress testing.

The diagnostic accuracy of any test is determined by the percentages of these false-positive and false-negative results. The *sensitivity* of a test is a measure of the percentage of patients with a particular abnormality that can be identified by an abnormal test result. For example, a test with 100% sensitivity will not have any false-negative results. The more false-negative results, the less sensitive is the test. The *specificity* of a test is a measure of the percentage of false-positive results. The more false-

positive test results, the less specific is the test. As just noted, both the sensitivity and the specificity of the ECG in diagnosing a variety of conditions, including MI, are limited. It is of great importance for those in clinical practice to be aware of these diagnostic limitations.

Following is a list of a number of important problems that *cannot* be excluded simply because the ECG is normal or shows only nondiagnostic abnormalities:

1. Prior MI
2. Acute MI*
3. Severe coronary artery disease†
4. Significant LVH
5. Significant RVH
6. Intermittent arrhythmias (such as ventricular tachycardia and complete heart block)
7. Acute pulmonary embolism
8. Pericarditis

UTILITY OF THE ECG: SPECIAL CASES

Despite these important limitations, the ECG is an extremely useful test that often helps in the diagnosis of specific cardiac conditions and sometimes can aid in the evaluation and management of general medical problems (such as electrolyte

---

*The pattern of acute MI may also be masked in patients with LBBB, Wolff-Parkinson-White preexcitation, or electronic pacemakers.
†A normal exercise tolerance test also does not exclude severe coronary artery disease.

disorders). The following list indicates some of the particular areas in which the ECG may be helpful:

1. Significant hyperkalemia, a life-threatening electrolyte abnormality, virtually always produces ECG changes, beginning with T wave peaking, loss of P waves, QRS widening, and finally asystole (p. 130).
2. LVH is seen in most patients with severe aortic stenosis.
3. Most patients with atrial septal defect have an RBBB pattern.
4. Persistent ST elevations several weeks after an MI should suggest a ventricular aneurysm.
5. Low QRS voltage in a patient with elevated central venous pressure (distended neck veins) and sinus tachycardia suggests possible pericardial tamponade.
6. Elevated central venous pressure in a patient with ECG evidence of acute inferior wall infarction suggests associated right ventricular infarction (Chapter 8).
7. Frequent PVCs and nonspecific ST-T changes, particularly in a younger patient, should prompt a search for mitral valve prolapse (click-murmur syndrome).
8. Unexplained atrial fibrillation should prompt a search for occult mitral valve disease, hyperthyroidism, or cardiomyopathy.
9. A new S_IQ_{III} or RBBB pattern, particularly in association with sinus tachycardia, should suggest the possibility of pulmonary embolism (Fig. 10-16).
10. Most patients with acute MI show diagnostic ECG changes (new Q waves, ST elevations, hyperacute T waves, ST depressions, or T wave inversions). However, in the weeks and months following an

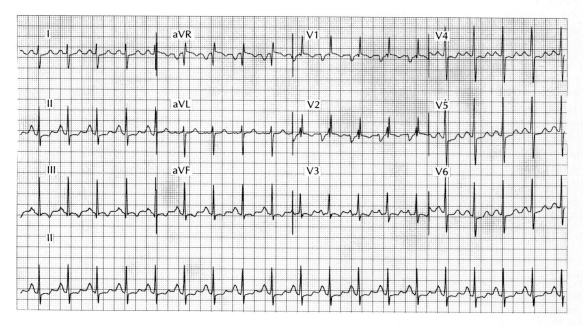

Fig. 19-1. This ECG from a 45-year-old woman with severe mitral stenosis shows multiple abnormalities. The rhythm is sinus tachycardia. Right axis deviation and a tall R in V_1 indicate right ventricular hypertrophy. The prominent biphasic P wave in V_1 indicates left atrial enlargment. The tall P waves in lead II may indicate concomitant right atrial enlargement. There are also nonspecific ST-T changes and an incomplete right bundle branch block. The combination of right ventricular hypertrophy and left atrial enlargement is highly suggestive of mitral stenosis.

acute MI these changes may become less apparent and, in some cases, disappear.

11. The combination of left atrial enlargement and right ventricular hypertrophy on the ECG should suggest the possibility of mitral stenosis (Fig. 19-1).
12. The combination of low voltage and sinus bradycardia should suggest possible hypothyroidism.
13. The combination of low voltage and poor precordial R wave progression is commonly seen with chronic lung disease.
14. The triad of relatively low limb lead voltage, prominent precordial voltage, and poor R wave progression suggests an underlying cardiomyopathy (Chapter 10).

COMMON APPLICATIONS OF THE ECG

The ECG may also provide very important clues in the evaluation of certain major medical problems, such as syncope, coma, shock, and weakness.

Syncope

Fainting can result from primary cardiac factors as well as from a variety of noncardiac causes. The noncardiac causes include vasovagal attack, orthostatic (postural) hypotension, brain dysfunction from vascular insufficiency or metabolic derangements (alcohol, hypoglycemia), and carotid sinus syndrome (vagal hyperreactivity). The cardiac causes can be divided into mechanical obstructions (aortic stenosis, primary pulmonary hypertension, atrial myxoma) and electrical problems (brady- or tachyarrhythmias).

Patients with syncope resulting from aortic stenosis generally show LVH on their resting ECG. Primary pulmonary hypertension is most common in young and middle-aged adult women. The ECG generally shows RVH. The presence of frequent PVCs may be a clue to intermittent ventricular tachycardia. A severe bradycardia (usually from heart block or sick sinus syndrome) in a patient with syncope constitutes the Stokes-Adams syndrome (p. 199). In some cases serious arrhythmias may be recorded only on longer rhythm strips or when 24-hour Holter monitoring is performed.

Syncope in a patient with ECG evidence of bifascicular block (such as RBBB with left anterior hemiblock) should prompt a search for intermittent second- or third-degree heart block. Syncope in patients taking quinidine may be caused by drug toxicity. These persons often have QT prolongation or prominent U waves and thus are prone to torsade de pointes, which may occur despite the fact that the serum quinidine level is in the "therapeutic" or even "sub-therapeutic" range.

Coma

An ECG should be obtained on all comatose patients. If coma is from MI with subsequent cardiac arrest, diagnostic ECG changes related to the infarct are usually seen. Subarachnoid hemorrhage may cause very deep T wave inversions (Fig. 9-10), simulating the changes of MI. Patients with coma associated with hypercalcemia will often show a short QT interval. Myxedema coma generally presents with ECG evidence of sinus bradycardia and low voltage. Widening of the QRS in a comatose patient should raise the possibility of drug overdose (phenothiazine or tricyclic antidepressant) or hyperkalemia.

Shock

An ECG should be obtained promptly on any patient with severe hypotension, because MI is a major cause of shock (cardiogenic shock). In other cases hypotension may be caused by a brady- or tachyarrhythmia. Finally, some patients with shock from noncardiac causes (for example, hypovolemia) may have myocardial ischemia and sometimes infarction as a consequence of their initial problem.

Weakness

An ECG may be helpful in evaluating patients with unexplained weakness. Elderly patients, in particular, may have relatively "silent" MIs with minimal or atypical symptoms, such as the onset of fatigue or general weakness. A prolonged QT interval may be an important clue to unsuspected hypocalcemia, an important metabolic cause of weakness. Hypokalemia may cause weakness along with characteristic ECG changes, including ST depression, T wave flattening, and prominent U waves. In other cases weakness may result from a brady- or tachyarrhythmia.

COMMON PITFALLS IN ECG INTERPRETATION

You can minimize errors in interpreting ECGs by taking care to analyze *all* the points listed on p. 253 in Chapter 21. Many mistakes result from the failure to be systematic (see box). Other mistakes result from confusing ECG patterns that are "look-alikes."

Some common pitfalls (caveats) in ECG interpretation are listed in the accompanying box.

1. Limb lead reversal. Inadvertent reversal of limb lead electrodes will cause diagnostic confusion unless recognized and corrected. For example (Fig. 19-2), reversal of the left and right arm electrodes will cause an apparent rightward QRS axis shift as well as an abnormal P wave axis that simulates an ectopic atrial or junctional rhythm. As a general rule, when lead I shows a negative P wave and a negative QRS, suspect that

---

SOME IMPORTANT REMINDERS

Check standardization

Exclude limb lead reversal (negative P with negative QRS in lead I suggests left/right arm electrode switch)

Look for hidden P waves: AV block, blocked PACs, PAT with block

Narrow-complex tachycardia at about 150/min: consider atrial flutter with 2:1 block

Group beating (clusters of QRS complexes): think of Wenckebach vs blocked PACs

Wide QRS with short PR: consider Wolff-Parkinson-White

Wide QRS without P waves or with AV block: think of hyperkalemia

---

the left and right arm electrodes have been reversed.

2. Failure to check standardization. Many an ECG is mistakenly thought to show "high" or "low" voltage when, in fact, the voltage

LEAD REVERSAL

ARM ELECTRODES
REVERSED

CORRECTED ECG

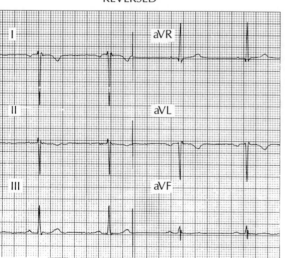
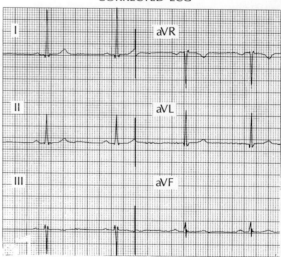

Fig. 19-2. Whenever the QRS axis is unusual, it is important to check for limb lead reversal. Most commonly, the left and right arm electrodes get switched so lead I shows a negative P wave and negative QRS complex.

is normal but the standardization marker is set at $2\times$ or $\frac{1}{2}\times$.

3. Atrial flutter with 2:1 block (conduction). This is one of the most commonly missed diagnoses. The rhythm is often misdiagnosed as either sinus tachycardia (mistaking part of a flutter wave for a P wave) or paroxysmal atrial tachycardia (PAT). *When you see a narrow-complex tachycardia with a ventricular rate of about 150/min, you should strongly suspect atrial flutter.* (See Fig. 13-2).

4. Coarse atrial fibrillation vs atrial flutter. When the fibrillatory waves are prominent (coarse), the rhythm is commonly mistaken for atrial flutter. However, with atrial fibrillation the ventricular rate is completely erratic and the atrial waves are not exactly consistent from one segment to the next. With atrial flutter, on the other hand, even when the ventricular response is variable, the atrial waves will be identical from one moment to the next (Fig. 19-3).

5. Wolff-Parkinson-White (WPW) pattern. The WPW pattern is frequently mistaken for a bundle branch block, hypertrophy, or infarction pattern because the preexcitation results in a wide QRS and may cause increased QRS voltage, T wave inversions, and pseudoinfarction Q waves (Fig. 10-20).

6. AV dissociation vs complete heart block. With AV dissociation the atria and ventricles become "desynchronized" and the QRS rate is the same as or slightly faster than the P wave rate (p. 201). With complete heart block the atria and ventricles also beat independently but the ventricular rate is much slower than the atrial (sinus) rate. AV dissociation is usually a minor arrhythmia, although it may reflect conduction disease or drug toxicity (for example, digitalis). Complete heart block is always a major arrhythmia and generally requires pacemaker therapy.

7. Normal variant vs pathologic Q waves. Do not forget (p. 104) that Q waves may be a normal variant as part of QS waves in leads aV_R, aV_L, aV_F, III, V_1, and occasionally V_2. Small q waves, as part of qR waves, may occur in leads I, II, III, aV_L, aV_F, and

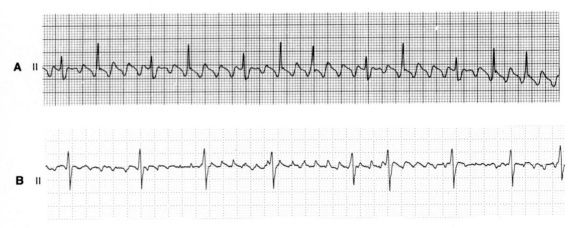

Fig. 19-3. Atrial flutter with variable block, **A,** and coarse atrial fibrillation, **B,** are often confused. Notice that with atrial fibrillation the ventricular rate is completely erratic and the atrial waves are not identical from segment to segment.

the left chest leads (V_4 to V_6). These "septal" q waves are less than 0.04 second in duration. On the other hand, small pathologic Q waves may be overlooked because they are not always very deep. In some cases it may not be possible to state definitively if a Q wave is pathologic or not.

8. AV Wenckebach. In this commonly missed diagnosis an important clue is the appearance of "group beating" (p. 195). The QRS complexes become grouped in clusters due to the intermittent failure of conduction.

9. Hidden ("buried") P waves. These may lead to mistakes in the diagnosis of a number of arrhythmias, including blocked premature atrial contractions (PACs), PAT with block, and second- or third-degree (complete) AV block. It is important therefore to search in the ST segment and T wave for buried P waves. (See Fig. 16-3.)

10. Multifocal atrial tachycardia (MAT) and atrial fibrillation. These are often confused because the ventricular response in both is usually rapid and irregular. With MAT, look for multiple different P waves. With atrial fibrillation, be careful not to mistake the fibrillatory (f) waves for actual P waves.

11. Left bundle branch block (LBBB). This may be mistaken for infarction because it is associated with poor R wave progression and often ST segment elevation in the right chest leads.

12. U waves. These are sometimes overlooked. While small U waves are a physiologic finding, large U waves (which may be apparent in only the chest leads) are sometimes an important marker of hypokalemia or drug toxicity for example, quinidine. Large U waves may be associated with increased risk of *torsade de pointes*, a potentially lethal ventricular arrhythmia (Chapter 14).

13. Severe hyperkalemia. Severe hyperkalemia must always be considered immediately in any patient with an unexplained wide QRS, particularly if P waves are not apparent. Delay in making this diagnosis has proved fatal, because severe hyperkalemia may lead to asystole and cardiac arrest while the clinician is waiting for the report from the chemistry laboratory (Figs. 10-5 to 10-8).

REVIEW

Like most clinical tests, the ECG yields both *false-positive* and *false-negative* diagnoses. For example, not all Q waves indicate MI and not all subjects with actual MI show diagnostic ECG changes. A normal or nondiagnostic ECG also does not exclude LVH, RVH, intermittent life-threatening brady- or tachyarrhythmias, pulmonary embolism, or pericarditis. Despite these limitations in sensitivity and specificity, the ECG does have major uses in a wide range of clinical situations. Besides its obvious utility in assisting cardiac diagnosis, the ECG may also help in evaluating some major medical problems (such as syncope, coma, weakness, and shock).

Questions

1. Which arrhythmias can lead to syncope (fainting)?

True or false (2 and 3)

2. A normal exercise tolerance test excludes significant coronary disease.

3. The more false-positive results associated with a particular test, the less sensitive the test is.

Answers

1. Syncope can be caused by a variety of brady- or tachyarrhythmias (including excessive sinus bradycardia, AV junctional escape rhythm, second- or third-degree AV block, atrial fibrillation with an excessively slow ventricular response, ventricular tachycardia, paroxysmal atrial tachycardia, atrial fibrillation with a rapid ventricular response, or atrial flutter).
2. False.
3. False. The sensitivity of a test is a measure of how well the test can detect a given abnormality. False-positive results (abnormal results in normal subjects) will lower the specificity, not the sensitivity, of the test.

20

Pacemakers: An Introduction

The purpose of this chapter is to provide a brief overview of an important aspect of clinical electrocardiography, electronic cardiac pacemakers. Particular emphasis will be placed on the different types of pacemakers, major indications for pacemaking, and recognition of pacemaker malfunction.

DEFINITIONS

Pacemakers are battery-powered devices designed to electrically stimulate the heart. Pacemakers are used primarily when the patient's own heart rate is excessively slow (bradyarrhythmias, Chapter 18).

A pacemaker has two major components: a battery, which serves as the power source, and a wire electrode, which attaches to the heart chamber being stimulated (usually the right ventricle).

There are two basic types of pacemakers: *temporary* and *implanted (permanent)*. With temporary pacemakers the pacing wire is connected to a battery outside the body. With long-term implanted pacemakers, the battery is inserted subcutaneously, usually under the chest wall. With both, the pacemaker wire is usually threaded through a vein into the right ventricular cavity so the pacemaker electrode can then stimulate the endocardium of the right ventricle (Fig. 20-1). Occasionally, *epicardial* pacemaker wires are used. In such cases the wire is sewn directly into the epicardium of the left or right ventricle and the battery is implanted under the skin of the abdomen. In addition, atrial pacing can be performed under special circumstances. Fi-

nally, some patients benefit from a *dual-chambered* pacemaker with electrodes in both the right atrium and the right ventricle.

PACEMAKER ECG PATTERNS

When a ventricular pacemaker fires, it produces a sharp vertical deflection (pacemaker spike) followed by a QRS complex (representing depolarization of the ventricle). Can you predict what the ECG will show with a functioning right ventricular pacemaker? The ECG should show an LBBB pattern (Fig. 7-8). Recall that the pacemaker is stimulating the right ventricle initially and therefore left ventricular depolarization will be delayed. Figs. 7-8 and 20-2 show examples of typical pacemaker tracings. The vertical line preceeding each QRS complex is the pacemaker spike, followed by a wide QRS with an LBBB morphology (QS in V_1 and wide R wave in V_6). What pattern would you predict with an epicardial pacemaker stimulating the left ventricle? It would be that of an RBBB.

An atrial pacemaker will produce a spike followed by a P wave (Fig. 20-3).

PACEMAKER BATTERIES

There are a variety of battery units that can be used to power implanted pacemakers. Early pacemaker batteries used mercury-zinc cells. However, because of their relatively short life span, these units have been supplanted by lithium batteries, which may last for 5 or more years. As the power cells of conventional pacemakers wear out, the pacemaker rate will usually start to slow.

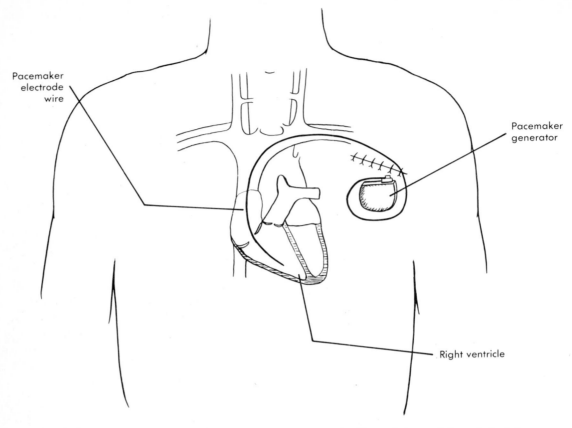

Fig. 20-1. Implanted pacemaker generator (battery) with a wire electrode inserted through the left subclavian vein into the right ventricle.

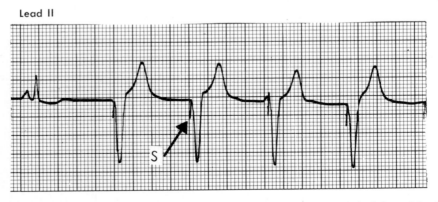

Fig. 20-2. Pacemaker beats. The first QRS is from a normal sinus beat. It is followed by four pacemaker beats. Notice the pacemaker spike *(S)* preceding each paced beat. Pacemaker beats are wide and resemble bundle branch block beats.

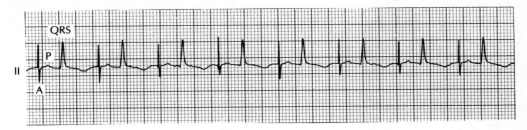

Fig. 20-3. With the pacemaker electrode placed in the right atrium, notice the pacemaker spike *(A)* before each P wave. The QRS is normal since there is no electronic ventricular pacemaker.

VENTRICULAR PACING: FIXED-RATE AND DEMAND PACEMAKERS

There are two modes of pacemaker function: (1) *fixed rate* and (2) *demand.* A fixed-rate pacemaker is one that fires at a specific preset rate, regardless of the patient's own heart rate. The earliest pacemakers were fixed-rate devices. Currently, virtually all pacemakers are demand units. A demand pacemaker literally functions "on demand," that is, only when the patient's heart rate falls below a preset number. Therefore, a demand pacemaker has two distinct aspects: first, a *sensing* mechanism designed so the pacemaker will be inhibited when the heart rate is adequate; second, a *pacing* mechanism designed to trigger the pacemaker when no intrinsic QRS complexes occur within a predetermined period. By contrast, fixed-rate pacemakers lack a sensing mechanism. Demand units can be temporarily converted to fixed-rate mode by placing a special magnet on the chest wall over the battery. The magnet test is routinely performed when the pacemaker rate is being checked. Most of the present day demand-type pacemakers are "programmable"; that is, the pacing rate can be adjusted once the pacemaker is implanted (p. 250). Adjustment of rate is accomplished by placing a special magnet on the chest wall to activate a switch inside the pacemaker unit.

There are actually two types of demand ventricular pacemakers: QRS (R wave) inhibited and QRS (R wave) triggered. The function of both units is essentially the same—to pace the heart when the intrinsic rate falls below some preset value. However, the circuitry of QRS-inhibited and QRS-trig- gered pacemakers is different, resulting in different ECG patterns.

QRS-inhibited pacemakers emit pulses only when the spontaneous heart rate falls below the escape rate of the pacemaker (for example, 70/min) (Figs. 20-4 and 20-5). The QRS-inhibited pacemaker does not emit pulses when the patient's spontaneous heart rate is faster than the escape rate of the pacemaker. Each time the pacemaker senses a spontaneous QRS complex, formation of a pacemaker pulse will be inhibited. Therefore a QRS-inhibited pacemaker will show pacemaker spikes only when the spontaneous heart rate is slower than the escape rate of the pacemaker. The spikes appear before each QRS complex.

The QRS-inhibited pacemaker also has a *refractory* period (for example, 0.4 sec), which begins whenever the pacemaker senses a QRS or emits a pulse (Fig. 20-6). During the refractory period the pacemaker cannot sense another R wave. However, if spontaneous ventricular beats or ventricular premature contractions occur during the refractory period, they will not be inhibited but will appear on the ECG. The refractory period is followed by an *alert* period, during which the pacemaker can sense an R wave. If no QRS is sensed by the end of the alert period, the pacemaker will emit another pulse (Fig. 20-6). However, if a spontaneous QRS occurs, the pacemaker will be recycled into another refractory period and then into another alert period. The escape rate and the refractory period may be externally adjustable on certain *programmable* pacemakers (p. 250).

QRS-triggered pacemakers emit a pulse when-

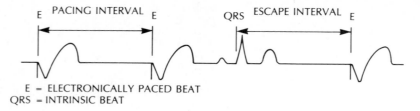

E = ELECTRONICALLY PACED BEAT
QRS = INTRINSIC BEAT

Fig. 20-4. A ventricular demand (QRS-inhibited) pacemaker will emit an electronic pulse only when the intrinsic heart rate falls below the escape rate of the pacemaker.

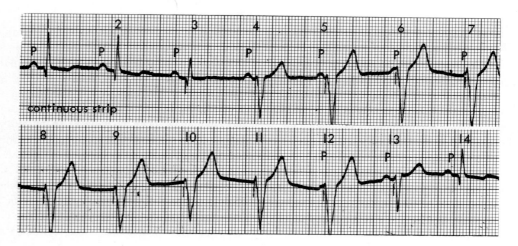

Fig. 20-5. QRS-inhibited pacing (lead II). In beats *1* and *2* the rhythm is regular sinus. In beat *3* the ventricular rate has slowed slightly so a pacemaker spike appears at approximately the same time as the regular stimulus spreads through the ventricles from the AV node. The result is a fusion beat. In beats *4* through *12* the pacemaker is functioning because the patient's spontaneous heart rate has slowed below the pacemaker escape rate (in this case, 70/min). Then the patient's spontaneous ventricular rate becomes more rapid, so beat *13* is a fusion beat and beat *14* again shows regular sinus rhythm. P waves merge into QRS complexes in beats *4* through *7* and then reemerge in beats *12* to *14*. (From Goldberger E: Treatment of cardiac emergencies, ed 4, St Louis, 1985, The CV Mosby Co.)

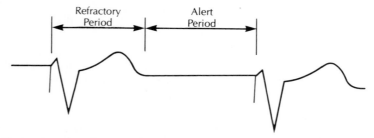

Fig. 20-6. During the refractory period a ventricular demand pacemaker will not sense any electrical activity. This is followed by the alert period. If no QRS is sensed by the end of the alert period, the pacemaker will emit an escape pulse.

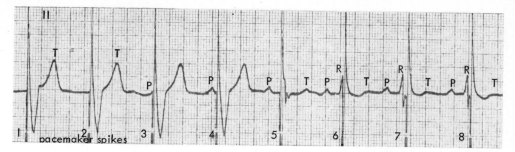

Fig. 20-7. QRS-triggered pacing (lead II). In beats *1* through *4* the patient's spontaneous ventricular rate has slowed below the escape rate of the pacemaker, which has started to form stimuli at a regular rate of 70/min. In the meantime the patient's spontaneous heart rate is increasing (notice P waves emerging), so beats *5* through *8* are spontaneous regular sinus beats with pacemaker spikes occurring in the QRS complexes. Notice how the shapes of the QRS complexes and T waves of beats *5* through *8* are different from their shapes in beats *1* through *4*. (From Goldberger E: Treatment of cardiac emergencies, ed 4, St Louis, 1985, The CV Mosby Co.)

ever the catheter tip senses a spontaneous QRS. The pulse is recorded on the ECG as a spike superimposed on the patient's own QRS (Fig. 20-7); hence, the term "QRS triggered." However, the pacemaker spike does not acutally "capture the ventricles" because the heart is refractory to further depolarization immediately after the QRS complex. Therefore the QRS-triggered pacemaker is actually in a *standby* stage as long as adequate spontaneous ventricular activity is present. When the patient's heart rate slows below the escape rate of the pacemaker, the spikes will appear *before* each QRS and the pacemaker will take over the function of pacing the heart. QRS-triggered pacemakers are confusing at first examination because the pacemaker spikes that come with the patient's spontaneous beat tend to distort the QRS and ST-T complexes (Fig. 20-7). Partly for this reason virtually all of the pacemakers currently in use are QRS-inhibited rather than QRS-triggered devices.

DUAL-CHAMBER PACING

In recent years there have been considerable advances in dual-chamber pacing, in which pacemaker wires are inserted into the right atrium as well as the right ventricle. With the most sophisticated models the circuitry permits sensing and pacing in both the atrium and the ventricle. Thus

the atrial lead is able to sense the patient's intrinsic P waves and, when the atrial rate becomes too slow, to stimulate the right atrium. The circuitry is designed to allow for a physiologic delay between atrial stimulation and ventricular stimulation. This *AV delay* (interval between the atrial pacemaker spike and the ventricular pacemaker spike) is analogous to the PR interval seen in normal conduction.

With the type of dual-chamber pacemaker that allows for both atrial sensing and atrial pacing as well as ventricular sensing and pacing, a variety of ECG patterns may be seen depending on the patient's intrinsic electrical activity. A schematic of these pacemaker patterns appears in Fig. 20-8.

Beats *1* to *5* show spontaneous atrial activity at a rate above the programmed atrial "escape" rate of the pacemaker. When these P waves are sensed by the atrial electrode, the atrial pacemaker will be inhibited. However, the spread of stimulus through the AV junction is slower than the programmed AV delay of the pacemaker; therefore the ventricular pacemaker will produce a wide QRS complex preceded by a pacemaker spike *(V)*.

In beat *6* a spontaneous P wave is also present and conduction through the AV junction is delayed as in the five preceeding beats; therefore a ventricular pacemaker spike will occur, but in this beat the spontaneous QRS occurs at the same time as

DUAL-CHAMBER (DDD) PACING

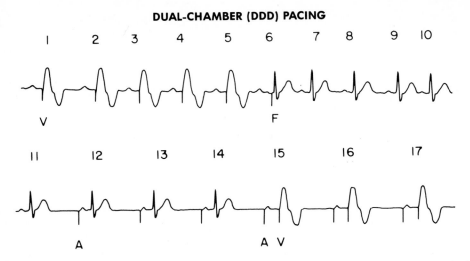

Fig. 20-8. Schematic of the different beats that may be seen with a properly functioning dual-chamber (DDD) pacemaker. (See text.) (Adapted from Zipes DP: In Current clinical applications of dual-chamber pacing. [Proceedings of a symposium in Dallas, November 15, 1981], Minneapolis, 1982, Medtronic Inc.)

the pacemaker spike, resulting in a so-called fusion beat *(F)*.

Beats *8* to *11* are normal beats, in which the atrial rate is above the escape rate of the atrial pacemaker and conduction through the AV junction is faster than the AV delay of the pacemaker; therefore, the pacemaker will be inhibited from discharging either atrial or ventricular stimuli.

In beats *12* to *14* the atrial rate has slowed; thus atrial pacemaker spikes *(A)* are now seen and the atrial electrode is pacing the atria. However, these paced P waves are conducted to the ventricles within the AV delay. Therefore, spontaneous QRS complexes occur.

In beats *15* to *17* the atrial rate has dropped below the programmed atrial pacemaker rate. In addition, the stimulus is delayed getting through the AV junction and this delay exceeds the programmed AV delay of the pacemaker. Therefore paced stimuli are delivered to both the atrium and the ventricle. Notice the pacemaker spike preceding the P wave and the QRS complex in these last three beats of the series.

PROGRAMMABILITY

In the early days of cardiac pacing the pacemaker rate was not adjustable once the unit had been inserted. A major advance was the introduction of programmable pacemakers, in which the pacemaker rate could be externally changed. In newer pacemakers multiple other parameters in addition to the rate can be externally programmed—including the voltage of the pacemaker discharge, the sensitivity of the electrode to the intrinsic beats, the pacemaker refractory period, and the duration of the pacemaker spike. For discussion of multiprogrammable pacemakers the reader is referred to the Bibliography.

INDICATIONS FOR CARDIAC PACING
Implanted (Permanent) Pacemakers

There are a variety of indications for electronic pacemakers. As noted before, *the major reason for implanting a pacemaker is the presence of a symptomatic bradyarrhythmia.*

For example, permanent pacemakers are indicated in patients with syncope, light-headedness, weakness, or congestive failure caused by complete heart block, second-degree AV block, marked sinus bradycardia or sinus pauses (sick sinus syndrome), slow junctional rhythms, or atrial fibrillation or flutter with an excessively slow ventricular response.

Temporary Pacemakers

There are three types of temporary pacemakers: transvenous, transthoracic, and external (pp. 213 and 215). With *transvenous* pacemakers the external battery is connected to a pacing electrode that has been threaded through a vein into the right ventricle. Sometimes, during cardiac arrest a *transthoracic* pacing wire will be inserted by trochar directly through the chest wall into the right ventricular chamber. Finally, *external* temporary pacing can be accomplished using specially designed electrodes pasted on the chest wall. Although this last technique is not successful in all patients and may cause some discomfort, it has proved of great use and may spare the patient the need for inserting a transvenous or transthoracic pacemaker.

Temporary pacemakers are often employed during cardiac emergencies (such as MI), when an extremely slow heart rate occurs. For example, patients with acute *anterior* wall MI in whom complete heart block develops always require a temporary pacemaker (and a permanent pacemaker later on) because of the markedly slow heart rate that occurs. On the other hand, second-degree and even complete heart blocks are not uncommon with *inferior* wall MI because of excessive vagal tone or AV junctional ischemia. AV block with inferior infarction tends to be transient, and the heart rate is often adequate without an electronic pacemaker. However, other patients with inferior MI and second- or third-degree AV block may require a temporary pacemaker if their heart rate becomes excessively slow, resulting in hypotension, angina, or congestive heart failure.

Temporary pacemakers are also often employed after open heart surgery. They may be required during cardiac arrest (Chapter 17), when the ECG

shows asystole or slow escape rhythm that does not respond to drug therapy. Occasionally they will be needed with digitalis toxicity, which may cause any of the major bradyarrhythmias.

As noted, temporary (and permanent) pacemakers are usually employed when the heart rate is too slow. Rarely one will be implanted to treat a tachyarrhythmia (such as atrial or ventricular tachycardia). The use of pacing in the treatment of atrial flutter is mentioned on p. 173.

As described in Chapter 15, temporary (transvenous or external) pacemakers are sometimes recommended prophylactically in patients with acute anterior wall MI in whom evidence appears of new bifascicular block (LBBB, RBBB with left anterior hemiblock, RBBB with left posterior hemiblock). Such patients have a high incidence of progressing to complete (trifascicular) heart block. On the other hand, as emphasized in Chapter 15, patients with *chronic* bifascicular block who are *without symptoms* do not require permanent pacemakers.

Dual-chamber pacing is helpful in maintaining physiologic timing between atrial systole and ventricular systole. When ventricular pacing alone is used, such physiologic timing will be lost. In some patients the loss of timed atrial contractions causes a marked reduction in cardiac output. Dual-chamber pacing will produce a significant improvement in the cardiac performance of these persons. It may also be desirable in selected patients in permitting a physiologic increase in ventricular rate during exercise. For example, consider the patient with complete heart block and underlying sinus rhythm whose ventricular rate with a ventricular pacemaker is constant (say, 72/min) regardless of the atrial (P wave) rate. With a dual-chamber pacemaker the ventricular rate will be able to increase in tandem with the atrial rate during exercise, further increasing cardiac output.

Dual-chamber pacemakers, however, are not without their disadvantages. Atrial electrodes are more likely than ventricular electrodes to become dislodged. Furthermore, dual-chamber pacemakers may induce tachycardias in some patients. In addition, they are considerably more expensive than simple ventricular pacemakers. Finally, atrial sensing or pacing is obviously of no use in the setting of atrial fibrillation or atrial flutter.

PACEMAKER MALFUNCTION

Pacemaker malfunctions occur when either the sensing or the pacing function is impaired.

For example, when the pacemaker battery runs down, the pacemaker rate generally slows and *failure to sense* may occur. Failure to sense can be diagnosed by observing pacemaker spikes despite the patient's own adequate QRS rate (Fig. 20-9). The most common causes of failure to sense are dislodgment of the pacemaker wire or excessive fibrosis around the tip of the pacing wire.

Pacemaker malfunction can also result from *failure to pace*. Failure to pace is diagnosed either by observing pacemaker spikes without subsequent

QRS complexes (failure to "capture") (Fig. 20-10) or by the complete absence of pacemaker spikes despite an excessively slow heart rate (Fig. 20-11). Failure to pace can also be caused by dislodgment of the pacemaker wire or by fibrosis around the tip of the pacing wire. In such cases pacemaker spikes will occur without associated QRS complexes. In other cases (particularly with a broken electrode wire, a short-circuit in the pacing circuit, or electrical interference from the muscles of the chest wall) failure to pace will occur without any pacemaker spike.

Pacemaker malfunction in patients with temporary pacemakers should always prompt a search for loose connections between the battery and the pacing wire, a faulty battery, or a dislodged wire.

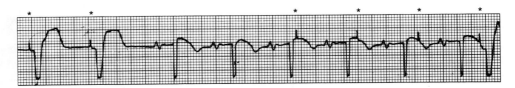

Fig. 20-9. Pacemaker malfunction: failure to sense. Notice that after the first two paced beats there is a series of sinus beats with first-degree AV block. Failure of the pacemaker unit to sense these intrinsic QRS complexes leads to inappropriate pacemaker spikes (*), which fall on T waves. Three of these spikes do not capture the ventricle because they occur during the refractory period of the cardiac cycle. (From Conover MH: Understanding electrocardiography, ed 4, St Louis, 1984, The CV Mosby Co.)

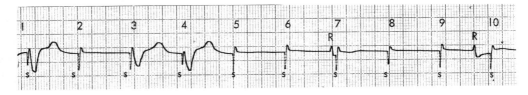

Fig. 20-10. Pacemaker malfunction: failure to pace. Notice that beats *1, 3,* and *4* show the pacemaker spikes *(s)* and normally paced QRS complexes and T waves. The remaining beats show only pacemaker spikes. *R* represents the patient's slow spontaneous QRS complexes. (From Goldberger E: Treatment of cardiac emergencies, ed 4, St Louis, 1985, The CV Mosby Co.)

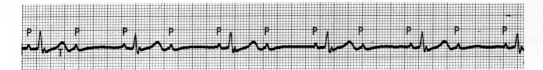

Fig. 20-11. Pacemaker malfunction: failure to pace (no pacemaker spikes). The underlying rhythm is 2:1 AV block (Mobitz type II). Despite a slow heart rate, the pacemaker fails to function. (From Goldberger E: Treatment of cardiac emergencies, ed 4, St Louis, 1985, The CV Mosby Co.)

COMPLICATIONS OF PACEMAKER THERAPY

Pacemakers are not without potential harm. Therefore careful thought should be given before inserting a temporary or, particularly, a permanent pacemaker. Infection may occur at the pacemaker site. The electrode may perforate the ventricular wall. The pacemaker itself may cause serious arrhythmias. For example, certain dual-chamber pacemakers may initiate runs of supraventricular tachycardia ("endless loop" arrhythmias). Occasionally the pacemaker will also pace the muscles of the chest wall or the diaphragm, resulting in patient discomfort.

DIAGNOSIS OF MI WITH PACEMAKERS

The ECG diagnosis of MI may be difficult or impossible in patients with functioning pacemakers in which all beats are paced. In such cases (with a right ventricular electrode) the ECG will show an LBBB configuration. As described in Chapter 8, LBBB generally masks both the QRS and the ST-T changes of MI. Therefore, unless you see spontaneous QRS-T complexes, the diagnosis of acute or prior MI may not be possible from the ECG alone.

Finally, it is important to recognize that pacemakers may also produce ECG changes simulating MI. Following periods of electronic ventricular pacemaking the ECG may show deep noninfarctional T waves in the patient's spontaneous beats. These *post-pacemaker T wave inversions* can be mistaken for primary ischemic ST-T changes.

APPENDIX: PACEMAKER CODE

A three-position pacemaker code is often used to describe what a particular pacemaker's functions and mode of response are. As shown below, the letter in the first position indicates the chamber(s) being paced—which may be the *atrium* (A), the *ventricle* (V), or *both* (D). The letter in the second position indicates the chamber(s) where sensing occurs—again the atrium (A), ventricle (V), or both (D). Finally, the letter in the third position refers to the mode of response of the pacemaker (p. 243). In the earlier, and in many current, pacemaker models the pacing mode was either *inhibited* (I) or *triggered* (T). The mode of response is labeled D *(double)* in the case of the newer, more advanced, *dual-chamber* pacemakers, which are engineered so the pacemaker responds to atrial electrical activity by delivering a ventricular spike (provided, or course, a spontaneous QRS has not already occurred).

There is a fourth mode of response, designated R, which stands for *reverse*. A pacemaker in the reverse mode will pace during periods of tachycardia rather than bradycardia. Such pacemakers are used for their antiarrhythmic action (p. 26 and Bibliography).

The most widely used pacemakers today are VVI units; that is, they are single-chamber pacemakers that both pace (V) and sense (V) exclusively in the ventricle and are inhibited (I) by the patient's own QRS complexes.

The most versatile pacemakers are DDD units. These are dual-chamber pacemakers that can pace the atrium or ventricle (D) and sense in the atrium or ventricle (D). In addition, the mode of response is double (D): atrial pacing can be inhibited by the patient's P waves and a ventricular pacer spike will be triggered by the patient's P waves if a native QRS does not appear within a preset time because of AV block.

Other types of dual-chamber pacemakers (for example, DVI and VDD models) have also been developed. The specific uses and limitations of these dual chamber units are discussed in references in the Bibliography.

The three-letter pacemaker code has recently been expanded to five letters, reflecting the rapid advances in pacemaker electronics over the past few years. The fourth letter indicates the *programming* features of the pacemaker. The fifth letter indicates *special antiarrhythmic features* that are available in certain pacemakers. Further discussion of these technical areas lies beyond the scope of this brief introduction.

Three-Position Pacemaker Code

Position	I	II	III
Category	Chamber(s) paced	Chamber(s) sensed	Mode of response(s)
Letters used	V–Ventricle	V–Ventricle	T–Triggered
	A–Atrium	A–Atrium	I–Inhibited
	D–Double*	D–Double	D–Double
			O–None
		O–None	R–Reverse

Double mode of response. This refers to dual-chamber pacemakers in which atrial pacing may be inhibited by the patient's own P waves and a ventricular spike may be triggered by the patient's P wave if AV block is present.

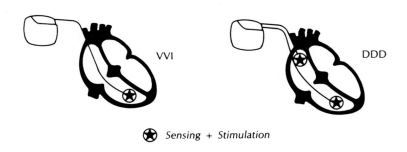

⊛ *Sensing + Stimulation*

REVIEW

Pacemakers are battery-powered devices used to stimulate the heart electrically, particularly in cases where the patient's own heart rate is excessively slow. When the pacemaker wire is attached to the right ventricular endocardium, the ECG will show an LBBB pattern as a result of delayed left ventricular stimulation. Each QRS will be preceded by a pacemaker spike. Cardiac pacing can be done in a *fixed-rate* or *demand* mode. Demand pacemakers are inhibited when the heart rate is faster than the escape rate of the pacemaker. There are two types of ventricular demand pacemakers: *QRS inhibited* and *QRS triggered*.

A temporary pacemaker is a unit with an external battery. Temporary pacing wires can be inserted during cardiac emergencies (for example, cardiac arrest caused by asystole or MI complicated by high-degree heart block or sinus arrest). An implanted permanent pacemaker, in which the battery is inserted subcutaneously, usually in the chest wall, is indicated for patients with symptomatic second- or third-degree AV block or other major bradyarrhythmias (such as sinus arrest or slow junctional escape rhythm) leading to inadequate cardiac output.

Dual-chamber (atrial and ventricular) pacemakers have been developed in recent years. They may be helpful in maintaining physiologic timing between atrial and ventricular contractions, thus increasing cardiac output.

When the pacemaker battery starts to run down, the pacemaker rate will slow. Dislodgment of the pacemaker wire or excessive fibrosis around the tip of the wire can cause failure to sense or failure to pace. Pacing failure in permanent units can also be caused by electrode fracture, short-circuits, or electrical interference from skeletal muscles.

Pacemakers may obscure the ECG diagnosis of MI. Conversely, following electronic pacing of the ventricles, deep noninfarctional T wave inversions may appear in spontaneous QRS complexes *(post-pacemaker T wave pattern)*.

Questions

1. The major indication for *permanent* pacemakers is
   a. History of multiple prior MIs
   b. Symptomatic bradyarrhythmias
   c. Digitalis toxicity
   d. Ventricular bigeminy
   e. Paroxysmal atrial tachycardia

2. The following rhythm strip shows
    a. Failure to sense
    b. Failure to pace
    c. Normal pacemaker function with a PVC
    d. Failure to sense and pace

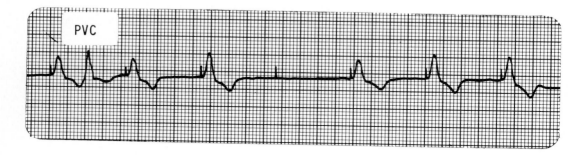

3. What does the following rhythm strip show?

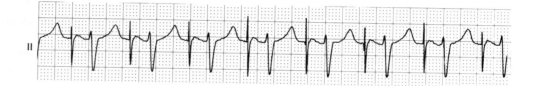

Answers

1. b.
2. b. This is an example of intermittent failure to pace, when the fourth pacemaker spike is not followed by a QRS. The two most common causes of failure to pace, with a pacemaker spike that does not capture, are dislodgment of the electrode wire and fibrosis around the pacing wire tip. Pacemaker failure may also occur in which no pacing spikes are seen (p. 248). Notice in Fig. 20-6 that the PVC falls within the refractory period of the pacemaker and is not sensed.
3. An atrial pacemaker. Notice the sharp pacemaker spike before each P wave followed by a normal QRS. (See Fig. 20-3.)

21

How To Interpret an ECG

In Parts I and II the fundamentals of the normal ECG and the major abnormal patterns and arrhythmias were described. Part III is a collection of test questions to help you review these topics. We will conclude Part II with a brief summary of how systematically to approach any ECG.

ECG INTERPRETATIONS

Accurate interpretation of ECGs requires, above all, thoroughness and care. Therefore it is essential to develop a systematic method of reading ECGs that is applied in every case. Many of the most common mistakes are errors of omission: failure to note certain subtle but critical findings. For example, overlooking a short PR interval may result in missing the important diagnosis of the Wolff-Parkinson-White pattern. Marked prolongation of the QT interval, a potential precursor of torsade de pointes (Chapter 14) and sudden death, often goes unnoticed. These and other common pitfalls in ECG diagnosis are reviewed in Chapter 19.

There are 14 points that should be analyzed on every ECG.

1. Standardization
2. Heart rate
3. Rhythm
4. PR interval
5. P wave size
6. QRS width
7. QT interval
8. QRS voltage
9. Mean QRS electrical axis
10. R wave progression in chest leads
11. Abnormal Q waves
12. ST segment
13. T wave
14. U wave

Standardization (p. 10). Make sure that the electrocardiograph has been properly calibrated so the standardization mark is 10 mm tall (1 mV = 10 mm).*

Heart rate (p. 16). Calculate the heart rate. If the rate is faster than 100 beats/min, then a tachycardia is present. A rate slower than 60 beats/min means a bradycardia is present.

Be particularly careful not to overlook hidden P waves, seen, for example, in some cases of second- or third-degree AV block, paroxysmal atrial tachycardia (PAT) with block, and blocked PACs. Also, whenever the ventricular rate is about 150/min, always consider the possibility of atrial flutter since the flutter waves may mimic the P waves of sinus or AV junctional rhythm.

PR interval. The normal PR interval (measured from the beginning of the P wave to the beginning of the QRS) is 0.12 to 0.2 second. A uniformly prolonged PR interval means *first-degree AV block* is present. A short PR interval (with a wide QRS and a delta wave) is seen with the Wolff-Parkinson-White syndrome. A short PR interval with a normal

---

*In special cases the ECG may be intentionally recorded at $^1/_2$ standardization (1 mV = 5 mm) or 2× standardization (1 mV = 20 mm).

width QRS may represent Lown-Ganong-Levine type of preexicitation. By contrast, a short PR with retrograde P waves (negative in lead II) generally indicates an ectopic atrial or AV junctional pacemaker.

P wave size. Normally the P wave does not exceed 2.5 mm amplitude and is less than 3 mm wide in all leads. Tall peaked P waves may be a sign of right atrial enlargement (P pulmonale). Wide P waves are seen with left atrial abnormality.

QRS width. Normally the QRS width is 0.1 second or less in all leads. The differential diagnosis of a wide QRS complex is described on p. 143.

QT interval. A prolonged QT interval may be a clue to electrolyte disturbances (hypocalcemia, hypokalemia), drug effects (quinidine, procainamide), or myocardial ischemia. Shortened QT intervals are seen with hypercalcemia and digitalis effect.

QRS voltage. Look for signs of right or left ventricular hypertrophy (p. 75). Remember that thin-chested people and young adults frequently show tall voltage without left ventricular hypertrophy. Do not forget about low voltage (p. 136), which may result from pericardial effusion, myxedema, emphysema, obesity, or myocardial disease.

Mean QRS electrical axis. Estimate the mean QRS axis in the frontal plane. Decide by inspection whether the axis is normal (between $-30°$ and $+100°$) or whether left or right axis deviation is present.

R wave progression in chest leads. Inspect leads V_1 to V_6 to see if the normal increase in R waves is seen as you move across the chest. Poor R wave progression may be a sign of myocardial infarction, but it may also be seen with left ventricular hypertrophy, chronic lung disease, left bundle branch block, and other conditions in the absence of infarction.

Abnormal Q waves (Chapter 8). Abnormal Q waves in leads II, III, and aV_F may indicate inferior wall infarction. Abnormal Q waves in the anterior leads (I, aV_L, and V_1 to V_6) may indicate anterior wall infarction.

ST segment. Look for abnormal ST segment elevations or depressions.

T wave. Inspect the T waves. Normally they are positive in leads with a positive QRS complex. They are also normally positive in leads V_3 to V_6 in adults, negative in lead aV_R, and positive in lead II. The polarity of the T waves in the other extremity leads depends on the QRS electrical axis. (T waves may be normally negative in lead III in the presence of a vertical QRS axis.)

U wave. Also look for prominent U waves, which may be a sign of hypokalemia or drug effect or toxicity (as with quinidine).

• • •

After you have analyzed these 14 points, you should formulate an overall interpretation.

The final ECG reading actually consists of two sections: (1) a list of notable findings and (2) an interpretive summary that attempts to integrate or explain these findings. For example, the ECG might show a prolonged QT interval and prominent U waves. The interpretation could state: ''Repolarization abnormalities consistent with drug effect or toxicity (quinidine, procainamide, etc.) or hypokalemia. Clinical correlation suggested.'' Another ECG might show wide P waves, right axis deviation, and a tall R wave in lead V_1 (Fig. 19-1). The interpretation could state: ''Findings consistent with left atrial abnormality (enlargement) and right ventricular hypertrophy. This combination is highly suggestive of mitral stenosis.'' In yet a third case the interpretation might simply be: ''Within normal limits.''

Thus the ECG is analogous to a newspaper account that consists, first, of the hard facts and, second, of the editorial comment. Like the editorialist, the ECG interpreter may sometimes offer suggestions, such as ''Serial tracings advisable to evaluate possible evolving ischemic T-wave changes.''

Fig. 21-1 illustrates this systematic approach to ECG reading. Part III contains other examples for practice.

Remember: Every ECG abnormality you identify should summon up a list of differential diagnostic possibilities. You should search for an explanation of every abnormality found. For example, if the ECG shows sinus tachycardia, then

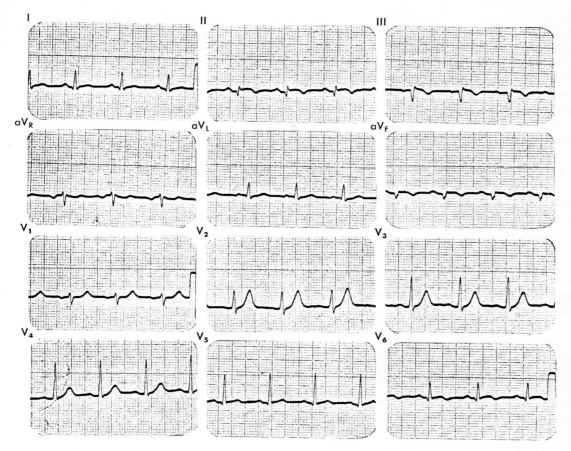

Fig. 21-1. ECG for interpretation:
1. Standardization: proper (1 mV = 10 mm); mark recorded at the end of leads I, V_1, and V_6 (The standardization mark need be recorded only once when taking an ECG.)
2. Heart rate: 88 beats/min
3. Rhythm: normal sinus
4. PR interval: 0.16 second
5. P waves: normal size
6. QRS width: 0.08 second (normal)
7. QT interval: 0.36 second (normal for rate)
8. QRS voltage: normal
9. Mean QRS axis: about −30° (biphasic QRS complex in lead II with positive QRS in lead I)
10. R wave progression in chest leads: early precordial transition with tall R in V_2
11. Abnormal Q waves: leads II, III, and aV_F
12. ST segments: slightly elevated in leads II, III, and aV_F
13. T waves: inverted in leads II, III, aV_F, and V_6
14. U waves: not prominent

Impression: This ECG is consistent with an inferolateral wall MI of indeterminate age. Comment: You cannot determine the age of an infarct from the ECG. The changes here (Q waves and ST-T abnormalities) could have been caused by an infarct that occurred the day before or the year before.

the next question to ask is what caused this arrhythmia? Is it a result of anxiety, hyperthyroidism, congestive heart failure, hypovolemia, sympathomimetic drugs, or other causes? If you find ventricular tachycardia, what are the diagnostic possibilities? Is it due to myocardial infarction or some potentially reversible cause such as hypoxemia, digitalis toxicity, toxic effects of another drug, hypokalemia, or hypomagnesemia? If you see signs of left ventricular hypertrophy, what is the likely cause: valvular heart disease, hypertensive heart disease, or cardiomyopathy? In this way the interpretation of an ECG becomes an integral part of clinical diagnosis and patient care.

Computerized ECG Interpretations

Use of computerized ECG systems is becoming increasingly widespread. These systems provide interpretation and storage of ECG records. In recent years the computer programs (software) for ECG analysis have become more sophisticated and accurate. They are now capable of storing and automatically retrieving thousands of ECGs.

However, despite these advances, computer ECG analyses have important limitations and, not infrequently, are subject to error. Diagnostic errors are most likely with arrhythmias or with more complex abnormalities. Therefore computerized interpretations (including measurements of basic ECG intervals and electrical axes) must never be accepted without careful review.

ECG Artifacts

This section will conclude with a brief discussion of some important ECG artifacts. The ECG, like any other electronic recording, is subject to numerous artifacts that may interfere with accurate interpretation. Some of the most common of these are described here.

60-Hertz (cycle) interference. Interference from alternating-current generators produces the characteristic pattern shown in Fig. 21-2. Notice the fine-tooth comb 60 hertz (Hz) artifacts. By switching the electrocardiograph plug to a different outlet or by turning off other electrical appliances in the room, you can usually eliminate 60 Hz interference.

Muscle tremor. Involuntary muscle tremor (Fig. 21-3) can produce undulations in the baseline that may be mistaken for atrial flutter or fibrillation.

Wandering baseline. Upward or downward movement of the baseline may produce spurious ST segment elevations or depressions (Fig. 21-4).

Poor electrode contact or patient movement. Poor electrode contact or patient movement (Fig. 21-5) can produce artifactual deflections in the baseline that may obscure the underlying pattern or be mistaken for abnormal beats.

Improper standardization. The electrocardiograph, as mentioned, should be standardized before each tracing so a 1 mV pulse produces a square wave 10 mm high (Fig. 2-5). Failure to standardize properly will result in complexes that are either spuriously low or spuriously high. Futhermore, most electrocardiographs are equipped with half standardization and double standardization settings. Unintentional recording of an ECG on either of these settings will also result in misleadingly low or high voltage.

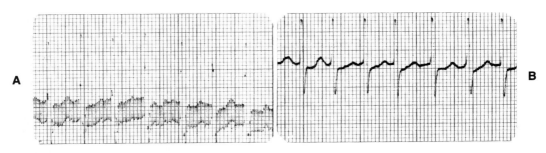

Fig. 21-2. A common ECG artifact is the produced by 60-hertz (Hz) interference. **A,** Fast oscillations of the baseline. **B,** Same pattern without the artifact.

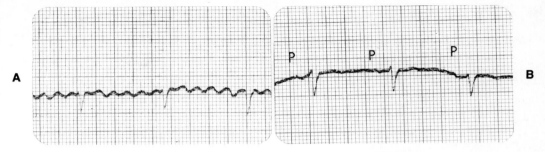

Fig. 21-3. Another common artifact is that produced by muscle tremor. **A,** Wavy baseline simulating atrial flutter. **B,** Same pattern without the artifact showing normal P waves.

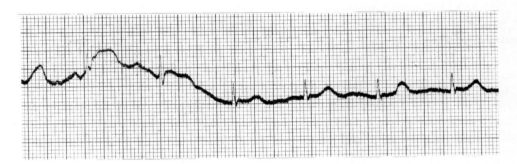

Fig. 21-4. Wandering baseline resulting from patient movement.

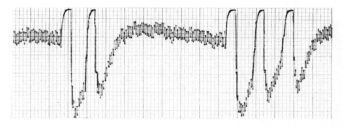

Fig. 21-5. Deflections simulating PVCs produced by patient movement. 60 Hz artifact is also present.

REVIEW

The following 14 points should be evaluated on every ECG:
1. Standardization
2. Heart rate
3. Rhythm
4. PR interval
5. P wave size
6. QRS width
7. QT interval
8. QRS voltage
9. Mean QRS axis
10. R wave progression in chest leads
11. Abnormal Q waves
12. ST segment
13. T wave
14. U wave

Any ECG abnormality should be related to the clinical status of the patient. The ECG can also be affected by numerous artifacts, including 60 Hz interference, patient movement, poor electrode contact, and muscle tremor.

Computer interpretations of ECGs are subject to error and must be carefully reviewed.

Self-Assessment Problems

This third and final section of the text is intended for self-assessment. Numerous review questions and practice examples are included based entirely on the material covered in Parts I and II. The review begins with a number of short-answer questions followed by actual ECGs for interpretation. Unless otherwise indicated, the ECGs have been standardized so 1 mV = 10 mm.

QUESTIONS

1. The P wave represents _____ _____ *(two words).*
2. The QRS complex represents _____ _____ *(two words).*
3. The T wave represents _____ _____ *(two words).*
4. The normal range of the PR interval in adults is between _____ and _____ _____ second.
5. Lead V_1 is obtained by placing the chest electrode to the right of the sternum in the _____ _____ intercostal interspace.
6. With hypocalcemia the QT interval _____.
7. A *delta* wave is seen in what syndrome?
8. Name a drug that may prolong the QT interval.
9. Name three causes of low-voltage QRS complexes.
10. Name at least three arrhythmias associated with digitalis toxicity.
11. A wide rSR' complex in lead V_1 with sinus rhythm most likely indicates _____.
12. Name three ECG patterns that may be seen with acute pulmonary embolism.
13. If the P wave in lead aV_R is -2 mm and the P wave in lead aV_L is -3 mm, then what must the amplitude of the P wave in lead aV_F be?
14. Two factors that may potentiate digitalis toxicity are _____ and _____ _____.
15. Digitalis *(increases? decreases? has no effect on?)* conduction of impulses through the AV junction.
16. What metabolic or drug-related factor may prolong the QRS duration?
17. Prominent U waves are often seen with what electrolyte abnormality?
18. Tall peaked P waves in leads II, III, and aV_F are suggestive of _____.
19. With normal sinus rhythm the P wave is virtually always negative in lead _____ and positive in lead _____ .
20. Draw the hexaxial diagram showing the six extremity (frontal plane) leads.
21. Normally the R/S ratio in lead V_1 (in adults) is less than _____.
22. Atrial fibrillation is sometimes seen in which endocrine disorder?
23. Name the three basic ECG patterns that may be seen in cardiac arrest.
24. Names three causes of sinus tachycardia.
25. Syncope associated with complete heart block or other profound bradycardias is called the _____ - _____ syndrome.
26. Define ventricular tachycardia.
27. Tall, peaked T waves are characteristic of which electrolyte disturbance?
28. Name three causes of ST segment elevations.
29. A patient experiencing typical angina pectoris with exertion may show what ECG pattern as a sign of subendocardial ischemia?
30. Right bundle branch block is always a sign of serious organic heart disease *(true or false).*
31. Atrial fibrillation is always a sign of serious organic heart disease *(true or false).*
32. Left bundle branch block is often a sign of serious organic heart disease *(true or false).*
33. The *early repolarization* pattern is a normal variant *(true or false).*

34. Prinzmetal's angina is characterized by ST segment elevations *(true or false)*.
35. With an acute *anterior* wall infarction, leads II, III, and aV$_F$ are likely to show ST segment _____.
36. Retrograde P waves are characteristic of _____ rhythm.
37. Draw a QS complex.
38. A wide (>0.12 sec) QS complex in lead V$_1$ is seen with _____.
39. Name five causes of ventricular ectopy.
40. A 20-year-old college student complaining of light-headedness and palpitations is found to have a regular tachycardia with narrow QRS complexes at a rate of 200 beats/min. The most likely diagnosis is _____.
41. A patient is found to have a pulse rate of 35 beats/min. The ECG is most likely to show one of five basic classes of rhythms. Name them.
42. Left axis deviation is defined as an axis more negative than − _____°.
43. Name three causes of sinus bradycardia.
44. Name three causes of atrial fibrillation.
45. Persistent ST segment elevations several weeks following a transmural myocardial infarct suggest a possible _____.
46. Which of the following tachycardias is most likely to terminate abruptly following carotid sinus massage: sinus tachycardia, atrial fibrillation, paroxysmal atrial tachycardia, or ventricular tachycardia?
47. A wide biphasic P wave in lead V$_1$ may indicate _____.
48. Which of the following drugs may shorten the QT interval: digitalis, quinidine, procainamide, furosemide (Lasix)?
49. Normally the QRS width is equal to or less than 0._____ second.
50. A qR complex is normally seen in which lead: V$_1$, V$_6$, or aV$_R$?

Define the Following Terms

51. "R on T" phenomenon (p. 184)
52. Ectopic beat (p. 160)
53. Current of injury (p. 95)
54. P mitrale (p. 67)
55. P pulmonale (p. 66)
56. Bifasicular block (p. 199)
57. Frontal plane leads (p. 30)
58. Horizontal plane leads (p. 30)
59. Hyperacute T wave (p. 95)
60. Vertical QRS axis, horizontal QRS axis (p. 44)

Draw the QRS-T Pattern You Would Expect to See in Lead V_6
(for nos. 61 to 65)

61. Normal pattern
62. Left bundle branch block
63. Right bundle branch block
64. Left ventricular hypertrophy with strain
65. Digitalis effect
66. What life-threatening metabolic abnormality caused the ECG findings in this patient?

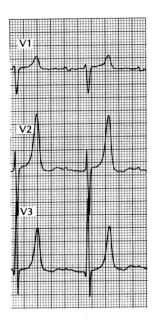

67. What drug could have produced these ST-T changes?

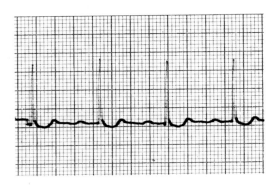

68. What ventricular conduction disturbance is present here?

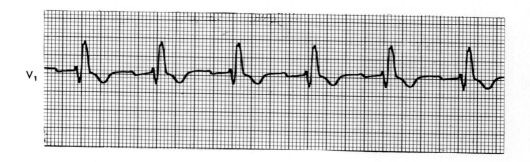

69. What is this heart rhythm?

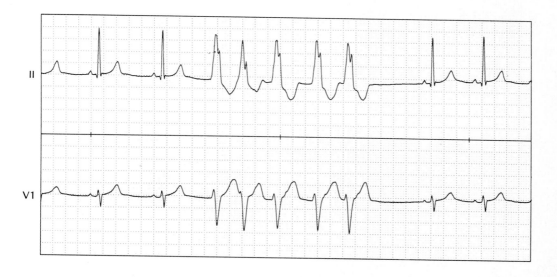

70. What is **X**?

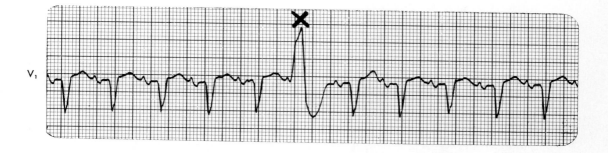

71. Calculate the mean QRS axis in *A* and *B*.

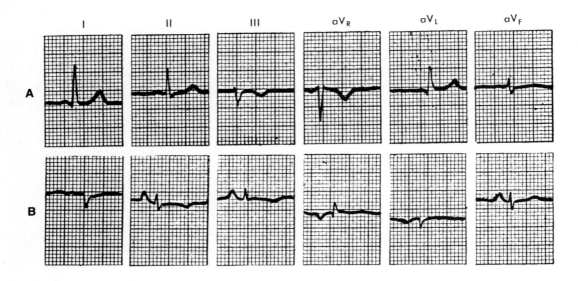

72. Calculate the mean QRS axis in these leads.

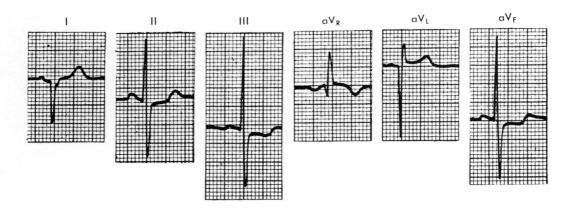

73. Is the mean QRS axis in this example normal, right, or left?

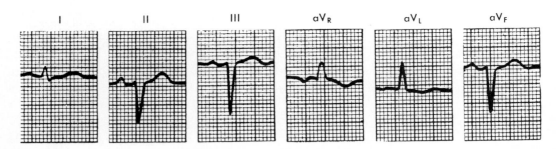

74. a. What is the major abnormality shown here?
    b. What factors can produce it?

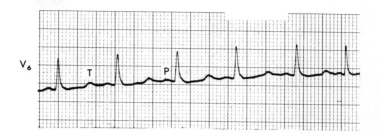

75. What is this heart rhythm?

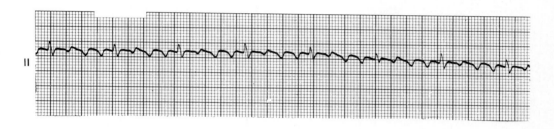

76. a. What is the approximate sinus (P wave) rate?
    b. What type of AV conduction disturbance is present?
    c. What abnormality is indicated by the P waves?

Holter monitor lead

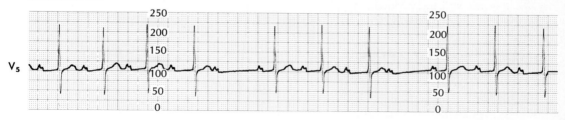

77. a. What is the approximate heart rate?
   b. What arrhythmia is present here?

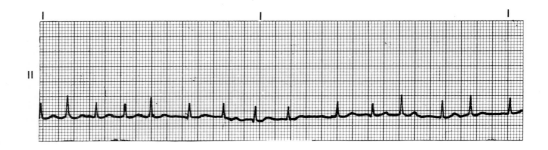

78. What type of AV conduction disturbance is present?

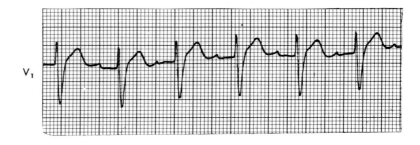

79. Identify beats *A* and *B*.

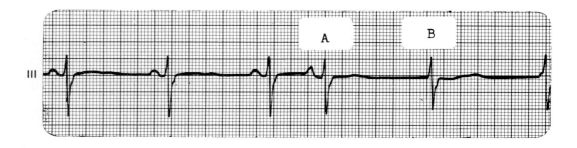

80. a. What arrhythmia is present?
    b. Of what symptom might this patient be complaining?

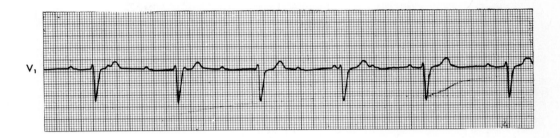

81. Look at the first and second halves of this rhythm strip. What are the rhythms? What syndrome do they suggest?

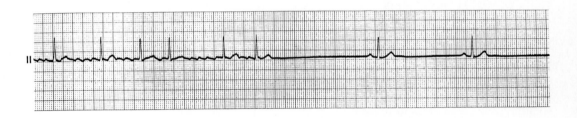

82. What type of conduction disturbance is present here?

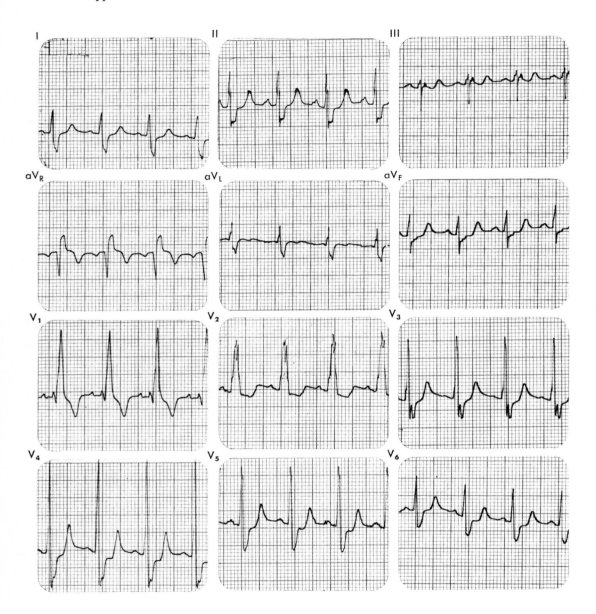

83. What is the arrhythmia shown here? Name three conditions that might lead to it.

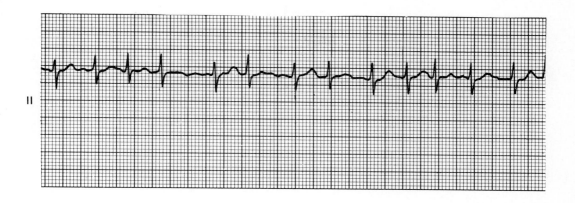

Identify the Rhythm in Each Case
(for nos. 84 to 111)

84.

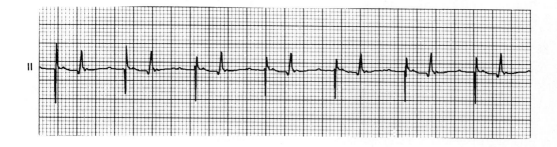

85.

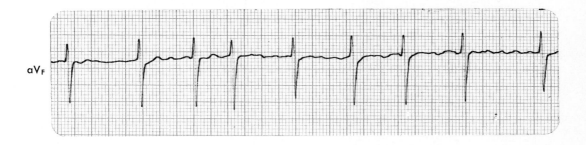

86.

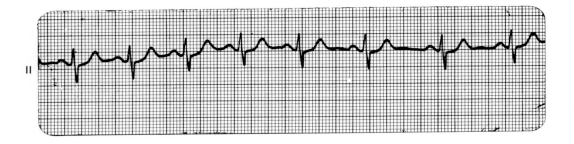

87.

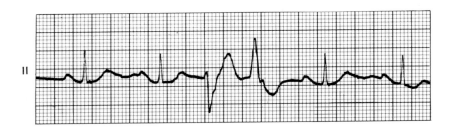

88.

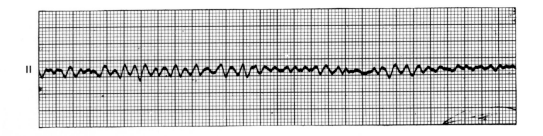

89.

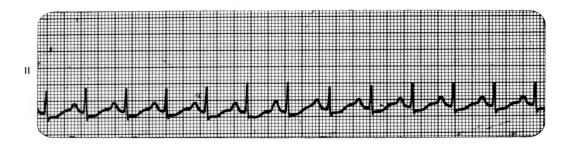

90.

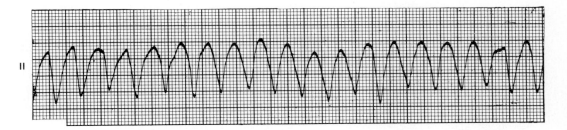

91.

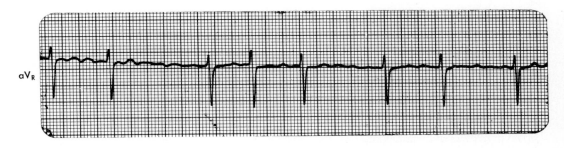

92.

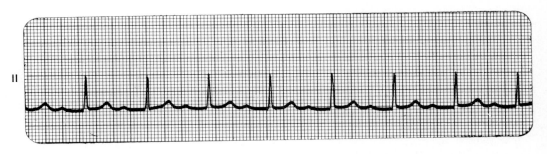

93.

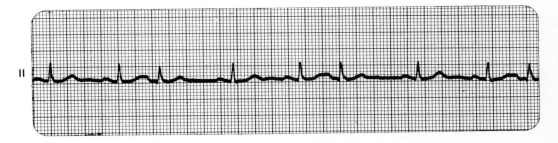

94.

Monitor lead

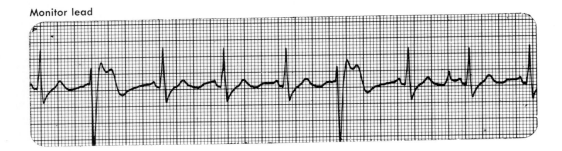

95.

II

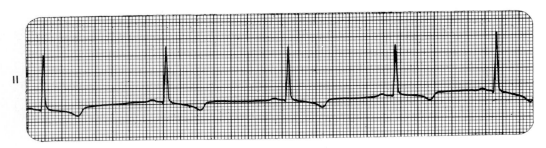

96.

aV$_R$

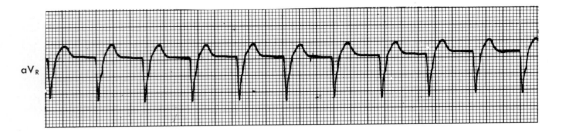

97.

II

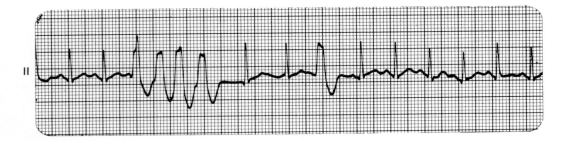

98.

Monitor lead

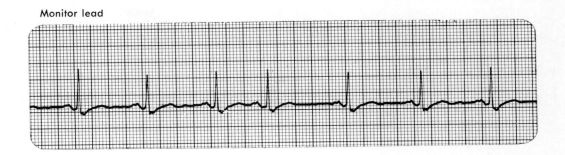

99.

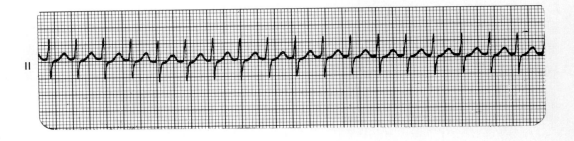

100.

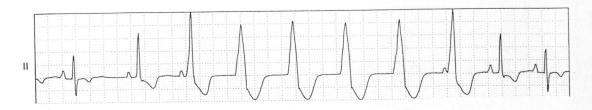

101.

Monitor lead

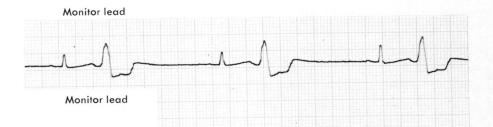

Monitor lead

102.

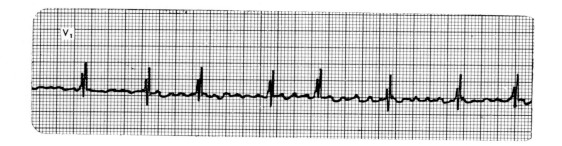

103.

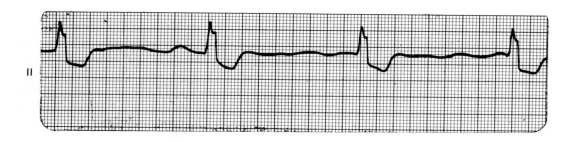

104.

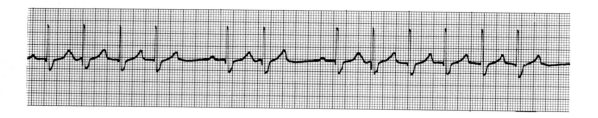

105.

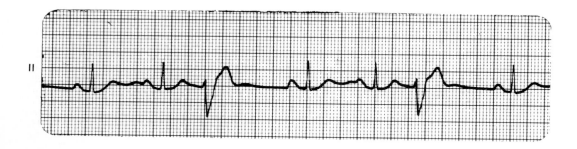

106.

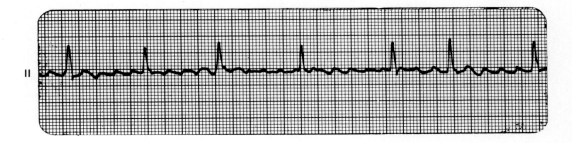

II

107.

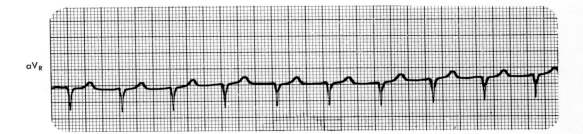

aV$_R$

108.

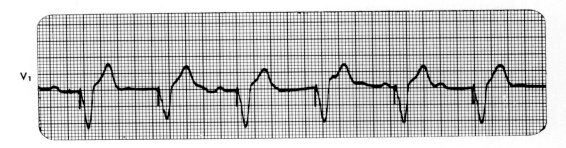

V$_1$

109.

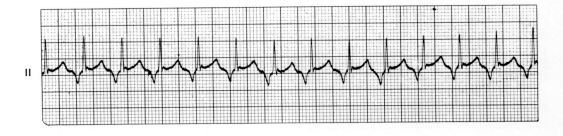

II

110.

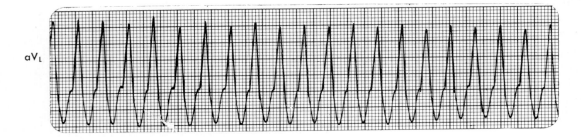

aV_L

111.

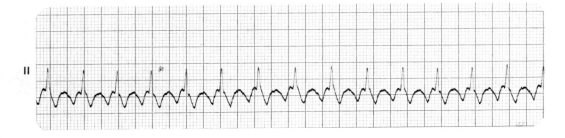

II

112. What two abnormalities are present here?

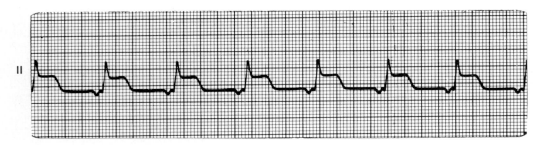

II

113. What two conduction disturbances are present?

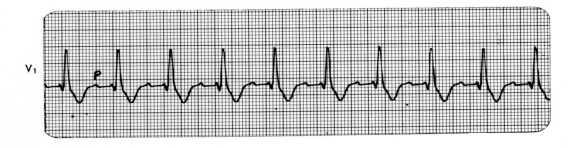

V₁

114. A 50-year-old patient complained of palpitations during the time this Holter monitor record was being obtained. What arrhythmia is shown?

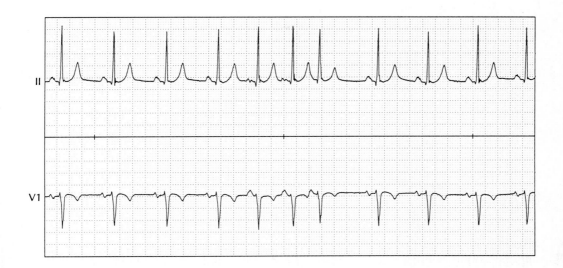

115. What abnormality is present here?

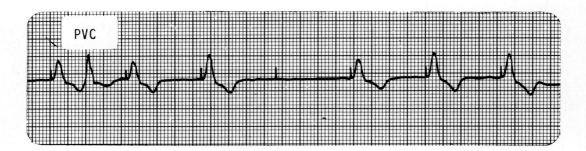

116. What conduction disturbance is present?

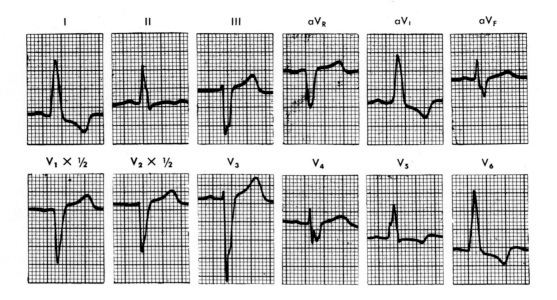

Interpret These ECGs Fully According to the Method Suggested in Chapter 21
(for nos. 117 to 121)

117.

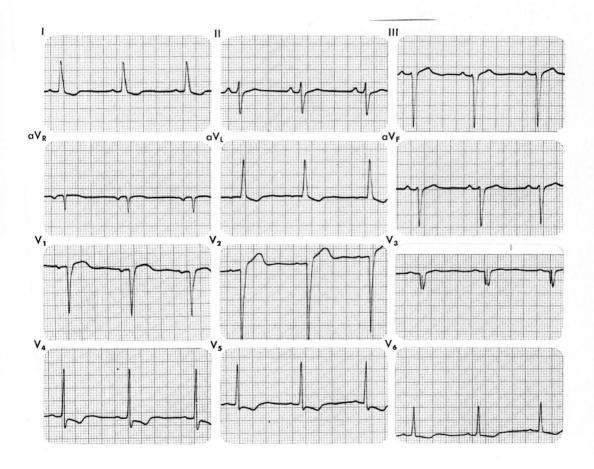

118.

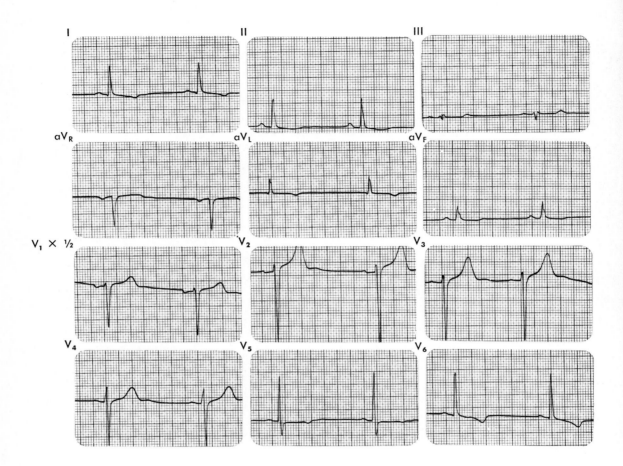

119.

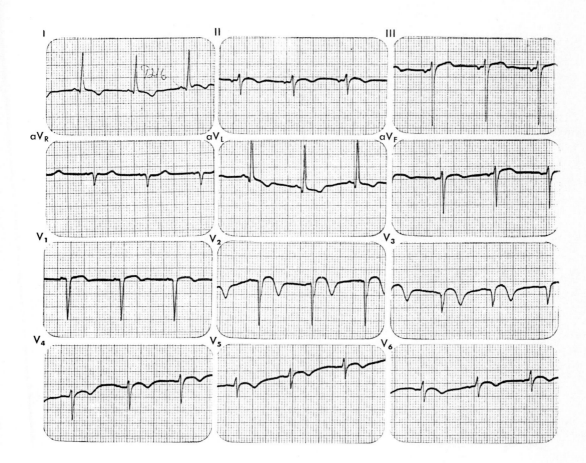

120.

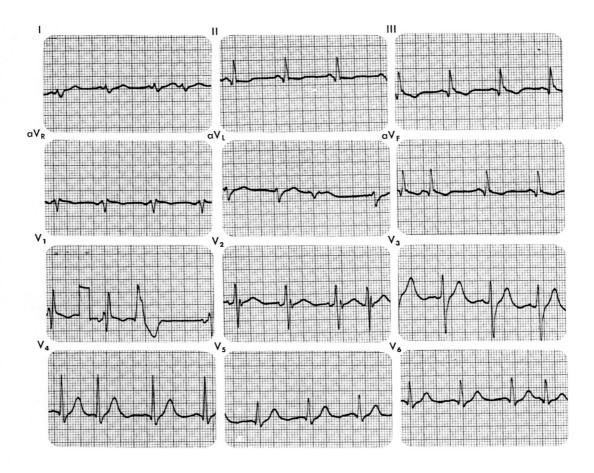

121.

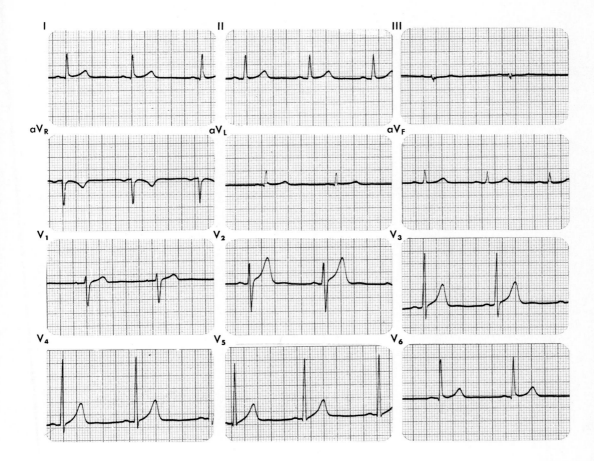

122. What is the major ECG diagnosis here?

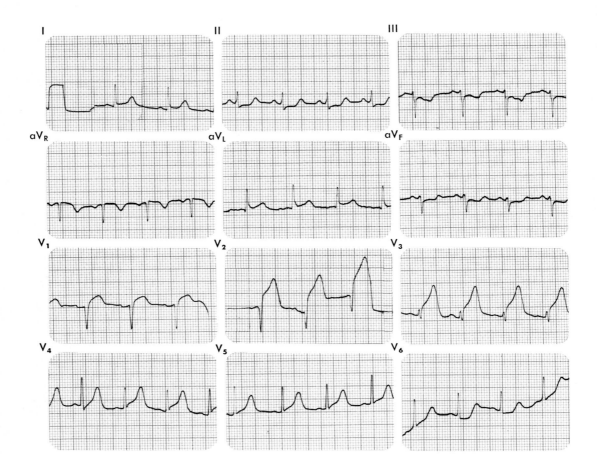

123. Answer these questions about the following ECG:
   a. Is it properly standardized?
   b. What is the heart rate?
   c. Is sinus rhythm present?
   d. What is the mean QRS axis?
   e. Is axis deviation present?
   f. Is the QRS voltage normal?
   g. What is the major abnormality?

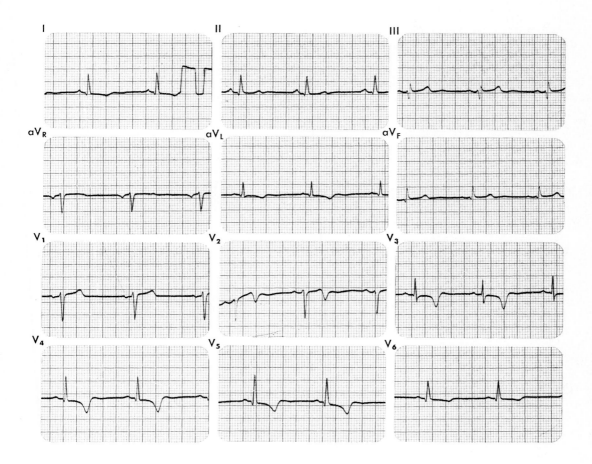

124. Answer these questions about the following ECG:
   a. What is the approximate heart rate?
   b. What evidence is there of myocardial infarction?

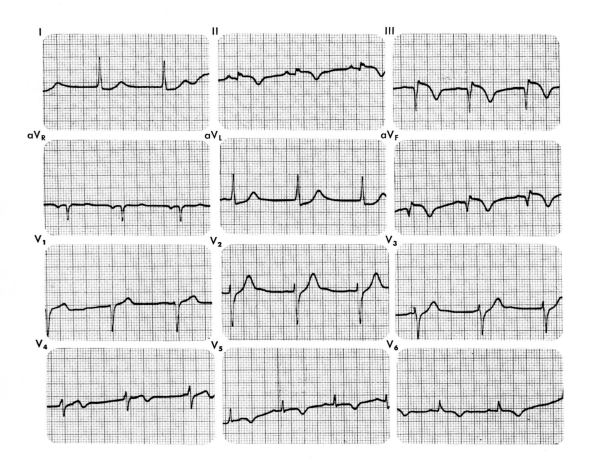

125. The following rhythm strip shows
   a. Sinus rhythm with frequent premature atrial contractions
   b. Sinus rhythm with complete heart block
   c. Sinus rhythm with 3:2 AV Wenckebach
   d. Multifocal atrial tachycardia
   e. Sinus arrhythmia

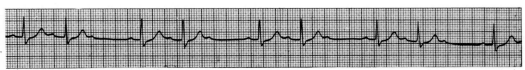

126. The following rhythm strip shows
    a. Atrial fibrillation
    b. Paroxysmal atrial tachycardia
    c. Multifocal atrial tachycardia
    d. Atrial bigeminy

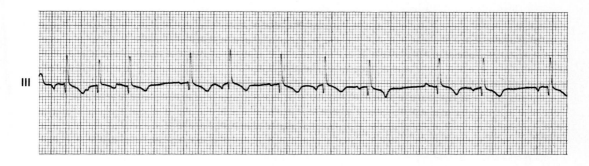

127. The ECG strip below, obtained during an exercise test, shows
    a. Ventricular tachycardia
    b. ST changes consistent with acute transmural infarction
    c. ST changes consistent with Prinzmetal's angina
    d. ST changes consistent with acute subendocardial ischemia

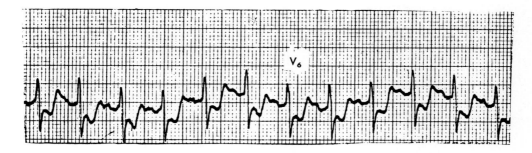

128. Answer these questions from the following ECG:
    a. What waveform is abnormally prominent here?
    b. What are the major causes for this finding?

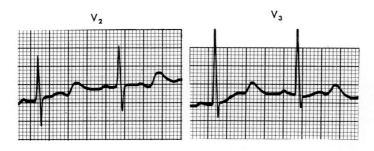

129. What wave does the arrow in V_5 point to, and what is the significance of this wave?

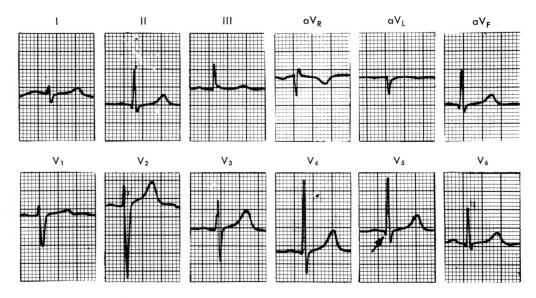

130. A patient complaining of severe chest pain had abnormally elevated cardiac enzymes. Using the ECG shown below, what is the clinical diagnosis?

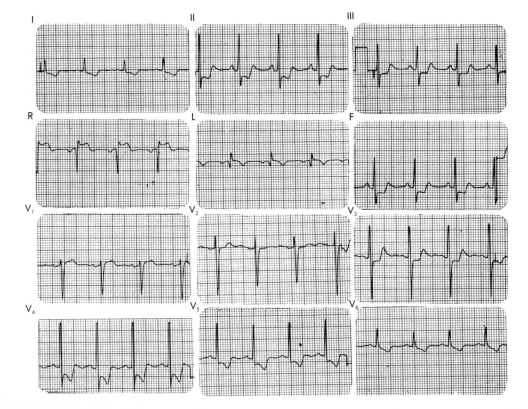

131. Answer these questions about the following ECG:
    a. What is the rhythm?
    b. What conduction disturbance is present?

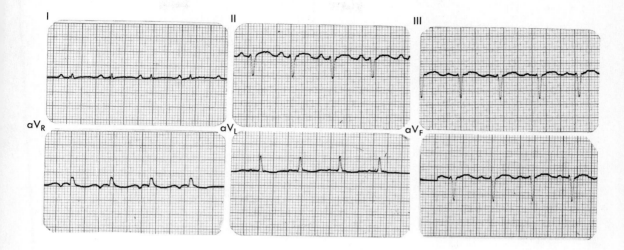

132. A 50-year-old man is complaining of chest pain. What is the likely cause of his complaint?

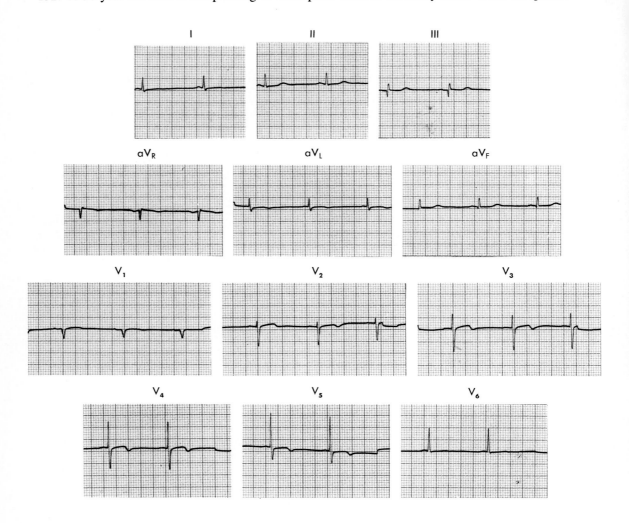

133. What is this rhythm?

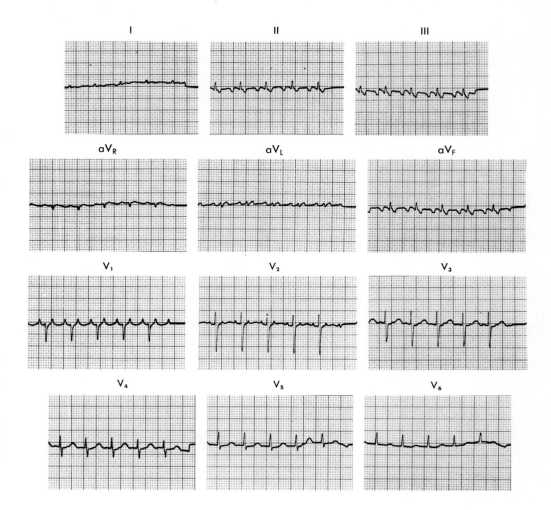

134. What arrhythmia is present here?

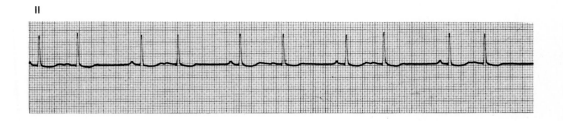

135. What is the major ECG diagnosis?

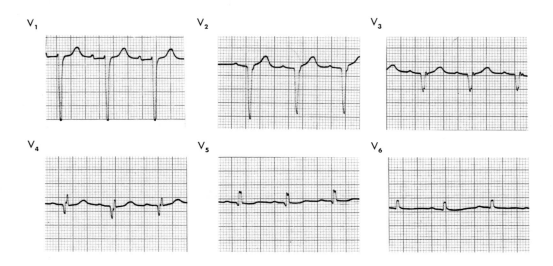

136. A patient presenting with palpitations received carotid sinus massage. What is the arrhythmia?

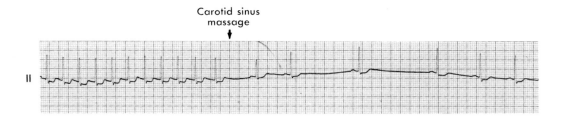

137. This patient's ECG was normal 3 days ago. What is the diagnosis from this repeat ECG?

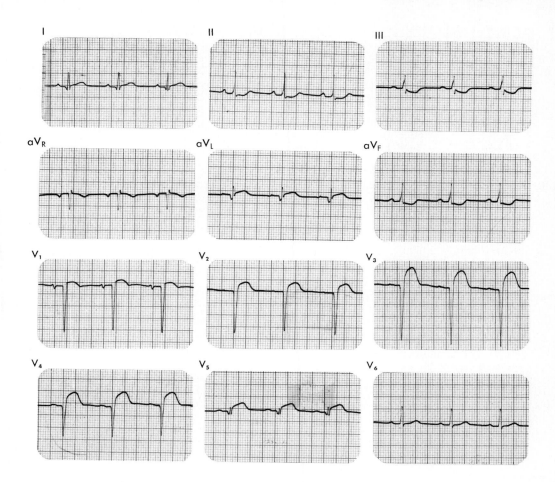

138. This lead II rhythm strip shows what three abnormalities?

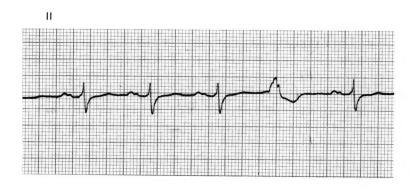

139. What is this subtle rhythm disturbance?

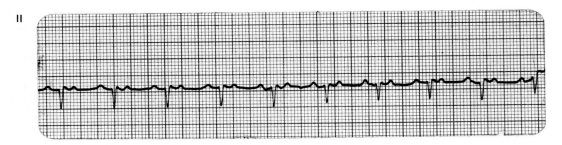

140. A 41-year-old man is complaining of "indigestion." What is the diagnosis?

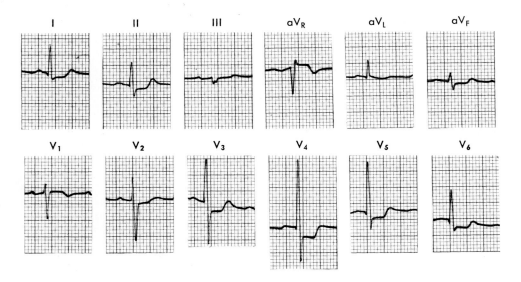

141. What is this rhythm?

Lead II: continuous

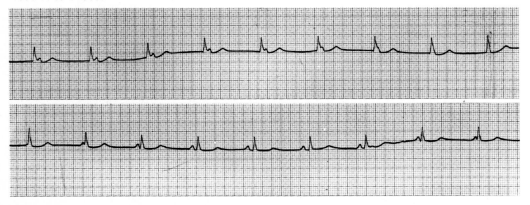

142. What is this rhythm?

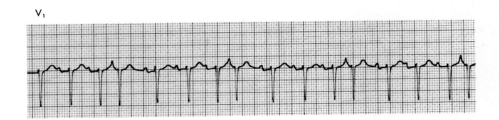

143. Name the major abnormalities here.

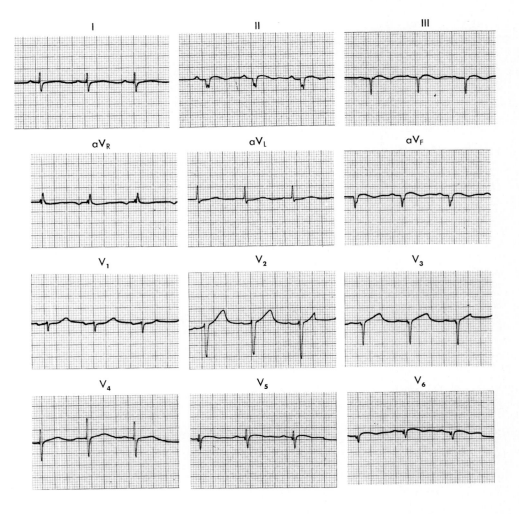

144. Name the major abnormalities here.

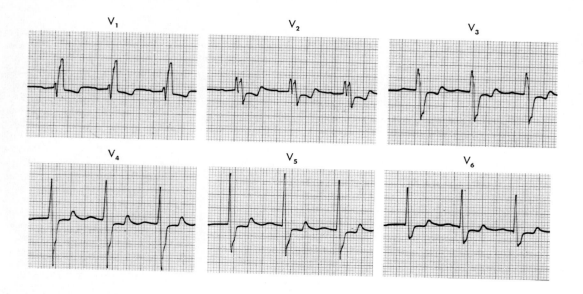

145. Name the major abnormalities here.

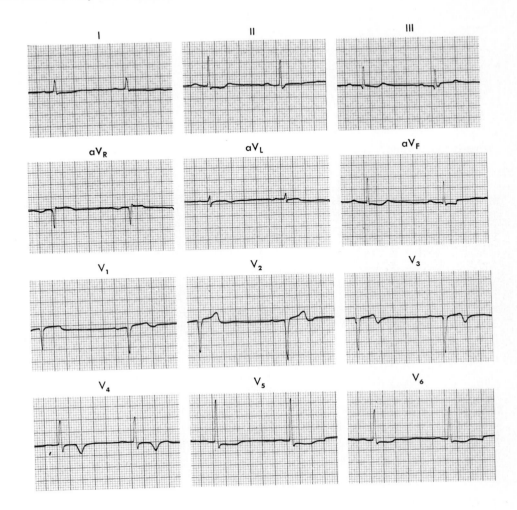

146. What is this arrhythmia?

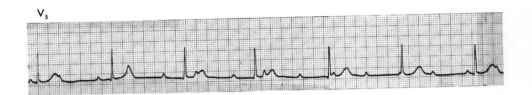

147. What is this arrhythmia?

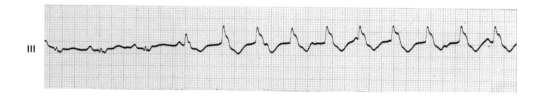

148. What is this rhythm?

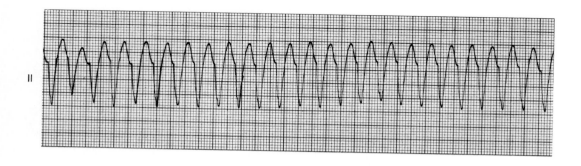

149. Following is the preoperative ECG of a 45-year-old man. What is the diagnosis?

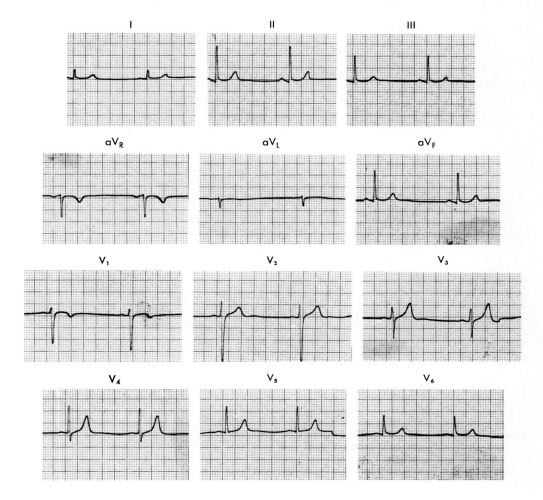

150. Following is the preoperative ECG of a 65-year-old woman. What is the diagnosis?

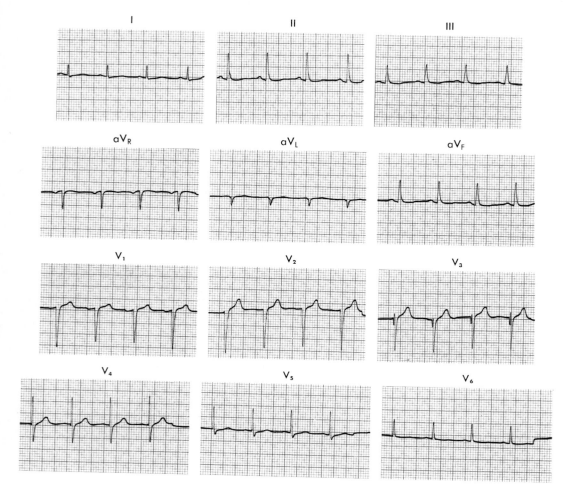

151. What caused this patient's syncope?

Monitor lead

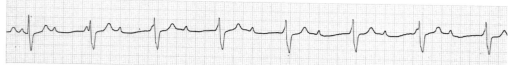

152. The following ECG is from a 60-year-old man with hypertension. What are the findings?

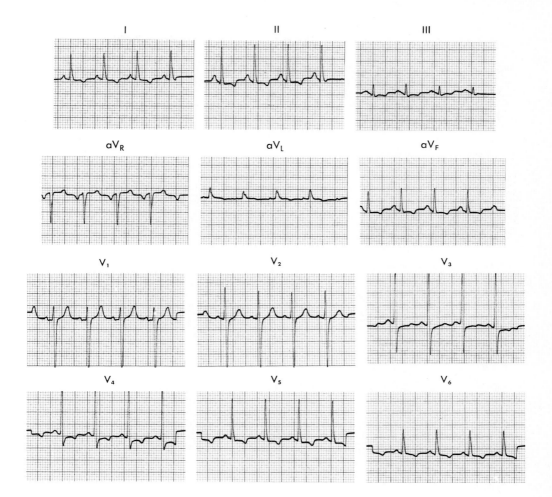

153. The following ECG is from a 24-year-old healthy male student. What is the diagnosis?

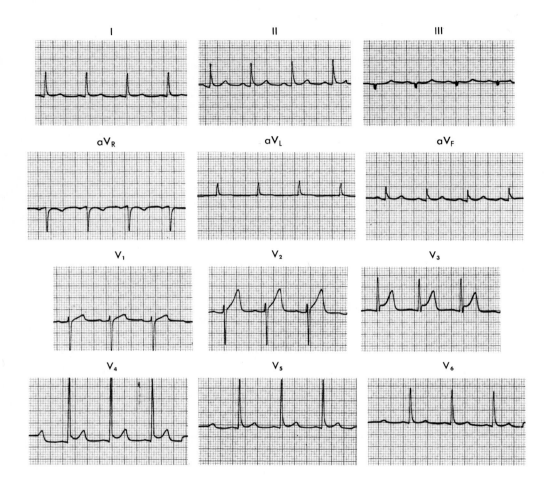

154. The following ECG is from a 50-year-old dialysis patient complaining of sharp pleuritic chest pain. What is the cause of his complaint?

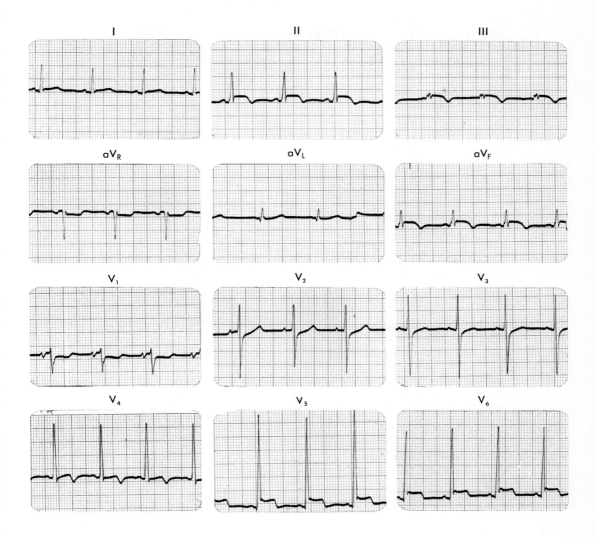

155. The following ECG is from a 62-year-old man. Describe the major abnormalities.

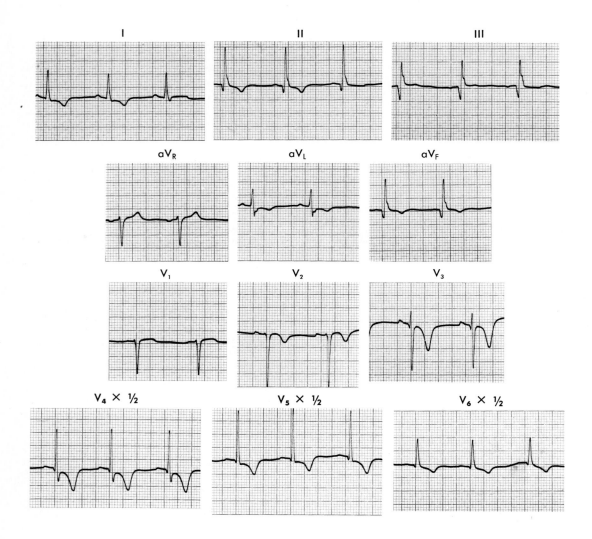

156. What arrhythmia is causing this patient's palpitations?

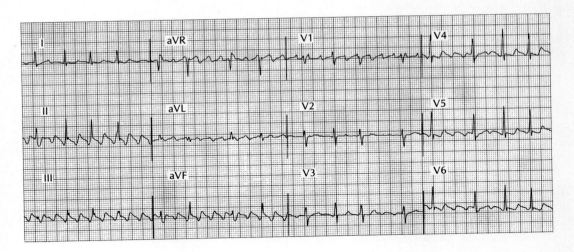

157. The following ECG is from a 59-year-old woman. Describe the major findings.

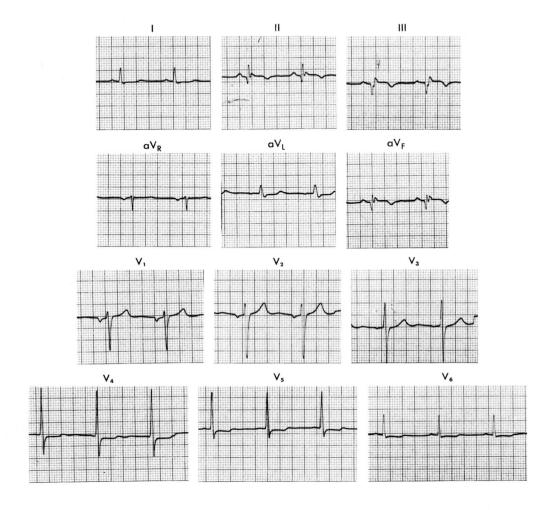

158. The following ECG is from a 50-year-old woman with suspected recurrent pulmonary emboli. What are the major abnormalities?

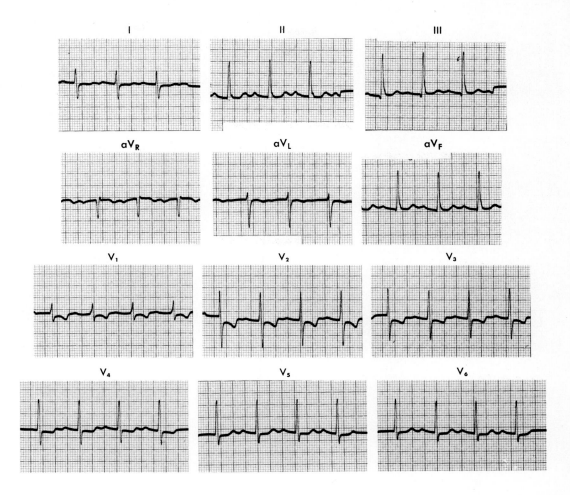

159. The following ECG is from a 20-year-old woman with chest pain. What is the diagnosis?

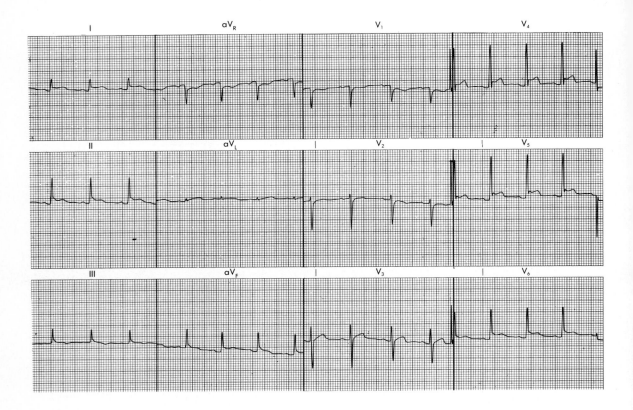

160. What abnormality might have caused the change from *A* to *B*?
     a. Hypocalcemia
     b. Hyperkalemia
     c. Hypokalemia
     d. Digitalis

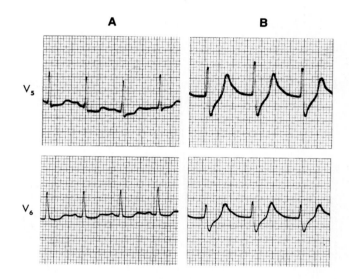

161. What is the cause of the wide QRS complexes?

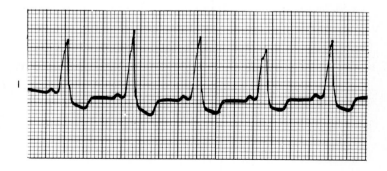

162. What is this rhythm?

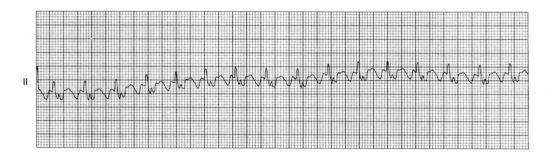

163. What are the notable findings here?

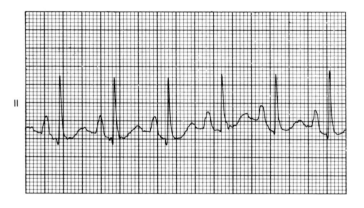

164. What is this rhythm?

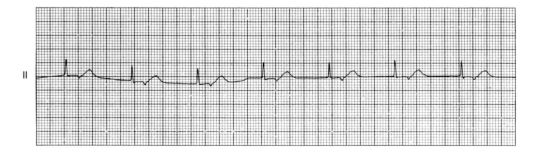

165. What is this rhythm and what clinical condition do you suspect?

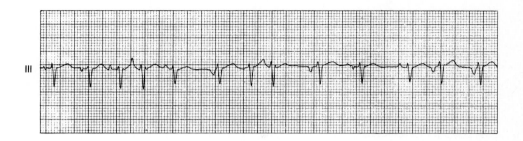

166. What is this rhythm and what clinical condition do you suspect?

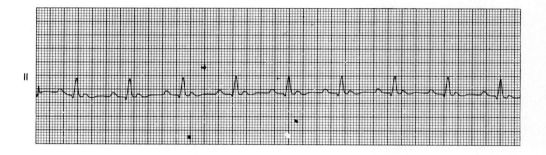

167. What metabolic problem was corrected in this patient, accounting for the marked change on the ECG from one day, *A*, to the next, *B*?

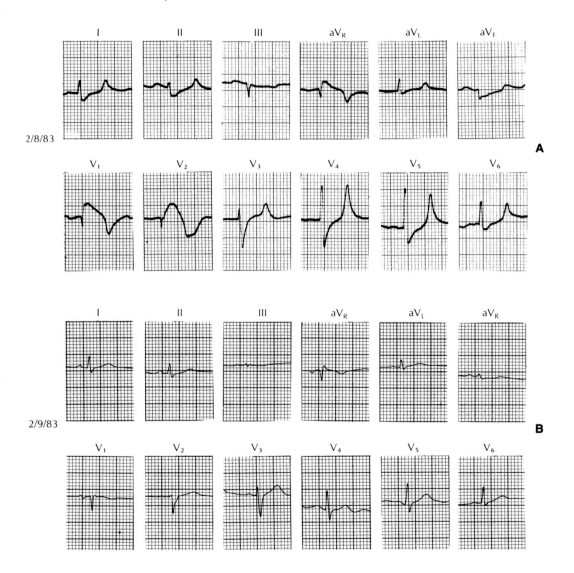

168. What type of conduction disturbance is present here?

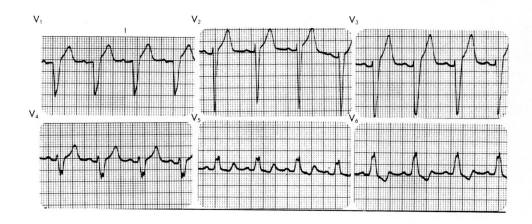

169. This patient's bradycardia is associated with what rhythm?

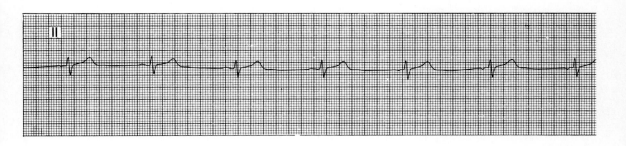

170. A patient with an evolving inferior infarction has intermittent wide QRS complexes. What are these beats?

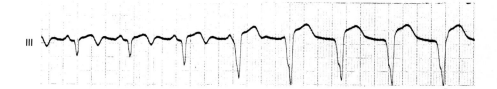

171. A 44-year-old woman with a history of intermittent atrial fibrillation complains of palpitations. What drug is she probably taking, and what is the arrhythmia?

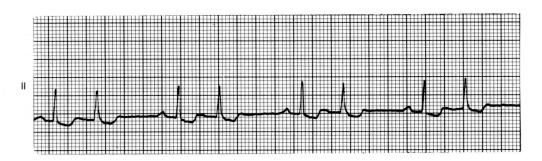

172. This patient with pulmonary edema that developed over 2 days is being seen in the emergency room. What are the major ECG findings?

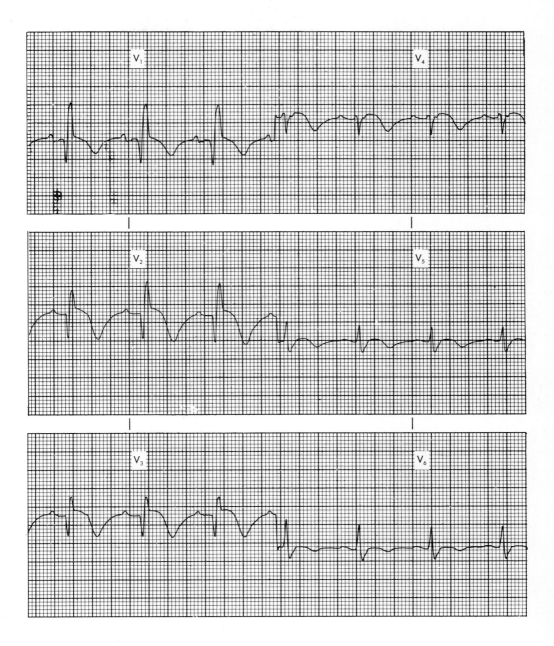

173. A 48-year-old man complains of intermittent palpitations. What arrhythmia does he have?

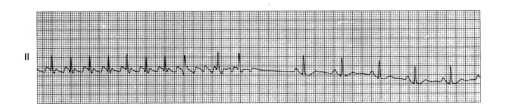

174. A 70-year-old man taking propranolol for hypertension comes to the emergency room complaining of light-headedness and weakness for the past week. What does his monitor lead rhythm strip show?

MONITOR LEAD

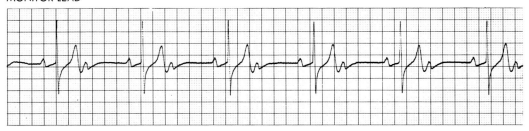

175. A 70-year-old man was given verapamil for treatment of angina. What does his rhythm strip show?

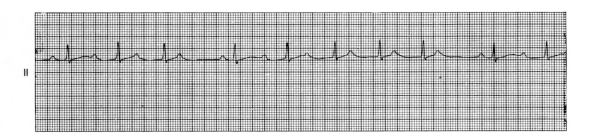

176. A 76-year-old woman complains that her "heart skips beats." What does her rhythm strip show?

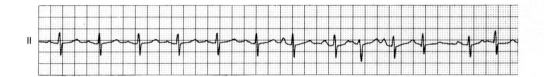

177. An acute left hemiparesis developed in a 72-year-old man. What etiology does his ECG suggest?

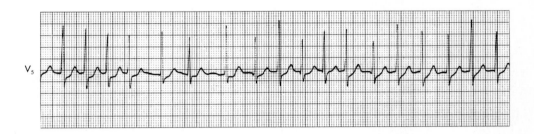

178. A 92-year-old man loses consciousness while eating dinner. What does his rhythm strip indicate?

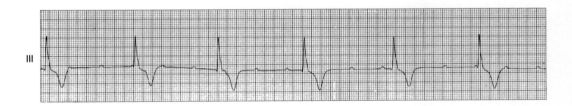

179. A 54-year-old psychiatrist complains of palpitations after an argument with a "significant other." What does his ECG show?

LEAD II

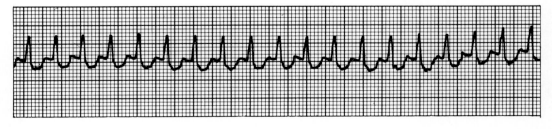

180. This ECG was initially misinterpreted as showing "accelerated idioventricular rhythm." What is the correct diagnosis?

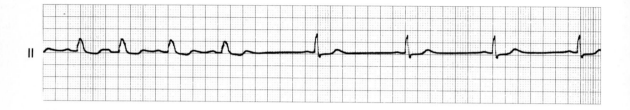

181. A 60-year-old man is admitted with severe congestive heart failure. His ECG is identical to one recorded 6 months earlier. Cardiac enzymes are normal. What is the likely diagnosis?

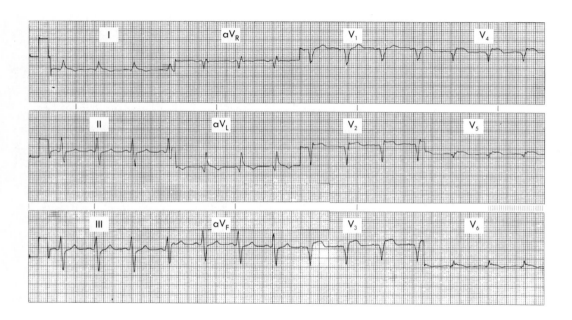

182. A 27-year-old man is told he has "congenital heart disease." Except for some mild exertional fatigue, he feels fine. He is not cyanotic on physical examination. A loud systolic ejection murmur is heard with fixed splitting of the second heart sound. What does his ECG show, and what is the likely clinical diagnosis?

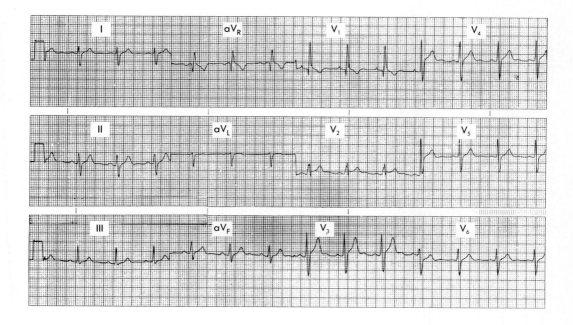

183. A 37-year-old man presents with intermittent palpitations. What does his ECG show?

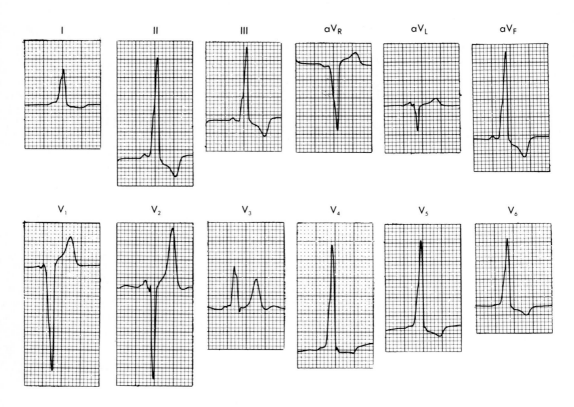

184. A 75-year-old woman treated with quinidine for atrial arrhythmias has a cardiac arrest 4 days later. This rhythm strip was obtained. What does it show?

MONITOR LEAD

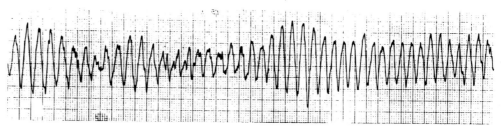

185. An 80-year-old woman complained of light-headedness. The following rhythm strip was obtained in the coronary care unit. What conduction disturbance is present?

MONITOR LEAD

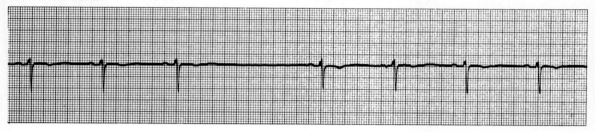

186. The following Holter monitor recording shows sinus rhythm with intermittent
    a. Ventricular tachycardia
    b. Left bundle branch block
    c. Accelerated idioventricular rhythm (AIVR)
    d. Wolff-Parkinson-White pattern
    e. Ventricular paced rhythm

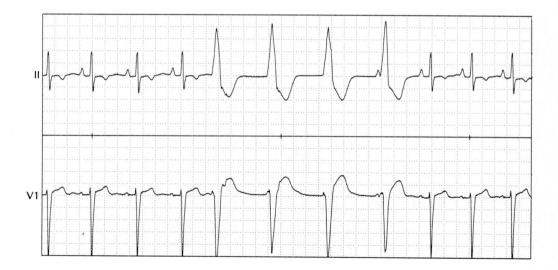

187. This ECG gives an important clue to a life-threatening metabolic abnormality. What is the likely diagnosis?

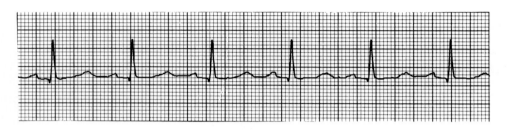

188. This ECG shows
   a. Sinus tachycardia
   b. Atrial flutter with 3:1 conduction
   c. Paroxysmal atrial tachycardia (PAT) with block
   d. Multifocal atrial tachycardia
   e. None of the above

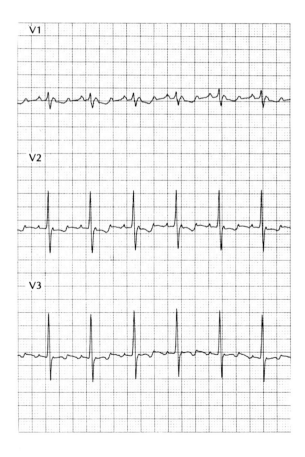

189. What life-threatening metabolic disturbance does this ECG strongly suggest?
    a. Hyperkalemia
    b. Hypokalemia
    c. Hypercalcemia
    d. Hypocalcemia
    e. Hyponatremia

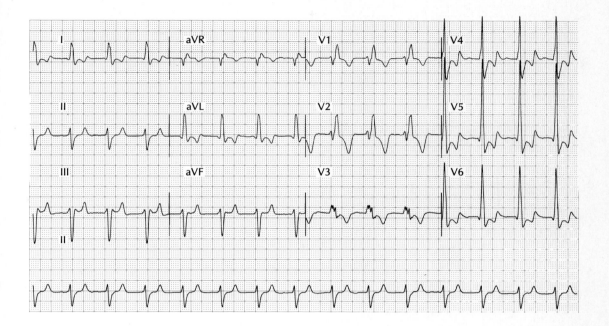

190. This patient was thought to have atrial fibrillation on examination. What is the actual finding accounting for the erratic pulse on this Holter monitor recording?

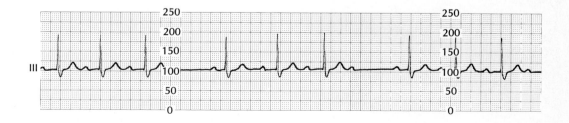

191. What does this patient have?

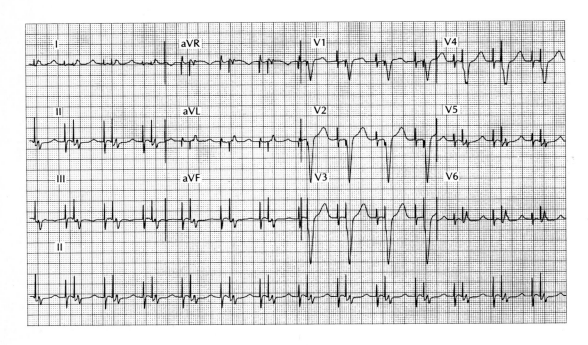

192. A 54-year-old woman complained of palpitations. The monitor lead recorded this episode. What is the diagnosis?

MONITOR
LEAD

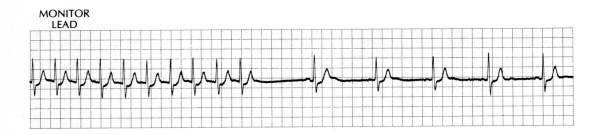

ANSWERS

1. Atrial depolarization (stimulation).
2. Ventricular depolarization (stimulation).
3. Ventricular repolarization (recovery).
4. 0.12 and 0.2.
5. Fourth.
6. Lengthens.
7. Wolff-Parkinson-White syndrome.
8. Quinidine, procainamide, and others.
9. Pericardial effusion, emphysema, and obesity. Also extensive myocardial fibrosis or infiltration with substances like amyloid. Low voltage may also be a normal variant.
10. Ventricular ectopy (PVCs, ventricular bigeminy, ventricular tachycardia, ventricular fibrillation, bidirectional tachycardia), sinus bradycardia and SA block, junctional rhythms, PAT with block, and so on. (See p. 207.)
11. RBBB.
12. Right axis shift, $S_I Q_{III}$ pattern, RBBB, sinus tachycardia and other arrhythmias, right ventricular strain. (See p. 139 for other patterns.)
13. $+5$ mm. Recall that the voltages of the P wave, QRS complex, and T wave in $aV_R + aV_L + aV_F$ must equal 0.
14. Hypokalemia and renal insufficiency; also hypoxia, hypercalcemia, hypomagnesemia, old age, and others. (See p. 207.)
15. Decreases.
16. Hyperkalemia, quinidine, procainamide, disopyramide, tricyclic antidepressants, phenothiazines, etc.
17. Hypokalemia.
18. P pulmonale (right atrial enlargement).
19. aV_R, II.
20. See p. 51.
21. 1.
22. Hyperthyroidism.
23. Ventricular fibrillation (and related ventricular tachyarrhythmias), asystole (with or without escape beats), and electromechanical dissociation.
24. Fever, excitement, and congestive heart failure. (See p. 154 for other causes.)
25. Stokes-Adams.
26. Three or more consecutive PVCs.
27. Hyperkalemia.
28. Acute myocardial infarction, acute pericarditis, Prinzmetal's angina; also ventricular aneurysm.
29. ST segment depressions.
30. False. Some normal people will have an RBBB pattern.
31. False. Atrial fibrillation, although often seen in people with organic heart disease (coronary, hypertensive, valvular, etc.), may occur in people with normal hearts.

32. True.
33. True. (See p. 137.)
34. True.
35. Depressions (reciprocal to the ST elevations seen in the anterior leads).
36. AV junctional or sometimes ectopic atrial.
37. See p. 12.
38. LBBB.
39. Myocardial ischemia, digitalis toxicity, hypokalemia, hypoxia, pulmonary embolism, and congestive heart failure. (See pp. 185-186 for additional causes.)
40. Paroxysmal atrial tachycardia (paroxysmal supraventricular tachycardia).
41. Sinus bradycardia, AV junctional rhythm, AV heart block (second or third degree) or AV dissociation, atrial fibrillation or flutter with a slow ventricular response, or idioventricular escape rhythm.
42. $-30°$.
43. Normal variant, beta blockers such as propranolol, calcium channel blockers (verapamil, diltiazem), digitalis toxicity, increased vagal tone caused by myocardial ischemia, and so on.
44. Coronary artery disease, hypertensive heart disease, and mitral valve disease.
45. Ventricular aneurysm.
46. Paroxysmal atrial tachycardia.
47. Left atrial enlargement.
48. Digitalis.
49. 0.1 second.
50. V_6.
51-60. See the pages listed.
61-65. See diagrams below.

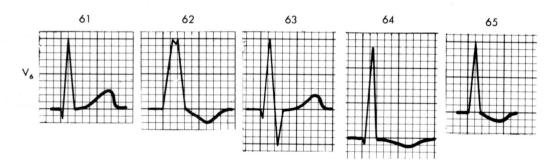

66. Hyperkalemia. Notice the tall "tented" T waves. First degree AV block is also present.
67. Digitalis.
68. RBBB is present with wide rSR' complexes in V_1. (In addition, first-degree AV block is present.)
69. Sinus rhythm with a five-beat run of ventricular tachycardia.
70. Ventricular premature contraction.

71. *A.* 0°.
    B. +180°.

    In both *A* and *B,* lead aV$_F$ shows a biphasic RS-type complex; thus the mean QRS axis must be directed at right angles to the axis of lead aV$_F$, which is +90°. In example *A* lead I shows a positive R wave deflection, so the axis must be pointed in that direction (at 0°). In example *B* the mean QRS axis is directed at right angles to aV$_F$, away from I, and toward leads III and aV$_R$, or at +180° (marked right axis deviation).

72. +150°. Lead II shows a biphasic RS complex; thus the mean QRS axis must be directed at right angles to the axis of lead II, which is at +60°. Therefore the axis must be either −30° or +150°. Obviously, since I is negative and II and aV$_R$ are mainly positive, the axis must be +150°. This indicates right axis deviation.

73. Left.

74. a. The QT interval is markedly prolonged (0.44 sec) with a heart rate of 94/min.
    b. QT prolongation may be caused by numerous factors including hypocalcemia, hypokalemia (often with large U waves), drugs such as quinidine or procainamide, and myocardial infarction (with deep T wave inversions).

75. Atrial flutter. Notice the characteristic sawtooth flutter waves. The atrial (flutter) rate is approximately 300 beats/min, while the ventricular (QRS) rate is about 75 beats/min; thus 4:1 flutter is present.

76. a. About 70/min.
    b. AV Wenckebach. Notice the repeating cycles in which the PR intervals get progressively longer until the P wave is not conducted. (The fifth and ninth P waves are not conducted.)
    c. The wide notched P waves indicate left atrial abnormality (enlargement).

77. a. About 130 beats/min. (There are 13 QRS cycles/6 sec.) (See p. 16.)
    b. Atrial fibrillation. Often, as in this case, with rapid atrial fibrillation, the fibrillation waves are not well seen. The diagnosis of atrial fibrillation is then made by finding a haphazardly irregular rhythm with no visible P waves.

78. First-degree AV block (PR interval about 0.22 sec). Notice that the QRS is somewhat wide, 0.11 second, indicating some type of intraventricular conduction disturbance as well.

79. *A* is a premature atrial contraction (PAC). *B* is a junctional escape beat.

80. a. Complete heart block. To analyze this arrhythmia, you need to label each P wave and each QRS complex. The ventricular rate is about 40 beats/min. Looking at the P waves (some of which are hidden by QRS complexes and T waves), you can see that the atrial rate is 90 to 100 beats/min and the PR intervals are completely variable. Therefore complete heart block is present. The QRS complexes are abnormally wide probably because the ventricles are being paced by an idioventricular focus located below the AV junction.
    b. The patient complained of light-headedness and fainting spells (Stokes-Adams syndrome).

81. The first part of the rhythm strip shows *coarse atrial fibrillation,* which then spontaneously converts to a marked *sinus bradycardia.* This sequence suggests the *brady-tachy variant* of the *sick sinus syndrome.*

82. RBBB.

83. Atrial fibrillation with a rapid ventricular rate. This may be due to multiple conditions, including coronary artery disease, hypertension, valvular disease, cardiomyopathy, alcohol consumption, and hyperthyroidism.
84. Atrial paced rhythm. Notice the pacemaker spike before each P wave.
85. Atrial fibrillation.
86. Sinus arrhythmia.
87. Sinus rhythm with multiform PVCs.
88. Sinus tachycardia. (Nonspecific ST-T changes are also present.)
89. Ventricular fibrillation.
90. Ventricular tachycardia.
91. Atrial fibrillation.
92. Sinus rhythm with first-degree AV block.
93. Sinus rhythm with premature atrial contractions. (The third, sixth, and ninth beats are PACs; therefore this is atrial *trigeminy*.)
94. Since rhythm with premature ventricular contractions. (The second and sixth beats are PVCs.)
95. Sinus bradycardia. (Notice also the abnormal ST-T segment because of left ventricular strain or ischemia.)
96. AV junctional rhythm (note the absence of visible P waves.)
97. Sinus tachycardia with short burst of ventricular tachycardia. (The ninth beat is also a PVC.)
98. Sinus rhythm with PAC (fourth beat).
99. Sinus rhythm with a run of accelerated idioventricular rhythm (AIVR). Notice that the second and ninth beats are *fusion* beats.
100. Paroxysmal atrial (or junctional) tachycardia
101. Ventricular bigeminy.
102. Coarse atrial fibrillation with incomplete RBBB (note the rSR′ in lead V₁).
103. Idioventricular (slow ventricular escape) rhythm.
104. Sinus rhythm with AV Wenckebach. Notice the group beating. Most of the P waves (under the dots) are partly hidden in the T waves.

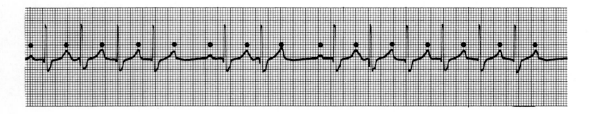

105. Ventricular trigeminy. Every second sinus beat is followed by a PVC.
106. Coarse atrial fibrillation.
107. Junctional rhythm. Notice the absence of visible P waves.
108. Paced rhythm. Notice the pacemaker spike before each QRS and the nonconducted P waves (some hidden). The latter indicate underlying complete heart block.
109. Junctional (or ectopic atrial) tachycardia, with retrograde P waves in II.

110. Ventricular tachycardia.
111. Atrial flutter with 2:1 block (atrial rate, about 300 beats/min; ventricular rate, about 150 beats/min).
112. Lead II rhythm strip showing marked ST elevations (caused by acute inferior wall infarction) with a junctional (or ectopic atrial) rhythm. (Notice the retrograde P waves preceding each QRS.)
113. First-degree AV block with RBBB. Notice the wide rSR' complex in V_1.
114. Sinus rhythm with a three-beat run of paroxysmal atrial tachycardia (PAT). Notice that beats 5 to 7 are premature atrial contractions (PACs).
115. Pacemaker rhythm with pacemaker malfunction. Notice the pacemaker spike in the center of the strip, which is not followed by a QRS (owing to pacemaker failure).
116. LBBB.
117. a. Analysis
     (1) Standardization: 1 mV = 10 mm (mark as shown).
     (2) Heart rate: about 60 beats/min.
     (3) Rhythm: normal sinus.
     (4) PR interval: about 0.16 second (normal).
     (5) P wave size: broad and biphasic in V_1, suggesting possible left atrial abnormality, although in other leads within normal limits.
     (6) QRS width: 0.1 second (upper limits of normal).
     (7) QT interval: about 0.4 second (normal for rate).
     (8) QRS voltage: R wave in aV_L is abnormally tall (15 mm).
     (9) Mean QRS axis: about $-60°$. The R wave in aV_L equals the S wave in aV_F, so the mean QRS axis must lie between the positive pole of aV_L ($-30°$) and the negative pole of aV_F ($-90°$). Therefore the mean QRS axis must be approximately $-60°$.
     (10) R wave progression in chest leads: poor, with QS complexes in V_1 to V_3.
     (11) Abnormal Q waves: V_1 to V_3 show abnormal QS complexes. Notice the bizarre **W**-shaped QS in V_3.
     (12) ST segment elevation in V_2 with slight depression in V_3 to V_6.
     (13) T waves: inverted in I, aV_L, and V_4 to V_6, with some scooping of the ST segment in I and aV_L.
     (14) U waves: normal.
   b. Interpretation
     Left axis deviation consistent with left anterior hemiblock.
     Abnormal QS complexes in V_1 to V_3 consistent with anteroseptal infarction of indeterminate age.
     Left ventricular hypertrophy by voltage.
     Left atrial abnormality.
     Abnormal ST-T changes consistent with left ventricular strain and/or ischemia, and possibly with digitalis effect (with scooping of ST-T in I and aV_L). (The ST-T changes on this ECG are somewhat complicated. As noted, the T wave inversions and slight ST depressions in V_3 to V_6 may reflect a combination of left ventricular strain and/or lateral wall ischemia. The scooping of the ST-T segment in I and aV_L may also reflect strain or ischemia but

are suggestive of the classic pattern of digitalis effect as well. Finally, notice the high takeoff of the ST segment in V_2, suggesting acute infarction. However, in cases of LVH the right precordial leads may show such ST elevation as a persistent finding in the absence of acute ischemia.)

118. a. Analysis
   (1) Standardization: 1 mV = 10 mm (mark not shown).
   (2) Heart rate: approximately 40 beats/min.
   (3) Rhythm: sinus bradycardia.
   (4) PR interval: about 0.18 second.
   (5) P wave size: biphasic in V_1, suggesting possible left atrial abnormality.
   (6) QRS width: 0.1 to 0.11 second.
   (7) QT interval: 0.52 second (within normal limits for rate).
   (8) QRS voltage: tall in chest leads (S_{V_1} + R_{V_6} = more than 35 mm).
   (9) Mean QRS axis: about + 30°. R waves are of equal amplitude in I and II so the mean QRS axis must be directed between these leads.
   (10) R wave progression in chest leads: delayed, with the transition zone between V_4 and V_5.
   (11) Abnormal Q waves: none.
   (12) ST segments: isoelectric.
   (13) T waves: inverted in I, II, aV_L, V_5, and V_6.
   (14) U waves: small in V_2 to V_4.
   b. Interpretation
   Marked sinus bradycardia.
   Left ventricular hypertrophy by voltage. ST-T changes are consistent with left ventricular strain and possibly ischemia.
   Possible left atrial abnormality.
   In this case the left ventricular hypertrophy and atrial abnormality resulted from hypertensive heart disease. The marked sinus bradycardia was caused by one of the drugs (beta blocker) that the patient was taking for high blood pressure.

119. a. Analysis
   (1) Standardization: 1 mV = 10 mm (mark not shown).
   (2) Heart rate: approximately 75 beats/min.
   (3) Rhythm: junctional or ectopic atrial. (Notice the retrograde P waves in II with biphasic P waves in aV_R.)
   (4) PR interval: 0.1 (short because of the junctional or ectopic atrial rhythm).
   (5) P wave size: normal.
   (6) QRS width: 0.08 second.
   (7) QT interval: 0.35 second (normal for rate).
   (8) QRS voltage: tall in aV_L (R wave = 16 mm).

(9) QRS axis: approximately $-45°$. The R wave in I is about equal to the S wave in aV_F. Therefore the mean QRS axis must lie midway between the positive pole of I ($0°$) and the negative pole of aV_F ($-90°$), making the axis $-45°$. Furthermore, by inspection, you can tell that left axis deviation is present (axis more negative than $-30°$), since lead II shows an rS complex with the S wave deeper than the r wave is tall. (See p. 57.)

(10) R wave progression in the chest leads: delayed with QS complexes in V_1 to V_3.

(11) Abnormal Q waves: QS complexes in leads V_1 to V_3. Abnormally wide in aV_L. (Notice that this Q wave is 0.04 sec wide, making it abnormal even though it is not very deep.)

(12) ST segments: slightly elevated in leads V_2 to V_4.

(13) T waves: deeply inverted and symmetric in leads I, II, aV_L, and V_2 to V_6.

(13) T waves: deeply inverted and symmetric in leads I, II, aV_L, and V_2 to V_6.

(14) U waves: normal.

b. Interpretation

Abnormal ECG.

Junctional or ectopic atrial rhythm.

LVH by voltage.

Left axis deviation consistent with left anterior hemiblock.

Abnormal Q waves and T wave inversions consistent with evolving anterior wall infarction. The exact age of the infarct cannot be deduced from the ECG. In this case it was 1 week old.

120. a. Analysis

(1) Standardization: 1 mV = 10 mm (mark shown in V_1).

(2) Heart rate: approximately 75 beats/min, with slight irregularity.

(3) Rhythm: normal sinus, with both premature atrial contractions (in leads I, aV_F, V_2, and V_6) and premature ventricular contractions (third beat in V_1).

(4) PR interval: 0.12 second (lower limits of normal).

(5) P wave size: broad and biphasic in V_1 (suggesting left atrial abnormality).

(6) QRS width: 0.12 to 0.13 second. The RSR' in V_1 suggests RBBB.

(7) QT interval: 0.36 second (normal for rate).

(8) QRS voltage: normal.

(9) Mean QRS axis: $+90°$. Biphasic RS wave in I.

(10) R wave progression in chest leads: normal.

(11) Abnormal Q waves in II, III, and aV_F.

(12) ST segments: normal.

(13) T waves: slight inversion in II, III, and aV_F.

(14) U waves: normal.

b. Interpretation

Abnormal ECG.

Sinus rhythm with atrial and ventricular ectopy.

RBBB.

Left atrial abnormality.

Inferior wall infarct of indeterminate age.

121. a. Analysis
    (1) Standardization: 1 mV = 10 mm (mark not shown).
    (2) Heart rate: 55 to 60 beats/min.
    (3) Rhythm: sinus bradycardia.
    (4) PR interval: 0.16 second.
    (5) P wave size: normal.
    (6) QRS width: 0.08 second.
    (7) QT interval: 0.4 second (normal for rate).
    (8) QRS voltage: upper normal limits.
    (9) QRS axis: $+30°$
    (10) R wave progression in chest leads: normal.
    (11) Abnormal Q waves: none.
    (12) ST segments: isoelectric in the extremity leads; slightly elevated J point in V_2 and V_3.
    (13) T waves: normal.
    (14) U waves: normal.
  b. Interpretation
    Normal electrocardiogram. The ST elevation in the chest leads represents a normal "early repolarization" variant.
122. Major finding is ST elevations and hyperacute T waves in the anterior chest leads (V_1 to V_5) with reciprocal ST depressions in II, III, and aV_F. (This patient was having an acute anterior wall infarction.)
123. a. Yes. (Notice that the standardization mark in I is 10 mm tall.)
  b. 60 beats/min.
  c. Yes.
  d. $+30°$
  e. No.
  f. Yes.
  g. Ischemic T wave inversions in I, aV_L, and V_2 to V_6. (Clinically the patient had an evolving MI.)
124. a. 60 beats/min.
  b. Prominent Q waves in II, III, and aV_F with ST segment elevations in those leads and reciprocal ST depressions in I, aV_L, and V_2 to V_3; deep T wave inversions in II, III, aV_F, and V_4 to V_6. (This pattern is consistent with an evolving inferolateral infarct.)
125. c.
126. c.
127. d.
128. a. Prominent U waves.
  b. The two major causes are hypokalemia and drug effect (particularly, quinidine, procainamide, and disopyramide). This patient was hypokalemic. Patients who have markedly prolonged repolarization with large U waves from any cause may, in addition, be at risk of the development of torsade de pointes (p. 191).

129. This is a normal "septal" q wave, representing left-to-right spread of septal depolarization forces. (Notice its low amplitude and short duration [less than 0.04 sec].)

130. Subendocardial infarction. (Notice the diffuse marked ST depressions [I, II, III, aV_F, and V_3 to V_6] with ST elevation in aV_R. These changes indicate subendocardial ischemia or infarction. The elevated enzymes confirm infarction.)

131. a. Sinus tachycardia.
     b. Left anterior hemiblock. Notice the marked left axis deviation, with normal duration QRS.

132. ECG showing abnormal T wave inversions in aV_L and V_3 to V_5, suggesting myocardial ischemia, with or without actual infarction.

133. Atrial flutter with 2:1 AV conduction. (The atrial rate is about 300/min, and the ventricular rate about 150/min. Notice the positive flutter waves in V_1 and the negative flutter waves in II. The classic sawtooth configuration may not be seen in all leads [for example, V_1 here]. Low voltage in the limb leads is also present.)

134. Atrial bigeminy.

135. Prior anterior wall MI. (There is a loss of normal R wave progression, with pathologic Q waves in V_2 to V_5.)

136. Paroxysmal atrial tachycardia (PAT) converting abruptly to normal sinus rhythm. (Notice the sudden slowing of heart rate and appearance of P waves.)

137. Acute anterior wall MI. (Pathologic Q waves in V_1 to V_5 and aV_L, with ST segment elevations in these leads and reciprocal ST depressions in II, III, and aV_F.)

138. a. Left atrial abnormality (enlargement).
     b. First-degree AV block (PR = 0.24 sec).
     c. One PVC. In addition, there is axis deviation. (Notice the RS complex in II with the S wave > R wave. Therefore the axis must be more negative than $-30°$ or more positive than $+150°$. You need two frontal plane leads to know if the axis is markedly leftward or rightward.)

139. PAT with 2:1 block. Notice the two P waves for every QRS, with an atrial rate of about 190/min and a ventricular rate of 95/min. This patient was suffering from digitalis toxicity.

140. Diffuse subendocardial ischemia. (Notice the horizontal or downward sloping ST segment depression, best seen in I, II, aV_F, and V_3 to V_6, with ST elevation only in aV_R.)

141. Isorhythmic AV dissociation. (The atrial and ventricular rates are about equal, with P waves moving "in" and "out" of the QRS.) (See p. 201.)

142. Sinus tachycardia with atrial quadrigeminy (that is, every fourth beat is a PAC).

143. a. Prior inferior and anterolateral MIs, with Q waves in II, III, aV_F, V_5, and V_6 as well as T wave inversions in the left chest leads.
     b. Borderline first-degree AV block (PR about 0.2 sec).
     c. QT prolongation. (The interval is 0.4 sec, which is long for a heart rate of about 77/min. The patient was taking quinidine, a drug that may prolong the QT.)
     d. Marked left axis deviation.

144. a. RBBB.
     b. Borderline first-degree AV block. (The PR is about 0.2 sec.)

    c. Nonspecific ST-T abnormalities. With "pure" RBBB you would expect to see T wave inversions in leads with an rSR′ complex, so-called *secondary* ST-T changes. However, the ST segments here are also abnormally depressed in I, II, aV_F, and V_3 to V_6. These *primary* ST-T changes are nonspecific and could have been caused by ischemia, digitalis effect, or some other condition. (See p. 79.)

145. a. Evolving anterior wall MI with Q waves in V_1 to V_3 and deep T wave inversions in V_3 and V_4. (The ST-T changes in the inferolateral leads are also suggestive of ischemia.)
    b. First-degree AV block.
    c. Probable left atrial abnormality (enlargement) with broad P waves.

146. Complete heart block. Notice the independent atrial and ventricular complexes, with an atrial rate of about 100/min and a ventricular rate of 43/min.

147. Accelerated idioventricular rhythm (AIVR). The first three beats are sinus, followed by a run of wide QRS complexes at a rate of about 110/min. Notice that the fourth QRS is actually a *fusion* beat resulting from simultaneous occurrence of a sinus beat and an idioventricular beat. AIVR is commonly observed during acute MI and is usually self-limited.

148. Ventricular tachycardia.

149. Normal ECG. (Remember, a "normal" ECG does not exclude significant underlying heart disease.)

150. Prior anteroseptal infarction. Abnormal Q waves in V_1 to V_3.

151. Complete heart block. (Notice the independent atrial and ventricular complexes, with the ventricles being paced by a slow indioventricular pacemaker [wide QRS]. The combination of heart block and syncope is called Stokes-Adams syndrome.)

152. LVH with strain. (Notice the prominent chest lead voltage [S_{V_1} and R_{V_5} greater than 35 mm] with "strain" pattern. P waves are prominent, broad, and notched in III [consistent with left atrial abnormality]. Notice also the relatively peaked P waves in II. In some patients with this pattern left atrial enlargement causes tall P waves simulating right atrial enlargement, the so-called "pseudo–P pulmonale pattern." In others biatrial enlargement is present.)

153. Normal variant "early repolarization." (Notice the ST segment elevations [without reciprocal ST depressions] in V_2 to V_4.)

154. Acute pericarditis. (Notice the ST elevations in I, II, III, aV_F, and V_4 to V_6, with T wave inversions in most of these leads. Diffuse distribution of ST elevations [present in I, II, and III] supports the clinical diagnosis of pericarditis. Notice also the LVH by voltage with left atrial abnormality. The patient was hypertensive as a result of chronic renal disease and had uremic pericarditis.)

155. a. Inferior wall MI of indeterminate age with Q waves in II, III, and aV_F and T wave inversions.
    b. Anterior wall MI of indeterminate age with loss of R waves in V_1 to V_3 and Q waves in V_3 to V_5, as well as deep ischemic T wave inversions in I, aV_L, and V_2 to V_6.
    c. LVH. (Notice the very prominent precordial voltage, with V_4 to V_6 recorded at one-half standardization.)

156. Atrial flutter with variable block.

157. a. Prior inferior wall MI.
    b. Probable left atrial abnormality.
    c. Nonspecific ST-T changes in V_4 to V_6 (consistent with ischemia or other causes).

158. a. First-degree AV block.
    b. Right axis deviation. (Notice the R wave in III greater than in II.)
    c. Right ventricular hypertrophy with strain (with a tall R wave in V_1 and T wave inversions in the right chest leads.)

159. Acute pericarditis. (Notice the diffuse ST segment elevations in I, II, aV_F, and V_4 to V_6. This pattern differs from the ST elevations of acute MI, which are more localized [anterior or inferior] with reciprocal changes. The pattern also differs from that of normal variant "early repolarization" [Fig. 10-15], which does not usually produce such marked ST elevations in V_5 and V_6 as are seen here. With normal variant early repolarization, the ST elevations are usually most prominent in V_3 and V_4. Notice also the subtle PR changes [Fig. 10-12].)

160. b. Hyperkalemia. (There is widening of the QRS with peaking of the T waves and loss of the P waves [junctional rhythm].)

161. Wolff-Parkinson-White pattern. (Notice the triad of wide QRS, short PR interval, and slurring on the QRS upstroke [delta wave].)

162. Atrial flutter with 2:1 conduction (block). Flutter waves at a rate of about 300/min *(arrows)*.

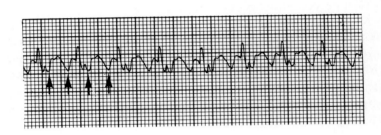

163. Sinus tachycardia and P pulmonale (right atrial enlargement).

164. AV junctional rhythm (retrograde P waves following the QRS).

165. Multifocal atrial tachycardia (MAT), which is most commonly associated with chronic obstructive lung disease.

166. Paroxysmal atrial tachycardia (PAT) with 2:1 AV block. Notice the P waves sitting on the T waves. (This arrhythmia is often, but not always, associated with digitalis toxicity.)

167. Severe hyperkalemia. The serum potassium was markedly elevated (8.1 mEq/L), and the ECG showed tall peaked T waves. (ST elevations in V_1 and V_2 may also be seen in this setting.) By the next day the serum potassium was normal (4.4 mEq/L).

168. Left bundle branch block.

169. Wandering atrial pacemaker. (Notice the subtle change in P waves.)

170. Accelerated idioventricular rhythm (AIVR).

171. The ST-T changes are consistent with digitalis effect, and the rhythm is atrial bigeminy.

172. Evolving pattern of anterior wall infarction and right bundle branch block. Left atrial abnormality is also seen (V_1).

173. Atrial flutter with spontaneous conversion to sinus rhythm. Initially there is atrial flutter with 2:1 conduction. The degree of block increases just before conversion.

174. Sinus rhythm with 2:1 AV block. Because the QRS is of normal duration here, this arrhythmia probably represents a Mobitz type I (Wenckebach) block and not a Mobitz type II, which is usually associated with a wide QRS. (See p. 195.)

175. Sinus rhythm with AV Wenckebach. Nonconducted P waves are present on the T wave of the third and eighth QRS-T complexes. AV Wenckebach may be caused by a variety of factors, including drug toxicity (for example, digitalis, beta blockers, and, in this case, verapamil).

176. Sinus rhythm with frequent premature atrial contractions (PACs) at the end of the strip. This type of rhythm may lead to sustained multifocal atrial tachycardia (MAT) or atrial fibrillation.

177. Atrial fibrillation may lead to left atrial thrombus formation and eventual embolization. An embolic-type cerebrovascular accident is therefore suggested. (Notice that with atrial fibrillation, fibrillatory waves may be hard to detect. The subtle changes in QRS complexes here from one beat to the next may reflect variability in ventricular conduction due to the fast rate.)

178. Complete heart block. Notice the independence of atrial (sinus) P wave activity (with a rate of about 88/min) and ventricular (QRS) complexes (at a rate of about 33/min). The combination of high-degree heart block and syncope is sometimes referred to as the Stokes-Adams syndrome. (This patient was treated with a permanent pacemaker.)

179. Paroxysmal atrial (or AV junctional) tachycardia (PAT).

180. Intermittent left bundle branch block. The first four beats are conducted with a left bundle branch block pattern, the last four with a normal QRS. In this case the bundle branch block was *rate related*. When the heart rate exceeded a critical value, the bundle branch block appeared. (Notice that all the beats are preceded by a P wave with a constant PR interval. Therefore the rhythm could not be accelerated idioventricular.)

181. Sinus rhythm, left axis deviation, and an intraventricular conduction delay (QRS duration = 0.12 sec). The major abnormality is extensive anterior wall infarction with pathologic Q waves in aV_L and V_1 to V_6. In addition, the ST segments are elevated in these leads. Persistent ST elevations following infarction suggests a *ventricular aneurysm*, which was the cause of the patient's heart failure in this case.

182. The ECG shows right bundle branch block and right axis deviation. This pattern, given the patient's history and physical examination findings, is most suggestive of an atrial septal defect (p. 235).

183. Wolff-Parkinson-White (WPW) pattern. The triad of short PR interval, wide QRS, and slurring of the QRS upstroke (delta wave) is best seen in II, III, aV_F, and V_4 to V_6. WPW is often associated with supraventricular tachycardias (in particular, PAT), which may have been the source of this patient's chief complaint of palpitations.

184. The classic pattern of *torsade de pointes,* a form of ventricular tachycardia characterized by oscillations in QRS amplitude and axis in the same lead. This potentially fatal arrhythmia is usually seen in the setting of abnormally prolonged ventricular repolarization, evidenced by a long QT interval or prominent U wave. Drugs such as quinidine may cause the arrhythmia (quinidine syncope). (See p. 191 for other causes.)

185. There is underlying sinus bradycardia with a 2.4-second pause following the third beat. This pause is almost exactly twice the underlying PP interval. Therefore this probably represents 2:1 SA block. Unlike 2:1 AV block (in which a P wave is not followed by a QRS), with 2:1 SA block an entire P-QRS-T cycle is "dropped". The patient had "sick sinus syndrome" and required a permanent pacemaker.

186. c.
187. Long QT (about 0.53 sec) at a heart rate of 70/min. The patient had severe hypocalcemia.
188. b. The atrial rate is about 300/min, which is diagnostic of flutter.
189. e. Notice the wide QRS complexes with absent P waves.
190. Sinus rhythm with AV Wenckebach.
191. A dual-chamber pacemaker. Notice the repeating sequence of atrial pacemaker spike, P wave, ventricular pacemaker spike, and wide QRS.
192. The first part of the rhythm strip shows a run of paroxysmal atrial tachycardia (PAT), probably due to AV nodal reentry. Alternative names for this arrhythmia are AV nodal (junctional) reentrant tachycardia or paroxysmal supraventricular tachycardia (PSVT). The tachycardia spontaneously breaks with the resumption of sinus bradycardia, raising the question of a brady-tachy syndrome.

Bibliography

Chapters 1 to 7

BASIC CONCEPTS AND PATTERNS

Burch GE, dePasquale NP: A history of electrocardiography, Chicago, 1964, Year Book Medical Publishers Inc.

Fisch C: Electrocardiography and vectorcardiography. In Braunwald EB, editor: Heart disease: a textbook of cardiovascular medicine, ed 3, Philadelphia, 1988, WB Saunders Co.

Flowers NC: Left bundle branch block: a continuously evolving concept, J Am Coll Cardiol 9:684, 1987.

Goldberger E: Unipolar lead electrocardiography and vectorcardiography, ed 3, Philadelphia, 1953, Lea & Febiger.

Goldberger E: How to interpret electrocardiograms in terms of vectors, Springfield Ill, 1968, Charles C Thomas Publisher.

Goldman MJ: Principles of clinical electrocardiography, ed 12, Los Altos Calif, 1986, Lange Medical Publications.

Lipman BS, et al: Clinical electrocardiography, ed 7, Chicago, 1984, Year Book Medical Publishers Inc.

Marriott HJC: Practical electrocardiography, ed 7, Baltimore, 1983, The Williams & Wilkins Co.

Murphy ML, et al: Sensitivity of electrocardiographic criteria for left ventricular hypertrophy according to type of cardiac disease, Am J Cardiol 55:545, 1985.

Surawicz B: Electrocardiographic diagnosis of chamber enlargement, J Am Coll Cardiol 8:1195, 1986.

Chapters 8 and 9

MYOCARDIAL ISCHEMIA AND INFARCTION

Cohn PF: Silent myocardial ischemia, Ann Intern Med 109:312, 1988.

Froelicher VF: Exercise and the heart, ed 2, Chicago, 1987, Year Book Medical Publishers Inc.

Goldberger AL: Recognition of ECG pseudoinfarct patterns, Mod Conc Cardiovasc Dis 49:13, 1980.

Goldberger AL: Myocardial infarction: electrocardiographic differential diagnosis, ed 4, St Louis, 1991, Mosby–Year Book.

Schamroth L: The electrocardiology of coronary artery disease, Oxford, 1975, Blackwell Scientific Publications.

Chapter 10

MISCELLANEOUS PATTERNS

Chou TC: Electrocardiography in clinical practice, ed 2, Orlando Fla, 1986, Grune & Stratton.

Douglas PS, et al: Extreme hypercalcemia and electrocardiographic changes, Am J Cardiol 54:674, 1984.

Goldberger A: A specific ECG triad associated with congestive heart failure, PACE 5:593, 1982.

Spodick DH: Diagnostic electrocardiographic sequences in acute pericarditis. Significance of PR segment and PR vector changes, Circulation 48:475, 1973.

Spodick DH: Electrocardiographic responses to pulmonary embolism, Am J Cardiol 30:695, 1972.

Surawicz B: Relationship between electrocardiogram and electrolytes, Am Heart J 73:814, 1967.

Surawicz B, Lasseter KC: Effect of drugs on the electrocardiogram, Prog Cardiovasc Dis 13:26, 1970.

Chapters 11 to 21

ARRHYTHMIAS, CONDUCTION DISTURBANCES, PACEMAKERS

Akhtar M, et al: Wide QRS tachycardia, Ann Intern Med 109:905, 1988.

Barrett PA, et al: The frequency and prognostic significance of electrocardiographic abnormalities in clinically normal individuals, Prog Cardiovasc Dis 23:299, 1981.

Brodsky M, et al: Arrhythmias documented by 24 hour continuous electrocardiographic monitoring in 50 male medical students without apparent heart disease, Am J Cardiol 39:390, 1977.

Chung EK: Principles of cardiac arrhythmias, ed 4, Baltimore, 1988, The Williams & Wilkins Co.

Cohen SI: Temporary and permanent pacemakers. In Grossman W, editor: Cardiac catheterization and angiography, ed 4, Philadelphia, 1990, Lea & Febiger.

Goldberger E: Treatment of cardiac emergencies, ed 5, St Louis, 1990, The CV Mosby Co.

Grauer K, Cavallaro D: ACLS: Certification preparation and comprehensive review, ed 2, St Louis, 1987, The CV Mosby Co.

Josephson ME: Clinical cardiac electrophysiology: techniques and interpretations, ed 2, Philadelphia, 1991, Lea & Febiger.

Josephson ME, Wellens HJJ, editors: Tachycardias—mechanisms, diagnosis, treatment, Philadelphia, 1984, Lea & Febiger.

Kastor JA: Atrioventricular heart block, I and II, N Engl J Med 292:462, 572, 1975.

Kennedy HL, et al: Long-term follow-up of asymptomatic healthy subjects with frequent and complex asymptomatic ventricular ectopy, N Engl J Med 312:193, 1985.

Mandel WJ, editor: Cardiac arrhythmias: their mechanisms, diagnosis, and management, ed 2, Philadelphia, 1987, JB Lippincott Co.

Moses HW, et al: A practical guide to cardiac pacing, Boston, ed 2, 1987, Little Brown & Co.

Roden DM, et al: Incidence and clinical features of the quinidine-associated long QT syndrome: implications for patient care, Am Heart J 111:1088, 1986.

Smith TW, et al: Digitalis glycosides: mechanisms and manifestations of toxicity, Prog Cardiovasc Dis 26:413, 1984.

Smith WM, Gallagher JJ: ''Les torsades de pointes'': an unusual ventricular arrhythmia, Ann Intern Med 93:578, 1980.

Textbook of advanced cardiac life support, Dallas, 1987, American Heart Association.

Vlay SC, editor: Manual of cardiac arrhythmias. A practical guide to clinical management, Boston, 1988, Little Brown & Co.

Ward DE, Camm AJ: Clinical electrophysiology of the heart, Baltimore, 1987, Edward Arnold (Publishers).

Winkle RA, et al: Long-term outcome with the automatic implantable cardioverter-defibrillator, J Am Coll Cardiol 13:1353, 1989.

Zipes D, Duffin EG: Cardiac pacemakers. In Braunwald EB, editor: Heart disease: a textbook of cardiovascular medicine, ed 3, Philadelphia, 1984, WB Saunders Co.

Zoll PM: External noninvasive temporary cardiac pacing: clinical trials, Circulation 71:937, 1985.

Index

n indicates footnote.

n indicates footnote.

n indicates footnote.